Nutritional Medicine

Nutritional Medicine

Dr. Stephen Davies and
Dr. Alan Stewart

Edited by Dr. Andrew Stanway

AVON BOOKS NEW YORK

AVON BOOKS
A division of
The Hearst Corporation
105 Madison Avenue
New York, New York 10016

Cover photograph courtesy *The Stock Market*
Published by arrangement with Pan Books Ltd.
Library of Congress Catalog Card Number: 89-91869
ISBN: 0-380-70733-0

First Avon Books Trade Printing: March 1990

Printed in the U.S.A.

OPM 10 9 8 7 6 5 4 3 2 1

Contents

Acknowledgments

I would like to acknowledge my parents, my family and all those who have given me such great support and assistance. I would also like to mention my daughter Sophie who, while I was writing this book, found her daddy unavailable for playtime. Trying to explain this situation to her, I showed her at the front of a number of different books how authors dedicate their books to members of their family. Ten minutes later she came back with a note, in her six-year-old handwriting, of what I should put at the beginning of this book. It stated (misspelled!): "To my dear famley most of all to my doughter Sophie who has wanted to spend time with me so much. I just want to say sorry."

I would like to thank in particular, biochemist Dr. John Howard, whose vision, dedication, experience, expertise, and love and care of his fellow man has been a true inspiration to me.

I would like to thank my clinic staff, past and present, for their support, hard work and contribution. Thanks also go to the following people whose skills resulted in the typing of a lengthy manuscript: Carmen Biggs, Karen Looij and Marina Boulding.

Thanks also to my wife, Shoura, for her support while I was writing my share of this book.

Dr. Stephen Davies

I would like to acknowledge Mrs. Judy Lehman and the staff of Brighton Postgraduate Medical Centre Library for their help in obtaining the hundreds of research papers that we have drawn upon to write this book. I would like to thank my secretary, Ann, whose nimble fingers have made light work of much of the text. Acknowledgment is also due to many practitioners local to me in Sussex, and our colleagues, whose support, and interest in nutrition, has made it clear to us that there is a definite need for soundly based practical advice on the use of nutritional methods in the management of illness. My wife, Maryon, and our two children, require special acknowledgment for their support and patience.

Dr. Alan Stewart

Joint Acknowledgments

We would both like to acknowledge our editor, Dr. Andrew Stanway, who had the mammoth task of translating, from medicalese into what we hope is comprehensible English, the original manuscript, which was three times the length of the final version. Thanks also to Annie Jackson, Judith Hannam and Hilary Davies of Pan Books for harassing us to get the book finished.

We would like also to thank our patients for teaching us so much and for bearing with us during those times when we have been unable to help them.

And finally, thanks go to all those physicians, scientists, colleagues and teachers who have been willing to teach us and to share their knowledge with us in such an unselfish way.

Note to Readers

You should always consult your own doctor before taking any nutritional supplements detailed in this book. You should always read any instructions and warnings in the text before embarking on a supplement program or diet.

The dosages given here may seem high to you and your doctor, but there is a scientific basis for each suggested supplement or dietary change. They should be followed exactly with your doctor's approval or supervision.

Abbreviations used:

g = gram
mg = milligram (1000 mg = 1 g)
mcg = microgram (1000 mcg = 1 mg)
IU = international unit
mmol/1 = micromols/liter

Case histories have been included to bring the real value of nutritional medicine into focus. In reading these, one should bear in mind that physical conditions can be caused by a whole range of different factors. Because a case history includes one particular treatment, it does not mean to say that this is the one and only treatment for any given condition. The names of the people have been changed.

Note to Doctors

This book is an edited version of a much longer, as yet unfinished, medical text with a bibliography of over three and a half thousand references. Considerations of space and practicality have caused us to include only a selection (approx. 650) of references, which constitutes only a tiny fraction of the scientific evidence upon which the nutritional-medical approach is based. Several of the concepts discussed in this book may initially seem unfamiliar, because doctors receive but a smattering of training in nutrition at medical school. The contents of this book represent a very viable approach to patient management; we hope that those of you who are dissatisfied with the drug-based approach to medicine will find it stimulating and helpful, and that you will find the nutritional approach professionally rewarding. We draw your attention to the introductory reading list for practitioners on page 442, which we hope you will find useful.

Foreword

As practicing doctors, we believe that medicine is based on a desire to help one's fellow man, the humane application of scientific knowledge, and the use of treatments that are safe and effective. Medicine has to move forward in order to meet the challenge that successive health-care problems bring. In the past, a fortune has been spent on excessive drug research and the use of only semi-effective methods in the care of the chronically mentally and physically ill. Medical and scientific expertise has been wasted, too. It is vital in these more frugal times that simpler, more economical solutions are found to the diseases and discomforts that affect our lives. It is our belief that nutrition is often an important but neglected answer to these problems, despite the large amount of excellent research already performed.

The term "nutritional medicine" has been coined to cover the application of nutritional methods in the treatment and prevention of disease. Over the past ten years there has been an explosion of interest in nutrition and how it relates to the diseases that affect the Western world. Each year some ten thousand medical and scientific papers covering the field of nutrition are published, and we have drawn extensively on these, as well as on our experience as medical practitioners, in writing this book. The first section examines the role of vitamins, minerals, other dietary factors and environmental pollution in health. The second and third sections deal with the management of a wide range of medical conditions by using specific diets and nutritional supplements, as well as adopting lifestyle changes.

The book is intended for members of the public as well as doctors and members of professions allied to medicine, such as dietitians, nurses and nutritionists. **If you feel that anything in the book applies to you, then we advise that you discuss it with your doctor.** The many technical references at the end contain the medical reasoning behind our recommendations.

With continuing research, nutritional medicine will undoubtedly progress from being the "orthodox alternative" to drug-based medicine, to become the mainstay of both prevention and treatment of many modern diseases. We hope that this book represents a step, albeit small, on the way to achieving a wider appreciation of just how effective a nutritional approach can be in dealing with a wide range of health matters.

Dr. Stephen Davies
Dr. Alan Stewart

Introduction

In order to understand just how fundamentally useful nutritional manipulation can be in maintaining health and improving the course of diseases, it is important to grasp a few basic principles.

Modern medicine has put far too little emphasis on nutritional treatments mainly, in our opinion, because of the failure of many professionals to grasp certain basic concepts which are outlined in this chapter.

SOME BASIC DEFINITIONS

These definitions are based on those of the British Society for Nutritional Medicine.

Nutrition Nutrition is "the sum of the processes involved in taking in nutrients, assimilating and utilizing them."

Nutrients Essential nutrients are those substances (proteins, carbohydrates, fats, vitamins and minerals) necessary for growth, normal functioning, and maintaining life; they must be supplied by foods because they cannot be made by the body. This definition can be extended to include other components that are necessary for human life. These could include oxygen and water, and some would even say emotional and psychological "nutrients" such as love. The main nutrients known to be essential for humans are:

- amino acids (proteins)
- carbohydrates
- essential fatty acids (fats)
- vitamins
- minerals
- others (fiber, oxygen, water, etc.)

Nutritional medicine "The study of the interactions of nutritional factors with human biochemistry, physiology and anatomy, and how the clinical application of a knowledge of these interactions can be used in the prevention and treatment of disease, as well as in the improvement of health."

FACTORS THAT INFLUENCE NUTRITIONAL STATUS

There are four main factors that influence nutritional status:

- the quality of the food we eat
- the quantity of the food we eat
- the efficiency of digestion, absorption and utilization
- biochemical individuality

The Quality of Food

The quality of the food we eat obviously influences our nutritional status. Food grown on nutrient-poor soil can be deficient in certain nutrients. Things which influence the quality of the soil, apart from natural variability in, for example, trace elements, are largely governed by farming policy. Has the soil been overworked? Have chemicals been added to it? Of the chemicals which have been added, can any influence the availability of the nutritional components in the soil, and in plants grown in the soil? Has the farmer added chemicals such as pesticides, insecticides and herbicides to his crops? Do these adversely influence the quality of the food? Can these chemicals influence the biochemistry of the body? Has the farmer given drugs and antibiotics to his livestock? Do these drugs find their way onto our plates? Can they influence the biochemistry of our bodies? Do certain processes that foods undergo during manufacture and storage influence their nutrient content? Do any food preparation procedures in the kitchens of our own homes influence the nutrient content of food?

The answer to all of these questions is often "yes." Indeed, there is a sound case for trying to choose foods that have been grown without any, or only with a minimum of, chemical additives.

The Quantity of Food

The quantity of food we eat, too, influences our nutritional status. In the West, *under*nutrition tends not to be a problem. It is, however, still a very real problem in developing countries. However, *mal*nutrition can occur anywhere as a result of wrong food choice and a dependence on large amounts of heavily refined foods. If nutrient-dense foods such as whole grains and unprocessed foods (including vegetables) are replaced by processed foods that have been stripped of essential nutrients, there will obviously be an alteration of the nutritional status of the person who eats them. The health-food "nuts" of the past who insisted on plenty of whole grains, fresh vegetables and so on have been proved right by modern science.

The Efficiency of Digestion

An individual whose digestive system, for whatever reason, is inefficient, is more likely to have a poor nutritional status than is someone with an efficient digestive system. This might seem obvious, yet it is widely overlooked by health professionals and public alike. An example of reduced digestive efficiency can be seen when the stomach fails to produce sufficient hydrochloric acid to allow the stomach enzyme pepsin to work properly. This leads to the impairment of other digestive enzyme activity.

The Efficiency of Absorption

As well as the process of digestion, in which intestinal juices act upon the food we eat, there is the actual process of absorption of digested food particles into the bloodstream. Certain conditions of the intestine reduce the efficiency with which digested foods are absorbed. Someone with absorption problems (see page 194) may *not* have gross signs of physical disease, but can still have a compromised nutritional status which, in turn, causes chronic disease.

An example of poor absorption is celiac disease. This is a condition in which a person is sensitive to gluten which is found in wheat, rye, oats and barley. This sensitivity results in a partial destruction of the absorptive surface of the small bowel, resulting in the inefficient absorption of nutrients. This can also happen in less severe forms of food sensitivity (see page 153).

The presence of other substances in the diet can prevent certain nutrients from being absorbed efficiently. For example, both tea and coffee reduce the absorption in iron and zinc, so iron and zinc intakes must be higher in the diets of tea and coffee drinkers. Certain types of fiber, for example bran, can reduce the absorption of calcium, iron and zinc, amongst other things. The problems involved in taking bran are discussed in more detail elsewhere (see page 126).

The Efficiency of Utilization

Once nutrients from food have been absorbed into the bloodstream, it is then a matter of how efficiently the body uses them. Someone who excretes large quantities of nutrients in the urine, for example, will have higher nutritional requirements than someone who uses nutrients more effectively. Some people may also have metabolic faults that prevent the body from efficiently utilizing nutrients that *are* there. This in turn reduces the functional nutritional status of that person. Such metabolic blocks can be caused by genetic factors, food intolerance, other nutrient deficiencies, toxins in food and environmental pollution (see page 89).

An example of poor utilization of an essential nutrient is seen in someone who has been exposed to pesticides belonging to the "hydrazine" group of chemicals. Chemicals in this group are potent vitamin B6 antagonists. If there are significant levels of any of this group of substances in the body, the body cannot utilize B6 properly, thus dietary requirements for B6 are increased substantially. There are also drugs used in treating tuberculosis and high blood pressure which can prevent the body's utilization of vitamin B6.

Biochemical Individuality

This is a fundamental concept in understanding the factors that determine whether an individual remains healthy or becomes ill. It is now becoming more widely accepted but, nevertheless, is seldom applied in an individual's nutritional assessment by doctors. Simply put, it is that each person has unique nutritional requirements. There is an optimum range of intake, for any one individual, for each of the forty-five or so essential nutrients. These ranges have not been clearly defined and we still do not know for certain how much any of us needs any of them. Just because one person needs 1–2 mg of vitamin B6 to maintain optimal health, it does not mean that everybody can get by with 1–2 mg of the vitamin. Some will be able to manage with less and others will require more.

But even allowing for the fact that we are all unique in our nutritional requirements, these are influenced by several factors. They include:

- age
- growth
- sex
- pregnancy and breast-feeding
- illness
- psychological and emotional stress
- activity level
- genetics
- other dietary considerations, toxic overload and drugs

AGE

As people get older, their nutritional requirements change. Elderly people are the highest users of medications and drugs, many of which interfere with the absorption, excretion and utilization of nutrients (see page 142).

GROWTH

Growing children have different nutritional requirements from adults. For example, a boy going through puberty will have zinc requirements that may well be higher than those of a man who went through adolescence a decade before. Essential fatty acid requirements are dramatically increased in rapidly growing infants, who, on a body weight ratio, may have higher requirements than an adult.

SEX

Certain nutrient requirements are very different between boys and girls and men and women—indeed, the nutritional requirements of women can vary throughout the menstrual cycle.

PREGNANCY AND BREAST-FEEDING

A woman who is pregnant or breast-feeding has very different nutritional requirements from one who is not. This might seem obvious, but is often overlooked in practice. This subject is covered in detail elsewhere (see page 326).

ILLNESS

Nutritional requirements vary greatly in health and disease. Certain diseases put pressure on, and result in considerable differences in, certain nutritional requirements. For example, zinc loss in someone with extensive skin burns may triple (or more) his or her normal zinc requirements.

PSYCHOLOGICAL AND EMOTIONAL STRESS

Psychological and emotional stress can influence food choice and appetite and thus nutrient intake. They can also increase requirements for B vitamins as well as minerals such as zinc and magnesium.

ACTIVITY LEVEL

The nutritional requirements of someone who leads a vigorous and physically active life are different from those of a person who sits behind a desk all day. Exercise increases nutrient requirements in some people and improves metabolic efficiency in others.

GENETICS

The influence of genetics on nutritional requirements cannot be overestimated. Though there is still a lot of scientific research to be done in this area, we already know that increased requirements for certain essential nutrients can run in families. In fact, there are certain inborn errors of metabolism that can be directly corrected by the administration of the appropriate nutrient in sufficient quantities.

OTHER FACTORS

Certain drugs (see page 142) and social habits such as drinking (see page 133) and smoking (see page 138) can also affect nutrient requirements. For example, drinking alcohol increases zinc, magnesium and vitamin B and C requirements, and smoking can increase vitamins C, B6 and zinc requirements. Tea (see page 131) not only inhibits the absorption of iron and zinc, but also contains a substance which reduces the utilization of thiamin (vitamin B1). Therefore, heavy tea drinkers, apart from requiring more dietary iron and zinc, also require more dietary vitamin B1. Similarly, coffee inhibits the absorption of iron and zinc.

THE NUTRIENTS WE NEED

There are known to be some forty-five nutrients essential for human life, in addition to carbohydrates, fats and proteins, and the relative proportions of these in the diet can influence health. The specific proportions and health effects of these food constituents are dealt with more extensively in Part One.

Each one of these forty-five can be present in ideal, insufficient or excessive amounts.

If any one nutrient is present in insufficient amounts, deficiency symptoms result, and if too much is present in the diet, toxic symptoms occur. In between these two extremes there is a range which can be thought of as "ideal."

But with only marginal deficiencies or marginal excesses, the effects on health may be subtle, insidious and only harmful after a prolonged period of time.

Obviously, the diagnosing of imbalances in the diet becomes easier the further away from the "ideal" one goes. This is why so many doctors and nutritionists find many of the concepts of nutritional medicine difficult to grasp or even to accept. Many still think of deficiency diseases as having to be very obvious clinically. Recent evidence is proving just how wrong this can be.

Out of this comes the concept of "optimum" nutrition; that is, that each individual should absorb into their system each nutrient in its optimum amount. This is, of course, a theoretically ideal state of affairs, and impossible to achieve in practice.

THE WESTERN DIET

With the advent of food processing at the end of the last century, it became possible for Man to interfere with natural foods in such a way as apparently to improve his nutrition. However, it has been clear for some years now that many of the effects of food processing can be detrimental to the nutritional quality of food and, more recently, that this has long-term consequences for health.

For example, the refining of flour not only removes dietary fiber, but also removes essential vitamins and minerals.

The idea behind food processing is to reduce its rate of deterioration (thus giving it a longer shelf-life); to make it easier to distribute; to produce "new" foods that would otherwise not exist at all; and, through the use of colorings and other additives, to make foods more "appealing." Many of the substances added to foods by food manufacturers can be harmful to certain susceptible individuals. It is hoped that increased public awareness will bring pressure on the food industry to produce foods that are less contaminated by artificial additives, many of which are petrochemical derivatives and unnecessary.

Undernutrition versus Malnutrition

It has been said that many people in the West are over*fed* yet under*nourished*. The concept behind this statement is that although our total energy intake is excessive, the quality of food is often so poor that the actual nutrient intake in terms of vitamins, minerals and certain amino acids is inadequate and can produce disease.

This is in contrast to certain developing countries, such as Ethiopia or Bangladesh, where there simply is not sufficient food of any kind to sustain healthy life. This is true *under*nutrition, which is seldom found in the West except in people with anorexia nervosa or certain severe illnesses. What *we* suffer from is *mal*nutrition, and throughout the book we shall be looking at how and why such malnutrition comes about, and the effects it can have on our health.

Many of the diseases from which we suffer in the West have been ascribed to excessive fat, excessive protein, or excessive refined carbohydrate intake. Refined carbohydrates are those carbohydrates that have been processed and have had the most nutritious components removed.

The pioneering work in the 1930s of an American dental surgeon, Weston Price, studied the dietary habits of thirty or so primitive cultures and observed that when they moved from their traditional diets and started consuming a typical "Western diet" they also started to suffer an increase in Western diseases—cancer, heart attack, dental decay, allergies and so on. This has now been confirmed by many other researchers, so the concept that nutritional factors cause those diseases that are mainly found in Westernized countries is no longer considered crazy or far-out.

Defusing Common Myths about the Western Diet

The idea that our Western diet is excellent and healthy needs to be debunked. Here are just a few truths that are still widely considered to be erroneous even by some doctors and nutritionists:

- animal protein is not necessary for optimum health
- nutrient deficiencies can and do exist in people on a so-called "healthy, balanced diet"
- sugar (as sucrose) is not an essential nutrient
- milk is not necessary to maintain adequate calcium balance
- food colorings and other additives can have adverse health effects in a percentage of individuals

So, in conclusion, the Western diet leaves a lot to be desired, and when compared with a theoretical "natural" diet, there are enormous differences. Put simply, it contains:

- too much animal fat
- too much salt
- too much sugar and refined flour
- not enough fiber
- too many processed foods
- potentially harmful insecticides, pesticides, herbicides and so on. Potentially harmful colorings and other food additives
- too much tea, coffee and alcohol

It is foolish to assume that giving any animal species a diet different from that which was present during the major part of its evolution would not result in certain individuals within that species running into health problems. But this is actually what we have done in the Westernized world over the last two centuries. We are now paying the price for this—the largest uncontrolled trial ever undertaken in human beings.

DISEASES OF CIVILIZATION

As repeated scientific studies have shown the importance of nutritional factors in the prevention and treatment of diseases, it is now taken for granted by doctors and scientists that diet is a major factor in the diseases of the Western world.

The problem now besetting health-care professionals and those involved in responsible government is one of nutrition education. Professor John Yudkin, emeritus professor of Nutrition at London University, expresses this succinctly:

I make no apology for saying that the health of the majority of human beings depends more on their nutrition than it does on any other single factor. However important and dramatic have been the advances in hygiene, medicine and surgery, it is still true that even more important will be the effects proper nutrition would have on human morbidity and mortality. For this reason, I believe that the ultimate objective of nutritionists must be the nutrition education of the public.

("Objectives and Methods in Nutrition Education—Let's Start Again," *Journal of Human Nutrition,* 1981.)

Yudkin points out that this viewpoint is based on the idea that man could be eating a healthier diet. Indeed, almost all Western populations are encouraged by governments and health education agencies to make dietary changes which many experts feel would result in reduced illness and mortality for the nation as a whole.

Some of the most common diseases of civilization include heart disease, high blood pressure (hypertension), dental caries, obesity, diverticulosis, gallstones, appendicitis, gout, varicose veins, strokes, diabetes and cancer. They are all more common in the Western world than elsewhere.

As well as these very serious conditions, many of the nonkilling diseases that beset technologically advanced countries may also be linked to food; these include asthma, eczema and other allergies; chronic degenerative diseases, such as osteoarthritis and rheumatoid arthritis; and mental illness. There is increasing, indeed, overwhelming evidence that many of these conditions can be prevented or treated by nutritional means. Many sectors of the public have been quick to catch on to the importance of nutrition in such conditions, but the medical profession as a whole has been somewhat slower. However, progress is now under way.

Nutritional Guidelines

In trying to establish advisory nutritional guidelines, we have to recognize that there is no single "optimal" diet for everybody. Ideally, we should be able to define the upper and lower limits of intake for each nutrient within which the individual would be "allowed" greater flexibility in eating patterns. However, at the moment the criteria for establishing these limits are poorly defined, and often depend on small studies of children or adults who rapidly develop biochemical abnormalities or disease while consuming a particular experimental diet.

A report by the UK National Advisory Committee on Nutrition Education (NACNE), published by the Health Education Council, London, in 1983, points out that several diseases prevalent in the UK have a major nutritional cause, and that these are mainly chronic diseases which develop from an excess intake, or an inappropriate ratio, of certain nutrients in the diet of those members of the community who are susceptible for genetic or other reasons. Despite some shortcomings, the NACNE report outlines desirable dietary goals which are the best we have to date. Simply summarized, the NACNE goals are as follows:

1. There should be a standard approach to dietary recommendations.
2. The choice of average intakes as population goals does not signify that there is a recommendation to which all people should conform.
3. Energy intakes should be defined in terms of those appropriate for the maintenance of an optimal body weight and activity level.
4. The risk of overweight should not be exaggerated in relation to the risk of continuing to smoke.
5. Fat intake should be on average thirty percent of total energy intake.
6. Saturated fatty acid intake should be on average ten percent of total energy intake.
7. No specific recommendation should be made on increasing polyunsaturated fatty acids.
8. No recommendation is made about lowering cholesterol intake.
9. Average sucrose (sugar) intake should be reduced to 20 kg per person per year (approximately half the current consumption).
10. Fiber intake should increase on average to 30 g from 20 g per person per day.
11. It would be desirable if salt intake on average fell by 3 g per person per day.
12. Alcohol intake should decline to four percent of the total energy intake.

13. Protein intake should not be altered, but a greater proportion of vegetable protein developing from other recommendations is appropriate.
14. Mineral and vitamin intakes which match the recommended daily allowance listed by the DHSS would generally be appropriate.
15. Special groups may require a further amount of information (e.g. the elderly, pregnant, or ill).
16. Fuller labeling of foods is long overdue and its health-educational as well as regulatory functions have to be recognized.

NACNE did not, however, address the problems of food additives or even vitamins and minerals—problems which concern us as nutritional physicians. There is an attitude, prevalent within the medical profession, that vitamin and mineral deficiencies are not common in the general population. This is not true, and recent dietary surveys in the US and UK have shown that the intakes of several nutrients, including folic acid, vitamin B6, vitamin C, iron and magnesium, can fall far short of what is optimal, even in people who imagine that they are eating a balanced diet. For example, at one recent conference one of us found that thirty-five percent of those present had white spots on their fingernails, suggesting they were zinc deficient—yet these were health visitors, dietitians, nutritionists and physicians—some of the better-informed members of the community.

CONCLUSION

1. Man's body is a complex, biochemical machine that has specific requirements for health, including specific nutritional requirements.

As well as proteins, fats, carbohydrates, calories and water, there are some forty-five different vitamins, minerals, amino acids and essential fatty acids required by our bodies if they are to be healthy. These are by no means the only requirements, as other essential ingredients include air (oxygen), warmth, shelter, sunlight and companionship. A deficiency of any essential nutrient will result in anything from mild, almost imperceptible, ill-health, to death. Isolated deficiencies are rare, but multiple deficiencies often occur, particularly in those who are already unwell. A Western diet is characterized by dietary excesses and shortages which have devastating effects upon body biochemistry and health.

2. Planet-wide dietary variations are enormous and the body's resilience is often remarkable.

On this planet there are billions of people, all of whom eat different diets and have different disease patterns. It is amazing that the health and lifespan of those who are underfed, or indeed overfed, are not worse than they are. The body is a remarkably tough machine that withstands, and has had to withstand, considerable changes in food supply. The human body has been able to tolerate, to a limited degree, some of the unwelcome changes in its food supply, and has still been able to maintain a succession of generations. Because it has been able to do so does not mean it has been doing anything more than just surviving on its so-called "healthy diet."

3. A truly healthy or optimum diet has never been fully defined.

It is probably true to say that no portion of the human race has lived on a completely healthy or optimum diet for any great length of time. Changes in climatic conditions, the presence of diseases affecting humans, animals and plants, and disruptions such as war and natural disasters, have meant that there has probably never been a long-lasting nutritional Garden of Eden. There has never been a supremely developed subsection of the human race, to serve as an example to scientists and nutritionists, of what a perfect, healthy diet is. There are, of course, very healthy sub-populations from whom important clues and, indeed, conclusions can and have been drawn about a healthy diet. But the majority of examples provided by both Eastern and Western communities have been of varying levels of nutritional disaster, and as a result, much of the dietary advice now being promoted is a series of "do nots," rather than "dos."

4. The rapidity of change in Western eating habits is unprecedented and undoubtedly accounts for many diseases affecting Western man.

The developed world has undergone momentous changes over the last 200 years; advances in technology have resulted in dramatic alterations in food supply and thus disease patterns, some for the good and some for the bad.

Dietary changes occurred only slowly before the development of modern technology, but now, botanical research and modern farming methods have made possible the introduction of new types and large quantities of foods into our food supply—many of which don't reach us in an unadulterated form. In the process of refining and processing, significant quantities of trace minerals and vitamins are lost; modern technology has led to the production of trans-saturated fats which are metabolically more like animal fats than their original vegetable origin—and so on. The more we interfere with food after it has been harvested, the greater is the potential for risk. On the other hand, the more we use scientific methods to enhance the quality of food before it is harvested, the greater the likelihood that we will benefit, apart, perhaps, from the use of pollutant chemicals.

This enormous change in the type of food we now eat, as compared to only two or three hundred years ago, put a "metabolic strain" on much of the biochemistry of the body. For example, a high sugar intake is associated with an increased risk of diabetes, dental caries, obesity, and perhaps even heart disease. Quite simply, we are just not used to eating sugar—sucrose—in such large amounts. Another example is the food additives which have too freely been added to foods. Some preservatives and coloring agents can cause asthma, eczema, or even hyperactive behavior in children. Not everyone is affected, so perhaps some of us have the metabolic machinery to deal safely with these additives, while others have yet to develop it. Subtle changes in food supply could probably be accommodated over a number of generations, but the rate of change has been too great for this to be achieved easily. So, as doctors, we keep an eye open for those people who have been unable to adapt to these changes and have become unwell.

5. The majority of diets are influenced by market forces and, in the West, by advertising rather than by scientific recommendations.

Food manufacturers have to make a profit. This means that they have to put the interests of their shareholders first, rather than altruistically providing the best foods for their customers. In short, they produce those foods which they know people will buy, and there's no guarantee that these are necessarily healthy foods. This does not make ogres of the manufacturers though, and many, if not most, of the large food companies are now sensitive to public pressures and those of the health community. A company will make the products that the public want to buy and if there is a demand for healthy products, then it will produce them.

The challenge now rests with those responsible for health care and health education to advise both the public on what is a healthy diet, and the food industry on what is an ethical product from which they can make a "healthy" profit. In this way the health of the nation will be served, the consumer will be satisfied, and the food industry will be profitable.

6. What is a healthy diet for one individual or population may not necessarily be so for other individuals or populations.

Individuals have different body chemistries and, after a time, whole populations may have grown accustomed to specific types of diets. A high salt intake, for example, is not universally associated with high blood pressure. Some individuals can smoke heavily, live to a ripe old age and die of a non-smoking-related disease. Another example is provided by kidney stones, which may run in families. People who are predisposed to kidney stones are particularly likely to form stones if they eat a diet high in sugar and low in fiber and magnesium. Such a diet in other people may be tolerated well and would not produce kidney stones. So there is real truth in the old saying, "One man's meat is another man's poison."

A failure to appreciate individual variation in biochemistry has resulted in many members of the medical profession dismissing diet as a factor in disease. For example, if diet is an important factor in diabetes and diabetes is more common because we consume a diet rich in refined carbohydrates, then why does everyone not have diabetes? The answer is probably that some people are *predisposed* to diabetes and others are not. This phenomenon is well known to the experimental scientist who uses particular strains of animals because they are known to be predisposed to certain types of disease. There are, for example, types of rats that rapidly develop high blood pressure when fed salt. There are almost certainly similar types of individuals in the human species and, conversely, others who are able to tolerate large quantities of salt without developing high blood pressure.

So, just because your neighbor, or even your doctor, is healthy on the diet that you eat, this does not mean that you will automatically enjoy the same good standard of health.

7. An "average" or normal diet is not necessarily a healthy one.

Many people believe that if they eat an average diet, they will be healthy. While for many this is undoubtedly true, it is not universally so, particularly in those who are already unwell. Repeated dietary surveys show that in many groups the intake of essential nutrients is low or borderline. The elderly are particularly at risk because of falling food intake and poor absorption—they easily develop nutritional deficiencies.

The food that we eat has not been selected by God or mother nature and is not necessarily related to our body's requirements. It is decided upon by personal preference, availability in stores, cafés and restaurants, advertising, and the influence of what our parents, friends and neighbors eat. Most of these people have little or no knowledge of what makes up a healthy diet. There is, as a result, considerable room for error. It is probably true to say that the majority of people who read this book could improve their diet a lot.

8. Anyone who is ill, or even who just has symptoms, is likely to have a nutritional deficiency or have a problem which may be amenable to dietary or nutritional treatment.

The presence of symptoms or of an illness is a sign that there is some sort of disturbance in metabolism. The individual with heart disease may have high cholesterol; someone with migraine, abnormalities of blood stickiness; and a child with eczema, food or other allergies. Increasingly, the specific biochemical abnormalities or nutritional deficiencies that can occur in certain disease states are becoming understood. This opens the door to powerful and sometimes curative treatment by simply using nutritional methods.

Nutrition is a far greater factor in man's biochemistry and health than is pharmacology. Indigestion is not caused by a deficiency of antacids; high blood pressure is not caused by a deficiency of beta blockers; and migraine is not the result of an aspirin deficiency, yet current medical prescribing would have us believe otherwise. A person who is ill or symptomatic has a disturbed body biochemistry and this disturbance may well be correctable by nutritional means. The appropriate and scientific application of nutritional methods in the treatment of disease is akin to an engineer repairing a machine by restoring its fundamental parts to working order. Drug therapy aims to do the same thing, but cannot because it introduces a new set of parts. Obviously, there are times when drugs and medications *are* extremely effective and, indeed, life-saving, and no doctor, including us, would want to do without them. But medicine is at a point where we are beginning to understand some very important truths, and one is that for too long we have chosen to make use of "unofficial spare parts" because we did not know the nature of the "true" or "official" spare parts that were needed to do the job properly.

This book is about these "official" spare parts and how we can use them to our advantage.

PART ONE

Nutrients and Anti-Nutrients

INTRODUCTION

The body requires dietary fatty acids, amino acids, carbohydrates, vitamins and minerals to function properly. The sections in Part One discuss them in some detail, showing how deficiencies and excesses affect physical and mental functions, how to recognize deficiencies and how to deal with them once they have occurred. These sections explain the theory on which the practical information in Parts Two and Three is based. In Part One we also discuss such things as drugs, toxic metals and other antinutrients (even such apparently harmless things as tea or eggs) which can compromise our nutritional status and cause both minor and major health problems.

RECOMMENDED DAILY ALLOWANCES

Recommended daily allowances (RDAs) are guidelines to the quantities of nutrients that should be taken daily. They are set by expert committees and are simply opinions based on the scientific evidence to hand; the recommendations are made on inadequate information, and they differ from one country to another.

All too often, unfortunately, doctors cite RDAs as though they were gospel. This is far from the case and highlights the fact that the mere existence of RDAs can lead to a misunderstanding of what is actually occurring with any individual.

The simple viewpoint that if one is on a "balanced, healthy diet" (whatever that is!), one will consume adequate amounts of nutrients to maintain health, is not true.

The fact is that recommended daily allowances change as the evidence changes and must therefore be seen as somewhat arbitrary.

The idea behind setting RDAs was to give at least some idea as to the likelihood of groups of individuals being deficient in a specific nutrient when considering their dietary intake. This has severe limitations because people not only have different, and unique fingerprints, but also different and unique nutritional requirements.

Whether or not an individual is deficient in one or more nutrients depends on a lot more than just the amount taken in the diet (see pages xviii–xxii).

The case for supplementation with vitamins and minerals and other micronutrients is sometimes criticized on the basis that "there are no double-blind, controlled experiments proving the value of supplementing a given nutrient over and above the RDA." This is not true; there are, in fact, a great number of studies indicating the contrary. It is also intellectually unsound because recommended daily allowances themselves are based on incomplete data, and are nothing more than an opinion, albeit an expert one. They, too, are not based on double-blind, controlled trials. Furthermore, much of the experimentation has been done on animals, or in short-term "acute" deficiencies in humans. The long-term effects of marginal deficiencies or excesses of one or more micronutrients has not been established.

However, from a medical point of view, if an individual has a clinical problem which resolves upon supplementation with either a multivitamin and mineral supplement, or with a single nutrient alone, then this is at least circumstantial evidence of a need for the supplement(s).

RDAs are often misused and are expected to provide more or different information than they were ever designed to give.

Thus, RDAs are not particularly useful, for example, when an individual is unwell, is on drugs, has a specific medical condition, has an unusual diet, and so on. Anyone in these categories should *not* be considered as *most* people.

So, in conclusion, while RDAs have a purpose and, for some, provide a point of reference, they are nothing more than guidelines. There are some doctors who consider that RDAs should not be referred to at all when treating patients, as they are too misleading and bear no relationship to the nutritional status of any one individual.

VITAMINS

Vitamins are dietary substances required by the body in very small amounts for normal biochemical function. There are two major groups: water-soluble vitamins (the B vitamins and vitamin C), and the fat-soluble vitamins A, D, E and K. Intensive research into their sources, their function and our requirements for them has been going on over the last sixty years or so and we now know a great deal about them. Unfortunately, much of this knowledge is not applied by medical doctors to their patients, and we hope that this chapter will, at least in part, help to bridge the gap that lies between the knowledge that exists and the application of that knowledge to helping people stay well or recover from illness.

Vitamin A

The term vitamin A covers several fat-soluble compounds including retinol, which is the most important component, and two lesser components, retinal and retinoic acid. Vitamin A is only found in animal products but various vitamin-A-type compounds, the most important of which is beta-carotene, are found in vegetables, and these are water-soluble.

All of them are fat-soluble, are sensitive to light and are easily oxidized.

Though the deficiency signs of vitamin A were recognized in ancient Egyptian times, it was only in this century that its chemical nature was elucidated. Two researchers recognized a substance described as "fat-soluble A" as being a growth-promoting factor in animals. Later it was shown that vitamin A activity was present in plants in the yellow pigments known as carotenes.

WHAT IT DOES

The most important and well-known role of vitamin A is in relation to eye function. Vitamin A is necessary to prevent drying of the eye (xerophthalmia) and corneal changes; also, the normal function of the retina, the part of the eye involved with vision, and particularly the function of the light-sensitive areas of the eye, are dependent upon there being sufficient vitamin A. In Third World countries, 500,000 people lose their sight every year because of vitamin A deficiency and some two thirds of these will die within a few weeks of developing deficiency.

Vitamin A is involved in a number of other bodily functions. It is important in maintaining the stability of cell membranes and this may be clinically important. Furthermore, beta-carotene is the most effective receptor of free radical oxygen (see page 146) and this may be relevant in situations involving cancer, inflammatory disease and atherosclerosis, in which free radical mechanisms are thought to play a part.

A connection between vitamin A and zinc metabolism has

been described by several researchers. It appears that in severe zinc deficiency the formation of the protein which carries vitamin A, retinol-binding protein, is decreased. Zinc is an important constituent of many enzymes, including one found in the retina that is involved in vitamin A metabolism. Night blindness which does not improve with vitamin A supplements has been described in zinc deficient individuals, particularly in alcoholics with liver disease who are often vitamin A *and* zinc deficient.

In diseases such as alcoholic cirrhosis, pancreatic disease and cystic fibrosis, zinc and vitamin A and other deficiencies also often occur together.

FOOD SOURCES

In the Western world, the major dietary sources are from animal products, which provides vitamin A—retinol—usually combined with a fatty acid. As vitamin A is stored in animal and fish livers, these provide the most concentrated sources. Others include kidneys, eggs, milk and butter. Good vegetable sources include any green, yellow or orange-pigmented produce; the darker the color, the higher the content of beta-carotene. Carrots, spinach, cabbage, and orange and yellow fruits are the best sources.

DIETARY REQUIREMENTS

Normal daily requirements for vitamin A are in the region of 1,000 mcg of retinol for adult males and 800 mcg for adult females. Pregnant women require 1,000 and lactating women 1,200 mcg. Infants and children have requirements ranging from 400–700 mcg. These figures are based on a WHO recommendation given in 1974.

DEFICIENCY SYMPTOMS AND SIGNS

Vitamin A deficiency is one of the most common and most serious world-wide nutritional deficiencies. Severe vitamin A deficiency is rarely seen in developed countries, but isolated examples occur in people who have malabsorption states. In particular, anyone with fatty stools caused by pancreatic disease, biliary obstruction, or small bowel disease, is at risk.

The earliest symptoms of vitamin A deficiency include night blindness (difficulty in seeing well in dim light) and dryness of the eyes.

Skin signs of vitamin A deficiency include follicular hyperkeratosis, a condition in which the whole hair follicle and its adjacent skin is raised by a plug of horny keratin. Dryness of the skin can be a feature of vitamin A deficiency but this may be due to an associate essential fatty acid deficiency or a deficiency of other micronutrients such a vitamin B complex, vitamin C and zinc involved in fatty acid metabolism. Deficiency can occur without skin signs.

In general, in developing countries, vitamin A deficiency is associated with poor growth and development, and impaired resistance to infection.

CONDITIONS WHICH MIGHT BEST BENEFIT FROM VITAMIN A

Skin conditions

Vitamin A has been advocated in the treatment of a number of skin conditions. Usually, high doses (100,000 IUs per day or more) are used, and the potential risk of side-effects when such high doses are administered over a long period of time has meant that vitamin A does not have an established place in the treatment of common skin complaints. It has been used, apparently successfully, in the treatment of acne (at dosages of 100,000–400,000 IUs daily over a period of several months) under medical supervision. Retinoic acid, the acid derived from retinol, has been used, both by mouth and directly on the skin, in a wide range of skin conditions. Oral retinoic acid appears to be of value in certain dry skin conditions and the application of retinoic acid directly to the skin may be of value in acne, and for dry skin.

Vitamin A and its plant-derived relative beta-carotene may also be of value in those whose skin is very sensitive to the sun.

Ulcers

Vitamin A has been used in the treatment of gastric ulcers and might also be of value in the prevention of stress-induced ulcers as well as those induced by taking steroid drugs.

Respiratory distress syndrome

Some preliminary research suggests that giving vitamin A to a mother during pregnancy might reduce the incidence of this syndrome in her baby, but further research is needed.

Gynecological conditions

Vitamin A in doses ranging from 50,000–300,000 IUs may be of value in such conditions as heavy periods, premenstrual syndrome and painful periods. Clinical trials on these conditions have involved the administration of vitamin A for fifteen days in the last half of the menstrual cycle. The dosage and duration of administration have varied. Premenstrual syndrome is probably better treated by a multifactorial approach which may involve some vitamin A supplements (see page 301). The dangers of taking too much vitamin A in pregnancy are discussed below.

Cancers

The role of vitamin A and beta-carotene in cancer prevention has been investigated by many researchers, and the increased incidence of certain types of cancer has been linked to poor vitamin A status. The results of these studies show that cancer of the lung in particular is associated with a poor dietary intake of vitamin A or carotene. Other cancers which have been similarly correlated include those of the larynx, naso-pharynx, esophagus, mouth, stomach, colon, prostate and cervix.

A report on diet, nutrition and cancer, from the National Academy of Science of the United States, has recommended an increase in the diet of vegetables rich in carotenes.

It is possible that the lack of Western diseases, such as many of the more common cancers, in Third World countries that have a relatively good nutritional state may well be due to their high intake of dietary vitamin A. The use in the West of low-carotene, high-fiber foods, in an attempt to improve health by increasing fiber, may result in a failure to include this important dietary constituent. It is notable that wheat and bran contain no retinol or carotene.

Recent research in Japan has found that those who eat green vegetables are less likely to suffer from cancers of many organs, even if they are in "at risk" groups.

The role of vitamin A and its analogues, the retinoids, in the treatment of cancer is, however, uncertain. It may be that vitamin A and beta-carotene are of value in situations where cancer cells are about to form. A study in the Philippines of local residents who chew betel nuts showed that the administration of retinol and beta-carotene for three months substantially reduced cellular abnormalities in the lining-cells from the cheeks. Vitamin A deficiency may also be important in cervical cancer.

It is likely that the majority of cancers are multifactorial in nature and that an individual's nutritional state during the earliest phase of cancer will be only one of several factors that will need to be considered.

RETINOIDS

The administration of large doses of vitamin A rapidly leads to toxic side-effects even in situations in which such a large dose might be clinically useful. Accordingly, the search for relatively nontoxic derivatives of vitamin A has been stimulated, with the result that certain derivatives are now used in clinical practice. Two major compounds have been developed. Etretinate (Tigason) has been used successfully in the treatment of psoriasis and some dry skin conditions. The second derivative, iso-retinoin (Roaccutane) has been successfully used in the treatment of severe acne and it may be of value in certain cancers. Trials are under way. Such powerful drugs are known to have many important and serious side-effects, particularly a risk of damaging the fetus. This means that women taking these agents must be sure not to become pregnant while, or for at least twelve months after, taking them.

DOSAGE AND TOXICITY

All the fat-soluble vitamins have the potential for being toxic because they are stored in the body and not excreted in the urine like the water-soluble ones. If too much vitamin A is taken it accumulates in the liver and eventually in other fatty tissues. Dosages of several hundred thousand IUs have been given without producing toxicity, but toxic levels have been described as occurring in doses as low as 15,000 IUs per day for several months in infants, and doses in the region of 30,000 IUs or more per day in adults, again administered for several months. Doses over 10,000 IUs per day should not be taken by anyone who is pregnant or likely to become pregnant; excess vitamin A has been shown to cause congenital malformations in animals.

Signs of vitamin A overdosage include fatigue, malaise, lethargy, headache, insomnia, restlessness, skin changes (including dryness and flakiness of the skin), loss of body hair and brittle nails. Bone changes may also occur. A common and relatively early sign is dryness and scaling of the skin. The most sinister symptom is a headache. **The presence of these means that urgent medical attention is essential.**

Introduction to the B Vitamins

The B group of vitamins is a collection of essential nutrients that have certain characteristics in common.

First, they are all water-soluble, and second, they are usually found in similar food sources such as brewers' yeast, animal meats, wholegrain cereals and vegetable proteins. While chemically distinct from one another, the ways they work in the body are closely interrelated. Folic acid and vitamin B12 metabolisms are closely connected; vitamin B2 is required for the activation of vitamin B6; and vitamin B3 can be manufactured from other dietary agents, provided there is adequate vitamin B6. So they are all interlinked.

It is extremely rare to see an isolated deficiency of any one of the B vitamins, except for that of vitamin B12. For example, someone with vitamin B2 deficiency may have red, greasy facial skin which might also be caused by a coexistent vitamin B6 deficiency. It is usual therefore, that when a deficiency of one of the vitamins is suspected, a B complex supplement is given.

There are certain people who are particularly susceptible to vitamin B deficiency. These include:

- Alcoholics, partly because of their poor diet and partly because of the effects of alcohol upon vitamin B metabolism.
- Those with poor dietary intakes. For example, those who eat a lot of junk food, or the elderly.
- Those with increased requirements, e.g. pregnant and breast-feeding women, growing children and adolescents.
- Those on long-term drugs such as anticonvulsants, certain antibiotics, and oral contraceptives.
- Those with a psychiatric history. Deficiencies of vitamin B1, B6, folic acid and vitamin B12 are particularly likely.

Symptoms such as a painful, sore, red tongue, cracking at the corners of the mouth and red, greasy facial skin, may all suggest deficiencies of any one of several B vitamins.

Someone can have symptoms of vitamin B deficiency for a considerable length of time before any outward signs become apparent. A chronic deficiency, particularly, may result in mental changes without there ever being any physical signs. So, if ever you, or anyone you know in any of the above situations, has a deteriorating level of health, or experiences mental changes, it is worth a trial of a substantial B complex supplement.

Vitamin B1 (Thiamin)

Thiamin was one of the first vitamins to be recognized, but although vitamin B1 deficiency has been described as occurring for thousands of years, it was not until the late nineteenth and early twentieth centuries that dietary factors were thought to play a role. In the Far East, consumption of "polished" or refined rice often led to vitamin B1 deficiency, as the discarded rice bran contained most of the vitamin B1. In the Second World War, many European prisoners-of-war held in the Far East developed vitamin B1 deficiency because of the poor diet they were fed. The term beri-beri (Singhalese for "extreme weakness") was used to describe the disease that occurred as a result of vitamin B1 deficiency.

WHAT IT DOES

Vitamin B1 is mainly found in skeletal muscle, heart muscle, brain, kidney and liver. It plays a crucial part in energy production and carbohydrate metabolism. Deficiency results in rapid deterioration in both heart and skeletal muscle function as well as brain and nerve function. The absorption of thiamin from the diet requires the presence of folic acid and a deficiency of folic acid may result in a thiamin deficiency. Substances which destroy thiamin are to be found in tea, coffee, certain raw, freshwater fish, and a number of fruits and vegetables including blackberries, blackcurrants, red beets, spinach and cabbage. Some of these dietary agents may be destroyed by heat, but others are not. On the whole they do not play an important part in influencing human needs unless consumed in excess.

FOOD SOURCES

Thiamin is widely distributed amongst foods of both vegetable and animal origin. Particularly good sources include whole grains, pork, beef, peas, beans, lentils and brown rice. Refined foods, particularly white rice and white flour, have substantially reduced levels.

DIETARY REQUIREMENTS

The requirements for thiamin depend upon calorie intake. With high carbohydrate, sugar or alcohol intakes, the requirements rise. They range from 1–1.8 mg per day for adults. The higher levels are needed during pregnancy, lactation and for those with high levels of physical activity and high calorie intake.

DEFICIENCY SYMPTOMS AND SIGNS

The body has very little in the way of vitamin B1 stores and a deficiency can occur within a few weeks if intake is substantially reduced. Initial symptoms include depression, irritability, failure to concentrate, and a deterioration of memory. In severe deficiency states (usually caused by alcoholism), mental confusion with marked deterioration of short-term memory is a feature. Such people confuse fact with fantasy, particularly when explaining recent events that they cannot remember accurately.

More commonly, thiamin deficiency shows up as a numbness and tingling in the hands and feet, with paralysis of muscles, leading to wrist- and foot-drop. The calf muscles may be particularly tender and this is sometimes a useful sign. The compression of muscles may lead to prolonged indentation of the muscle for several seconds. Again, this is an early sign of vitamin B1 deficiency. Other features include reduced pain tolerance, reduction in manual and foot dexterity and an increase in reaction times, personality changes, insomnia, disturbed sleep, fatigue, night sweats, abdominal and chest pains and even fever of unknown cause.

In the elderly a deficiency of vitamin B1 may affect the heart. Cardiac failure with a rapid pulse, shortness of breath and ankle swelling can sometimes be due to vitamin B1 deficiency and is particularly likely to be seen in alcoholics. Such individuals often have a ruddy complexion and warm hands and feet.

THOSE WHO MIGHT BEST BENEFIT FROM THIAMIN

Several groups of people are particularly at risk from vitamin B1 deficiency. They include:

- those with a moderate to high alcohol consumption
- the elderly
- those who pass large volumes of urine, such as diabetics
- those on diuretics (water tablets) or digoxin (a drug used in heart failure)
- those recovering from heart failure
- those who consume a lot of refined carbohydrates or junk food
- psychiatric patients, particularly those suffering from depression and anxiety
- women on the Pill or estrogen replacement therapy
- those with liver or thyroid disease
- people suffering or recovering from infections
- elderly people after operations
- those with recurrent vomiting, such as in pregnancy; those with stomach diseases; and those with cancer

DOSAGE AND TOXICITY

Vitamin B1 is usually given in doses of 10–50 mg or more per day, which should be adequate to correct most mild to moderate deficiencies. The severely ill and those who have a high alcohol intake can be given their large doses of vitamin B1 by injection and not by mouth.

Toxicity from vitamin B1 is very rare, but severe reactions have occasionally been described in those receiving repeated injections of vitamin B1 intravenously.

Heart failure and vitamin B1 deficiency

Mr. S.J., a seventy-eight-year-old retired former naval captain, had been confined to his bed for over a month because of heart failure. He was short of breath, with markedly swollen ankles, and the lack of oxygen had resulted in his lips becoming blue and his becoming increasingly mentally confused. He had responded only partially to treatment with powerful diuretic drugs. His wife told me that he had been eating poorly over the last few months and that his diet consisted mainly of white bread with honey or golden syrup, numerous cups of tea with sugar, and he always had his two shots of rum at night. I suspected that he might well be short of vitamin B1—thiamin. His wife wanted to stop his drugs and treat him with some "natural remedies." I strongly advised her against this, and asked her to continue with his drugs and add some high-dose vitamin B. Within two weeks his ankle swelling had reduced, he became markedly less breathless, and he returned to being the mentally alert man that his wife had known. Sugar and alcohol were forbidden in his diet henceforth. He improved so much that he returned to driving his car a few months later. Unfortunately, his vitamin supplements were stopped and he again developed an episode of heart failure. This case illustrates how vitamin B deficiencies may be particularly likely to occur in the elderly, especially those who have a high intake of alcohol or refined carbohydrates, including table sugar.

Heart failure which is unresponsive to diuretic drugs is a feature of vitamin B1 deficiency, and mental confusion can be caused by deficiency of almost any of the B vitamins. Ill, elderly patients should, as routine, receive multivitamin supplements.

Vitamin B2 (Riboflavin)

Vitamin B2 was first discovered in the 1930s when it was isolated from yeast extract.

WHAT IT DOES

Riboflavin plays a crucial role in the formation of a number of enzymes that are mainly found in the liver. These enzymes allow the removal of molecules of hydrogen and the introduction of oxygen. By this process certain substances are metabolized and energy is released. It is surprising that people who are deficient in vitamin B2 do not suffer from severe metabolic disturbances or a lack of energy. This is probably because liver-stores of vitamin B2 are maintained even in deficiency states. Vitamin B2 plays a major role in the metabolism of proteins, fats and carbohydrates, as well as in the oxidation of many other substances. Requirements are increased at times of growth and high protein intake. It also enhances the metabolism of vitamin B6. This is why some people with vitamin B2 deficiency have vitamin B6 deficiency symptoms and signs.

FOOD SOURCES

Major food sources of riboflavin are milk and other dairy produce, cereals, meats, and some green, leafy vegetables. Riboflavin is fairly stable with heat but deteriorates on exposure to light.

DIETARY REQUIREMENTS

Requirements vary considerably depending upon the amount of growth. Infants require approximately 0.6 mg per day, and this increases up to 1.8 mg per day for teenagers. Adults require 1.2 mg per day, and up to 1.6 mg per day are needed for pregnant women. Lactating women may require 2.0 mg per day because of their increased needs.

DEFICIENCY SYMPTOMS AND SIGNS

Perhaps because of the interrelationship between vitamins B2 and B6, the physical signs of deficiency are very similar for both these nutrients. Soreness and burning of the lips and tongue are early features and can also occur in vitamin B6 deficiency, but dryness, cracking and peeling of the lips is characteristic of a lack of vitamin B2. The skin of the face becomes red, greasy and scaly, particularly at the sides of the nose. Unlike vitamin B6 shortage, there may be changes in the eye such as a dislike of light, excessive tear production, and eye irritation. "Burning feet" can be caused by lack of this vitamin.

THOSE WHO MIGHT BEST BENEFIT FROM RIBOFLAVIN

- children during growth spurts (especially adolescence)
- pregnant and breast-feeding women
- those who consume moderate to large amounts of alcohol
- the elderly
- women on the Pill or on estrogen replacement therapy

DOSAGE AND TOXICITY

Deficiencies of vitamin B2 can easily be corrected by taking 10–20 mg of vitamin B2 daily. Toxicity is almost unheard of. However, there are practically no reasons for taking more than 20 mg of the vitamin a day.

You may notice a yellow coloration of the urine when you take supplements of vitamin B2. This is completely normal.

Vitamin B3 (Nicotinic Acid and Nicotinamide)

There are several forms of vitamin B3. Nicotinic acid (which is also known as niacin) is very closely related to the other compound nicotinamide, or niacinamide. They all have vitamin B3 activity but nicotinic acid has rather specific effects on cholesterol metabolism.

Although vitamin B3 was discovered in 1911 its full role as a vitamin was not appreciated until 1937. Classical deficiency of vitamin B3 produces pellagra—a condition characterized by dermatitis, diarrhea and dementia. This was described in Italy in the eighteenth century and was endemic in the southern states of the USA at the end of the last century and the beginning of this. Nicotinic acid, like many of the other B vitamins, was first isolated from yeast.

WHAT IT DOES

Vitamin B3 plays an important part in the formation of certain enzymes that are involved in the transport of hydrogen, and in this respect it is similar to vitamin B2, riboflavin. The majority of enzymes helped by vitamin B3 are involved in glucose and carbohydrate metabolism.

FOOD SOURCES

Major food sources include meat, particularly beef, milk, fish and whole grains. Maize corn can be a poor source of nicotinic acid. Populations that rely heavily upon corn as a major source of protein are likely to be at risk of developing vitamin B3 deficiency. Vitamin B3 can also be synthesized from the amino acid tryptophan: 60 mg of tryptophan provides 1 mg of vitamin B3. Many foods are therefore described as having a "niacin equivalent," which is dependent upon their content of both niacin and tryptophan.

DIETARY REQUIREMENTS

Dietary requirements of vitamin B3 vary from 12–18 mg per day for adults. Higher levels are required by men, those who are more physically active, and during pregnancy and lactation. There may be a need for even more during periods of rapid growth.

DEFICIENCY SYMPTOMS AND SIGNS

A deficiency of vitamin B3 probably occurs less frequently than do deficiencies of vitamin B1 or B6. Severe deficiency states are rarely seen.

B3 deficiency is more likely to develop in those with a low protein intake, particularly if they also have a high alcohol consumption. The alcoholic is perhaps the most obvious person likely to develop this deficiency. Mental changes such as irritability, headache, loss of memory, and emotional instability are early features. Skin changes are characteristic and consist of redness, scaling and pigmentation of the skin in light-exposed areas, particularly on the backs of the hands and face. This contrasts markedly with skin that is covered by clothing. Changes in the gastrointestinal tract are an important characteristic. The tongue is often sore, painful and fissured. This can look like the dried-up bottom of a river bed, or the tread of a car tire. Other changes in the gastrointestinal tract include diarrhea, and an impairment of acid production by the stomach which may further upset the individual's nutritional state. Mental changes due to deficiency can occur without any other signs and may pass unrecognized in the elderly.

THOSE WHO MIGHT BEST BENEFIT FROM NICOTINIC ACID

- those who have a moderate or large intake of alcohol
- those with a poor protein intake
- those with thyrotoxicosis (overactive thyroid gland), Crohn's disease (see page 213), those on certain anti-cancer drugs
- **high doses may be helpful in reducing elevated blood fats, schizophrenia and arthritis—but this needs medical supervision**

Nicotinic acid, but not nicotinamide, will produce powerful and sometimes uncomfortable flushing of the skin, particularly on the face and hands, and this can be associated with tingling. This is much more likely to occur when nicotinic acid is taken in dosages in excess of 25 mg and especially if it is taken on an empty stomach. Nicotinic acid has been used in the treatment of chilblains in dosages of approximately 50 mg three times a day, sometimes with success. It has an acknowledged place in the treatment of those who have elevated levels of cholesterol and another group of blood fats, the triglycerides, which may be associated with increased risk of heart disease. The dosages used in such cases can be very high, up to 6 g of nicotinic acid per day. This is some 400 times the normal recommended daily allowance. It is effective in lowering elevated cholesterol levels, reducing them by about twenty percent or considerably more if combined with certain cholesterol-lowering drugs. Elevated triglycerides may be lowered by anything from twenty-three to forty-six percent and this effect can be further improved by the addition of other agents.

Another possibly important role for nicotinic acid has been in the treatment of schizophrenia. It was noted in 1951 that there was a similarity between the mental changes caused by vitamin B3 deficiency and the mental changes in schizophrenia. A number of studies seem to demonstrate the value of the vitamin in certain patients with schizophrenia, particularly when combined with other vitamins; other studies, however, have not confirmed these findings. The use of nicotinic acid in such a way was one of the first examples of "megavitamin" therapy.

Large doses of nicotinic acid (not nicotinamide) have been used as part of a successful broad-spectrum megavitamin program to reduce total body burdens of organic herbicides and pesticides, polychlorinated biphenyls and their related compounds polybrominated biphenyls.

Finally, nicotinamide has been reported to benefit some cases of osteoarthritis of the knees, but this has never been formally tested.

There are relatively few indications for general vitamin B3 supplementation. Vitamin B3 is often incorporated with other B vitamins and this is a wise precaution. However, the number of conditions that respond to vitamin B3 is relatively low and should not be confused with the specific conditions for which high-dose vitamin B3 is appropriate.

DOSAGE AND TOXICITY

Nicotinic acid or nicotinamide in doses of 50–100 mg per day will correct a deficiency state. High doses of nicotinic acid and nicotinamide can alter liver function tests, changes which quickly reverse when treatment is stopped or the dosage reduced. Sometimes diabetics can be worsened by high-dose nicotinic acid. There have been no permanent long-term effects from high-dose nicotinic acid administration. Nicotinamide in high doses can sometimes cause depression.

Vitamin B5 (Pantothenic Acid)

Pantothenic acid is one of the lesser B vitamins. It was given the name pantothenic acid because it is widely distributed in food (*pantothen* is the Greek word for "from all sides").

WHAT IT DOES

Pantothenic acid plays a crucial role in many of the reactions involving carbohydrates, fats and amino acids.

FOOD SOURCES

Pantothenic acid is widely distributed. Particularly high levels are found in eggs, wholegrain cereals, and meat.

DIETARY REQUIREMENTS

The exact requirements are unknown but are probably in the region of 5–10 mg per day.

DEFICIENCY SYMPTOMS AND SIGNS

A deficiency of pantothenic acid has been produced experimentally and such symptoms as fatigue, headaches, weakness, emotional swings, impaired muscle coordination, numbness and tingling, muscle cramps and gastrointestinal disturbance including nausea, vomiting and abdominal cramps were observed. However, this severe deficiency was produced only under extreme conditions.

THOSE WHO MIGHT BEST BENEFIT FROM PANTOTHENIC ACID

Pantothenic acid deficiency has been described as occurring in ten to twenty percent of alcoholics. Such individuals are more likely to be deficient in folic acid, vitamin B6, vitamin B1, nicotinic acid and vitamin B2, but pantothenic acid deficiency is simply a part of the spectrum. Substantial B complex vitamins are essential for such individuals and it seems a wise precaution to include adequate quantities of pantothenic acid. Painful, burning feet also sometimes respond to pantothenic acid supplements.

Vitamin B6 (Pyridoxine)

Vitamin B6 was discovered in the 1930s when its necessity for animal life was first demonstrated. A deficiency of vitamin B6 does not produce such a "classical" picture as do the deficiencies of vitamin B1 and B3. It is, however, one of the most widely consumed supplements of the vitamin B complex because of the range of conditions that appear to be influenced by it.

WHAT IT DOES

Vitamin B6 comes in three closely related forms: pyridoxine, pyridoxal and pyridoxamine. These are all converted to the active compound pyridoxal-5-phosphate. Most of the vitamin B6 taken as tablets is in the form of pyridoxine hydrochloride. In the diet, the three varieties of vitamin B6 are often found together. The conversion of these dietary forms to the active pyridoxal-5-phosphate apparently requires the presence of vitamin B2 and magnesium. This is yet another example of the interrelationship of the B vitamins.

Vitamin B6 plays a major part in the metabolism of protein and its constituent amino acids. Vitamin B6 requirements are very much related to protein consumption: the more protein we eat, the higher our requirement for vitamin B6.

It is worth noting that a large hamburger from a fast-food chain provides only 0.02 mg of vitamin B6 (one to two percent of the daily dietary requirement) while providing a very substantial quantity of protein—so, to metabolize the protein of the hamburger, vitamin B6 must be obtained from another source!

Vitamin B6 is also involved in the metabolism of certain essential body chemicals including histamine, hydroxytryptamine and serotonin. This latter compound is particularly important in normal brain chemistry, so a deficiency of vitamin B6 may have profound effects upon mood and behavior.

Vitamin B6 is involved in sugar metabolism, and the metabolism of essential fatty acids which play an important role in inflammatory diseases, skin diseases and disorders of the immune and cardiovascular systems. Vitamin B6 is necessary for the formation of vitamin B3 (niacinamide) from the amino acid tryptophan.

Vitamin B6 is also important in the metabolism of certain minerals, particularly magnesium; also, absorption of zinc might be impeded in people with vitamin B6 deficiency. Smoking, some drugs and possibly some food additives may increase requirements of vitamin B6, while exercise may improve the conversion of vitamin B6 to its active form in the body.

FOOD SOURCES

Good food sources of vitamin B6 include most meats, fish, egg yolk, wholegrain cereals, bananas, avocados, nuts, seeds and some green, leafy vegetables. Low levels are to be found in cottage cheese, often the staple food of dieters. No wonder they are often troubled with "combination skin," the red, greasy, scaly, facial skin that is found with vitamin B6 deficiency.

DIETARY REQUIREMENTS

Adult men and women require about 2 mg of vitamin B6 a day. The exact requirement will increase if protein consumption is high. 2.5 mg a day during pregnancy and breast-feeding is recommended. Higher doses, in the region of 5–10 mg, may be required by pregnant or breast-feeding women to correct some of the biochemical abnormalities which occur in these conditions.

It is worth pointing out that considerable losses of vitamin B6 occur during cooking. Also, exposure to light speeds up the destruction of this vitamin.

DEFICIENCY SYMPTOMS AND SIGNS

It must be remembered that as with all the B vitamins, deficiency symptoms will appear before physical signs, so people usually complain of mental changes such as irritability, nervousness, insomnia and weakness, before skin problems and other visible signs appear.

The most common physical sign of vitamin B6 deficiency is the development of a seborrheic dermatitis in the areas of the nose, corners of the eyes and mouth, and the development of an acne-like rash, particularly on the forehead. The skin is red and greasy, but there may also be scaling and flaking of the skin. There is a considerable similarity between the presence of vitamin B6 and B2 deficiency as far as skin signs are concerned. The tongue may also become sore and the taste buds prominent and easily seen, particularly at its tip. In more severe cases, loss of appetite, weight loss, a reduced resistance to infection, anemia and nerve damage develop. Very often an individual suffers from multiple vitamin B deficiencies, rather than just one.

THOSE WHO MIGHT BEST BENEFIT FROM PYRIDOXINE

- Women on estrogen-containing oral contraceptives.
- Women on hormone replacement therapy.
- Pregnant women for nausea, diabetes and pre-eclamptic toxemia.
- Women who suffer from premenstrual syndrome.
- Pregnant and breast-feeding women.
- People suffering from psychological problems, e.g. depression, anxiety, schizophrenia, insomnia.
- Hyperactive or autistic children.
- People with kidney disease; kidney stones, kidney failure, bladder cancer.
- Diabetics.
- People with carpal tunnel syndrome.
- Those with increased need, e.g. alcoholics; those with poor nutritional intake.
- People with allergies to monosodium glutamate and tartrazine.
- Sufferers from cardiovascular disease, to prevent excessive clotting of the blood.

Vitamin B6 may occasionally be of value in sickle cell disease, vertigo, peptic ulcers, acne, seborrheic dermatitis, skin light-sensitivity, herpes infections during pregnancy, epilepsy, Parkinson's disease and radiation sickness.

Some drugs act against vitamin B6: especially penicillamine, L-dopa, isoniazid, hydralazine and Amiodarone.

DOSAGE AND TOXICITY

Vitamin B6 should always be taken with vitamin B complex.

Don't take more than 50 mg per day unless advised by a physician.

Recently it has been appreciated that taking large doses of vitamin B6 can result in significant side-effects. One study has reported on incidents of nerve damage developing as a result of the long-term administration of high-dose vitamin B6. This evidence makes it sensible not to take high doses of vitamin B6. There are conditions that genuinely do require treatment with high doses of vitamin B6, but people with such conditions should always be under the care of a physician. More recently, some reports suggest that doses as low as 100–200 mg a day may have adverse effects, but this has yet to be confirmed.

Vitamin B12

In the late 1920s it was found that the serious and often fatal disease of pernicious anemia responded when victims ate massive quantities of liver or had injections of liver extract. Vitamin B12, sometimes called cyanocobalamin, was finally isolated in the 1950s and found to be the agent effective in the treatment of pernicious anemia.

WHAT IT DOES

Vitamin B12 is found only in animal-based foods. It is originally produced by bacteria but is essential to man if he is to be healthy. Vitamin B12 in the diet is absorbed by the small intestine but requires the presence of a compound known as intrinsic factor, produced by the stomach. This combines chemically with vitamin B12 enabling it to be absorbed in the lower part of the small intestine. Vitamin B12 is transported to the liver where it is stored. The actions of vitamin B12 are very similar to those of folic acid.

Conditions affecting the stomach and the lower part of the small intestine can cause a vitamin B12 deficiency. However, as body-stores of vitamin B12 can last for anywhere from three to six years, the production of a clinically obvious deficiency takes some time.

FOOD SOURCES

The best sources of vitamin B12 are liver, organ-meats, meat and, to a lesser extent, fish, dairy products, eggs and brewers' yeast. Strict vegetarians—vegans—who eat only vegetables may be risking vitamin B12 deficiency in the long term.

DIETARY REQUIREMENTS

The requirements for vitamin B12 are minimal, particularly as the body conserves most of the vitamin. Requirements are in the region of 1 mcg per day, rising to 3–4 mcg per day for pregnant and breast-feeding women.

DEFICIENCY SYMPTOMS AND SIGNS

Those short of vitamin B12 often have anemia, with symptoms such as exhaustion, shortness of breath on exertion, pale skin and mucous membranes. There are also characteristic changes in the nervous system, including numbness and tingling in the hands and feet, clumsiness and difficulty with walking. The walking difficulty is often particularly obvious at night when the person is unable to see where he or she is going and has to rely upon an awareness of the position of their legs. Early treatment is vital to prevent serious and permanent damage to the nervous system.

A lack of vitamin B12 can also affect mental functions, and elderly, confused, depressed or mentally deteriorating individuals should be suspected of having vitamin B12 deficiency; vitamin B12 levels are often measured routinely in all elderly patients admitted to the hospital. Pernicious anemia tends to run in families, and also to be associated with blue eyes and premature graying of the hair.

THOSE WHO MIGHT BEST BENEFIT FROM VITAMIN B12

- Those with pernicious anemia.
- People who have had their stomachs removed.
- Vegan, pregnant or breast-feeding women.
- Those with small bowel disease, e.g. Crohn's Disease, or those who have had a part of the small bowel removed.
- Those with bacterial bowel overgrowth.
- People with tobacco blindness (see page 282).
- People complaining of tiredness.
- Sufferers from other conditions, including diabetes (with or without neuropathy), multiple sclerosis, trigeminal neuralgia, post-herpetic neuralgia, diabetic retinopathy, seborrheic dermatitis, discoid lupus erythematosis, asthma, senile dementia,

various mental problems, types of nerve damage, and those on certain types of drugs (see page 143).

In the first four conditions, there is an impaired absorption of vitamin B12 from the gastrointestinal tract. The vitamins therefore have to be given by injection and such people usually receive regular injections of vitamin B12. Many people can inject themselves with their vitamin B12, just as diabetics give themselves injections of insulin.

Certain drugs can adversely affect vitamin B12 levels. Prolonged use of the antibiotic neomycin; certain antidiabetic drugs; potassium chloride supplements, and the cholesterol-lowering agent cholestyramine can all do so.

DOSAGE AND TOXICITY

Vitamin B12 is generally given by injection. The usual dosage is 1 mg given at weekly or three-monthly intervals, depending on the clinical situation.

Toxicity is practically unknown, but the vitamin B12 preparation cyanocobalamin is best avoided, particularly in certain eye

Vitamin B12 deficiency

Hilda, a sixty-nine-year-old woman, had noticed that she was becoming increasingly unsteady on her feet. Characteristically, she said that she was never troubled during the day, but was almost unable to walk if she got up at night from her bed. It seemed that when she was in the dark, her walking became particularly difficult. Examination showed her to have a marked loss of balance, due to decreased sensation in the feet and legs. This is very characteristic of vitamin B12 deficiency, which indeed she proved to have. It is particularly likely to occur in the elderly, and may be associated with thyroid disease and diabetes, as well as being more common in patients with blue eyes and white hair. In Hilda's case it was in fact due to abnormal bacteria in the bowel, which was the cause of her long-standing rumbling and gastric stomach. Treatment with a course of antibiotics cleared her bowel symptoms, and she continues with vitamin B12 injections, once a month, for life. Lack of vitamin B12 should be considered in any elderly patient with unsteadiness in walking, loss of sensation in the legs, or deteriorating mental function. It is a preventable and treatable cause of all of these symptoms.

conditions that require vitamin B12. Hydroxycobalamin is now the preferred supplemental form of B12. A normal serum-B12 level does not exclude deficiency.

Folic Acid

Folic acid is another member of the B vitamin group. Different forms of folic acid, the folates, are found in foods. Folic acid was isolated in the 1930s from yeast and liver, but its name is derived from the word foliage because it is so frequently found in green, leafy vegetables.

WHAT IT DOES

The metabolism of folic acid is closely linked with that of vitamin B12 and is vital for the workings of the central nervous system.

Folic acid is absorbed from the diet mainly from the first part of the small intestine. It is then transported to the liver where it is metabolized and stored. The body has approximately three to six months' store of folic acid.

FOOD SOURCES

The best sources of folic acid include liver, green vegetables, kidneys, eggs, and wholegrain cereals. Dairy produce contains relatively little folic acid. The vitamin can be destroyed by cooking, but its breakdown appears to be protected by vitamin C. The absorption of folic acid from different sources of food varies considerably.

DIETARY REQUIREMENTS

The requirement for folic acid varies from 400–800 mcg per day for adults. The higher level is required during pregnancy and lactation. The average diet probably contains only borderline levels of folic acid.

DEFICIENCY SYMPTOMS AND SIGNS

Mild deficiencies of folic acid may be very common in the general population. Only the more severe folic acid deficiencies show up as anemia. Those with a lack of either folic acid or vitamin B12 will eventually become anemic, which produces symptoms such as lethargy, tiredness, shortness of breath on exertion, and pallor of the skin and mucous membranes. Cracking of the corners of the mouth has recently been described as being due to folic acid deficiency; however, this can also be caused by a lack of iron, vitamin B2 or vitamin B6.

Folic acid deficiency can produce a painful, sore tongue which has a smooth almost bald appearance. Similar symptoms are found with a shortage of vitamin B12 and iron. Very often a deficiency of folic acid will be diagnosed, not by the presence of symptoms or signs, but because a blood test has shown an anemia of a type that can be caused by its lack. While iron deficiency is the most common cause of anemia, shortages of folic acid or vitamin B12 are the next most likely nutritional causes. Mild deficiency may cause depression, and more severe ones can lead to damage to the nerves—peripheral neuropathy.

INCREASED REQUIREMENTS

Increased requirements occur at certain times of life. The main ones are:

- during pregnancy
- during breast-feeding
- in premature infants

Goats' milk, which is given to children who have cows' milk allergy, is a particularly poor source of folic acid and supplementation may be required in these children.

Folic acid is a vitamin that is particularly required at times of increased growth and stress. A deficiency is most likely to occur at the extremes of life and in women who are pregnant or breast-feeding.

It appears that a folic acid deficiency is especially common in those with a psychiatric illness. Those who are depressed, or even schizophrenic, can be markedly deficient, and correcting the folic acid deficiency has been shown not only to improve the patient's mood, but also to reduce his or her stay in the hospital. Considering how cheap folic acid is, the potential financial savings are considerable. Very often such patients are also deficient in other B vitamins, so we think that appropriate supplementation should be considered in all psychiatric patients, as well as in the elderly who are showing signs of mental deterioration.

Folic acid deficiency can occur even with normal blood levels.

One of the most remarkable discoveries in the last few years has been the effect of folic acid supplementation on the prevention of neural-tube defects such as spina bifida. Spina bifida is a condition in which the spinal column of the developing fetus fails to form properly, with resultant damage to the nervous system. Such a child can be born severely deformed and may die either before or after birth. Many require considerable long-term medical treatment.

Any woman who has had a child with spina bifida or other severe abnormality of the nervous system should consult her general practitioner *before* trying for a baby again. Her nutritional state, including that of folic acid, should be carefully assessed (see page 322).

DOSAGE AND TOXICITY

Many multivitamin supplements contain small quantities of folic acid in the range of 100–200 mcg. This is adequate to ensure satisfactory levels of folic acid for most people. It is important to include in the diet foods that are high in folic acid, such as green, leafy vegetables. Our experience shows us that people who live alone almost never eat green, leafy vegetables regularly. The bother of buying, preparing and cooking them seems to be too much for just one person. Linked to this way of life, the widespread use of convenience foods almost certainly means a borderline intake of folic acid. There really is no substitute for an adequate intake of lightly cooked green, leafy vegetables or salads. Eat your greens!

Biotin

Biotin is one of the lesser known B vitamins. It is widely distributed in meats, dairy produce, and wholegrain cereals.

In adults, a deficiency of biotin may cause the development of a scaly dermatitis, with weakness and tiredness. Severe cradle cap in infants can also be due to biotin deficiency. It is possible to become deficient in biotin by eating large numbers of raw egg whites, or taking long-term antibiotics. Lower levels are also found in athletes.

Choline

Choline is known to be essential in animal and human nutrition. As the production of choline probably occurs satisfactorily in humans, true deficiency states have not been described. However, its action is related to that of other B vitamins in man. Choline, together with glycerol and certain fatty acids, is a constituent of lecithin. Choline also helps to form acetyl-choline which is essential for electrical conduction of nerve impulses in the whole nervous system. So it is clearly an important biological compound, but not, strictly speaking, a vitamin.

Choline has also been tried as a supplement in a number of neurological diseases including Alzheimer's disease, Huntington's chorea, and a condition called tardive dyskinesia which can be a side-effect of long-term anti-schizophrenia medication. Doses of up to 12 g a day have been given **but this level of dosage must be done under medical supervision.**

Lecithin, a dietary fat which contains choline, has been used in the treatment of cholesterol problems, but there is little good evidence to support its use in this respect.

Lecithin, together with *cholic* acid (a constituent of normal bile) has been given to people with gallstones, causing the stones to dissolve.

Inositol

Inositol is an essential factor in the diet of certain animals, but it is so widespread in food that a deficiency has not been described in man. Like choline, it appears to be involved in fat metabolism, particularly in relation to the liver. In people with kidney disease and diabetes, high levels of a type of inositol have been found in the blood, and some abnormality of metabolism of this compound is thought to occur. It may play a role in the disease of the nerves seen in diabetics.

Vitamin C

A lack of vitamin C produces scurvy. Scurvy was the scourge of the British navy in the seventeenth and eighteenth centuries. Long sea voyages meant eating stored foods in which fruit and vegetables played little or no part. Dr. James Lind, physician to the British navy, conducted what is thought to be one of the first controlled experiments, administering citrus fruits to one group of sailors in addition to their standard diet, while another group ate just the standard diet. His results were published in 1753, but it was not until 1795 that his observations were accepted.

Vitamin C was isolated in 1928 and one of the original workers, Dr. Szent-Gyorgyi, received a Nobel Prize for his work. In the early 1930s the chemical structure of vitamin C was discovered, and in 1933 it was synthesized. Vitamin C is now the most widely consumed nutritional supplement.

WHAT IT DOES

Vitamin C appears to have a number of important roles. These include the maintenance of healthy connective tissue and bones (a deficiency often leads to bleeding and poor wound healing), the normal metabolism of cholesterol, and the production of cortisol by the adrenal gland. It is biochemically active in the production of collagen (found both in skin and bones), in the metabolism of various brain chemicals, and in the synthesis of a hormone, noradrenalin, which has powerful effects upon pulse rate and blood pressure. It is a powerful anti-oxidant and can be used as a food preservative. It also has antiviral and antibacterial properties.

Its exact role in these reactions, and indeed the mechanics by which a deficiency produces the classical signs of scurvy are still not fully understood.

FOOD SOURCES

Good food sources include most fruits, green vegetables (including broccoli, brussels sprouts, and cauliflower), liver, kidney, and potatoes. Particularly high levels are found in rosehips and certain exotic fruits, but these rarely form a substantial part of anyone's diet. Potatoes, because we eat so much of them, particularly in winter months, play a very important part in maintaining dietary levels of vitamin C, particularly in the elderly. Vitamin C is usually destroyed by exposure to the atmosphere and by prolonged cooking, and there is a moderate reduction when foods are stored.

DIETARY REQUIREMENTS

The recommended intake in the UK is in the region of 30 mg per day for adult men and women, rising to 60 mg a day during pregnancy and lactation. Elsewhere, in the USA, Canada and many European countries, for example, levels of 45 mg or higher have been recommended. Only 10 mg per day is necessary to prevent or treat scurvy, but some authorities have suggested figures as high as 200 mg per day. However, it is not clear whether individuals consuming less than this amount suffer any long-term adverse effects and there is probably considerable individual variation.

Infants, the elderly, and those who eat poorly have traditionally been thought to be particularly at risk, usually because they eat so few fresh vegetables and fruit.

Vitamin C enhances the absorption of iron as well as protecting the deterioration of folic acid in foods. So ensuring that you get enough vitamin C may help two other important nutrients.

Unlike most other mammals, man lacks the ability to synthesize vitamin C. During stress, infection and certain other conditions, there is an increased need for vitamin C which our metabolisms cannot supply. Supplements may then be desirable.

DEFICIENCY SYMPTOMS AND SIGNS

The classical picture of scurvy can still be seen these days in the elderly and severely ill. The signs are bleeding, swollen gums, easy bruising, and a dry, scaly skin. People with scurvy can die from massive bleeding unless they are treated promptly.

Far more common than this is a mild or not clinically obvious deficiency state. The early features of vitamin C deficiency include depression, hysteria, and hypochondriasis. Early physical signs include finding the hair follicles on the limbs and trunk plugged with skin scales. Each hair as it leaves the skin may be coiled or distorted. The hair follicle is raised by the horny plug and can be surrounded by a red halo of bleeding.

MEDICAL REASONS FOR GIVING VITAMIN C

First of all we should point out that there are different levels of vitamin C administration. Someone with scurvy obviously needs a rapid correction of this deficiency and doses of 100–1,000 mg per day produce an improvement very quickly.

Second, is the question of dietary vitamin C intake in relation to the recommended daily allowance. As we have already pointed out, some doctors feel that the UK recommended daily allowance is only about fifty to sixty percent of the ideal. The question then arises as to whether certain groups of people should routinely take a moderate supplement such as 50–150 mg per day. This may be particularly relevant in the elderly, or in those who have increased needs. The latter include women on the Pill, those taking aspirin, antibiotics, appetite-suppressants or anticonvulsants, and those on steroid drugs. Alcoholics also have increased needs for vitamin C, as do smokers.

There is a strong case, in our view, for the elderly, those on poor diets, those who are taking any of the above drugs on a long-term basis and those who drink and smoke heavily, to take a moderate supplement of vitamin C, e.g. at least 100 mg per day, every day.

Finally, there is a question as to whether large doses of vitamin C are of benefit in treating a number of medical conditions. Vitamin C in doses of several hundred milligrams to several grams per day can be used as a pharmacological agent—as if it were a drug. It is at this level that medical opinion begins to get confused and confusing, but available evidence quite clearly shows that vitamin C *is* a very useful pharmacological agent when given in doses in excess of 600 mg per day. In such large doses vitamin C can have occasional adverse effects. For more details, see below.

THOSE WHO MIGHT BEST BENEFIT FROM VITAMIN C

Those with heart disease

Vitamin C helps lower raised cholesterol levels. It apparently has little or no effect upon normal cholesterol levels, but in individuals who have an elevated level of cholesterol, particularly if they are on a diet with a borderline intake of vitamin C, taking 300–1,000 mg of vitamin C a day significantly lowers their cholesterol levels.

The risk of having a stroke appears to be reduced in those who consume higher than average quantities of fruit and vegetables. This may be a simple and safe way of reducing the incidence of this common and devastating condition. The beneficial effects may be a result of a higher intake of vitamin C, but this is not yet entirely clear. Elderly people with high blood pressure, who have signs of vitamin C deficiency, should probably take vitamin C if they are unable to increase their dietary intake of vegetables and fruit. Proper control of the high blood pressure is also important.

Those with infections

Dr. Linus Pauling has become well known because of his research on, and enthusiasm for, the use of vitamin C in the treatment and prevention of the common cold. For the prevention of colds, doses in the region of 1–2 g per day are needed when symptoms develop. Controlled studies have been carried out to see whether taking vitamin C actually prevents the onset of colds. The results are not very convincing, though it appears that some individuals benefit. We are not surprised that the response is so unpredictable. The adequacy of intake of B vitamins, zinc, iron and other nutrients, as well as adverse effects of refined carbohydrates on resistance to infection, need to be taken into account on an individual basis. Vitamin C is much more likely to help those individuals who have borderline or obvious deficiency states to start with.

Vitamin C in massive doses has been used with some success in the treatment of viral hepatitis and even poliomyelitis. **Treatments such as these must, of course, be carried out under the guidance of a specialist.** A number of other viral infections have been reported as responding to high-dose vitamin C, including measles, mumps, inflammation of the testes, viral pneumonia, shingles, and viral encephalitis. Japanese researchers found that hepatitis following blood transfusion can be almost completely abolished by the taking of 2–6 g of vitamin C per day in the weeks following the transfusion, but not all studies have supported this.

Those with cancer

Linus Pauling, together with his co-worker, Dr. Ewan Cameron, advocates the use of vitamin C in the treatment of cancer. A number of reports, mainly in patients who had inoperable or untreatable terminal cancer, suggest that taking significant doses of vitamin C helps in maintaining well-being as well as improving survival times. Again, the response seems to be varied and this may well depend upon the pre-existing nutritional state of the patient. Some researchers suggest that cancer patients have markedly increased demands for vitamin C. The administration of several grams of vitamin C per day may well be worth a try, particularly if the person is unable to eat an adequate diet (see page 398). One study found that women with abnormal cervical smears were more likely to have a lower intake of dietary vitamin C than normal women. Smoking is a known risk factor for cervical cell abnormalities and is also known to lower vitamin C levels. It is possible that there is a connection between smoking, low levels of vitamin C and cervical cancer.

Also, cancer of the stomach has been linked with the increased ingestion of certain dietary agents, especially nitrites and nitrates (preservatives found in bacon and other foods). These are converted into carcinogenic nitrosamines in the stomach. Sufficient vitamin C in the diet may inhibit the formation of these substances, and giving vitamin C to those at risk probably makes sense.

The elderly

A deficiency of vitamin C is particularly likely to occur in the elderly, especially those who are in an institution or live alone.

Low levels of vitamin C have been linked to an impaired ability to think, mental deterioration, a reduced resistance to infection, poor wound-healing and easy bruising. Taking vitamin C (1 g per day) produces significant increases of body weight and blood proteins, as well as reductions in the frequency of bruises and hemorrhages.

Diabetics

Diabetics are at risk of developing serious eye damage because of hemorrhages in the eye. Taking vitamin C has been found to reduce the fragility of the tiny blood vessels that predispose to this.

Drug addicts

Large doses of vitamin C have been used in the treatment of drug addiction. A dietary support program with the use of high-dose vitamins (particularly vitamin C) may be of great assistance to a person coming off drugs. Addicts on methadone are known to have depressed levels of the natural steroid hormone cortisol, and this could theoretically be due to vitamin C deprivation, either because of the methadone itself, a poor diet, or heavy smoking.

Those with heavy metal poisoning

In the long term, vitamin C, particularly along with zinc, helps reduce lead and possibly cadmium toxicity. Vitamin C has the advantage of being a cheap and safe agent in this respect. One of the arguments for increasing the intake of vitamin C significantly above the recommended daily allowance is its effectiveness in reducing body burdens of toxic minerals generally.

Those with wounds and leg ulcers

It appears that in certain situations, high doses of vitamin C (500–3000 mg per day) enhance the healing of certain wounds. The elderly often have significant falls in blood levels of vitamin C after an operation. This is more likely to occur with major operations, and particularly in those who have a borderline nutritional state beforehand. It is probably a wise precaution to take a good multivitamin supplement, high in vitamin C, in the week before an operation, especially if you are old.

Those who are on other nutrients

Vitamin C enhances iron absorption, as well as preventing the destruction of folic acid in foods. Its effects on other nutrients, including other trace minerals, are unknown, but it may have potential adverse effects upon copper, zinc and possibly vitamin B if taken in very high doses for a long time.

Those with rheumatological conditions

Vitamin C, when taken in high doses (4 g per day), increases the excretion of uric acid in the urine and could *theoretically* increase the formation of uric-acid stones in the kidney, or precipitate attacks of gout. However, if an individual with gout has no evidence of kidney damage, or uric-acid kidney stones, then vitamin C may be helpful because of its effect on lowering the levels of uric acid in the blood by increasing its loss in the urine. Thus, in the long term, vitamin C may reduce the risk of attacks of gouty arthritis. Doses that have proved useful are in the region of several grams per day and treatment must be combined with other dietary methods of gout control (see page 256).

Some people with rheumatoid arthritis can, however, experience a worsening of their condition by taking vitamin C.

Those exposed to toxic chemicals

Vitamin C helps the detoxification and excretion of a wide range of toxic chemicals.

DOSAGE AND TOXICITY

Clearly, the dose of vitamin C that you can take varies enormously. Be guided by the above list.

Vitamin C has been shown to have a number of adverse effects.

- Long-term administration can reduce the availability of certain trace minerals, such as copper and zinc, as well as the amino acids lysine and cysteine.
- Vitamin C, at a dose of 1 g a day, biochemically alters the effects of a low-dose contraceptive pill into those of a high-dose pill, thus possibly enhancing the adverse effects.
- The excretion of oxalic acid, as well as uric acid, common causes of kidney stones, is increased in certain individuals consuming high doses of vitamin C. A personal or family history of kidney stones is a warning that you should not take high doses of vitamin C in the long term. **Consult your doctor about this.**
- A blood disease, glucose-6-phosphate-dehydrogenase deficiency, can be worsened by taking high-dose vitamin C. **If you**

have this condition, take supplements of vitamin C only under medical supervision.

- Certain tests to determine the presence of blood in the stool can produce false negatives if high doses of vitamin C are being taken.

Vitamin D

Though it is widely accepted that vitamin D is essential for normal calcium metabolism, there are many misconceptions about the role of vitamin D, and, indeed, the frequency of vitamin D deficiency. Vitamin D is said to be a vitamin because it used to be thought that trace quantities were required in the diet to prevent a deficiency occurring. However, in people who are exposed to adequate amounts of sunlight, it is now considered that there is no need for any oral intake of vitamin D because vitamin D is synthesized naturally in the skin.

Historically man has always obtained the majority of his vitamin D from sunlight exposure, just as he does today. The oral intake of vitamin D has only become of interest as the less sunny regions of the world have become inhabited. So as to obtain increased amounts of vitamin D from decreased amounts of light, man's skin has lost pigmentation. Eskimos are an exception. They still have skin of a medium-dark color, but their diet is very high in vitamin D (from fish oil products) and as a result it has not been necessary for them to lose their skin pigmentation in order to maintain their vitamin D production.

Vitamin D in food is absorbed from the intestine into the lymphatic system. This requires the presence of bile, pancreatic enzymes and a functioning small bowel. Vitamin D formed by the action of sunlight is released from the skin at a slow and regular rate into the bloodstream and then finds its way to the liver.

WHAT IT DOES

Vitamin D has its main effects on calcium metabolism and bone, but also has an important part to play in the health of other tissues. The actions of vitamin D are:

- In the gastrointestinal tract. Vitamin D increases the absorption of calcium and phosphate from the food we eat.
- In bone. Vitamin D is essential for calcification of newly formed bone which is present at the growing end of the bones.

- In kidney metabolism. Vitamin D enhances the reabsorption of calcium and phosphate from the urine so that it is not lost in the urine.
- In lead absorption. There is some evidence to suggest that vitamin D supplements can enhance the toxic effects of lead so people with lead poisoning or at risk of developing lead poisoning (see page 90) should take vitamin D supplements very cautiously.
- In bone marrow. The presence of vitamin D appears to encourage the replacement of bone marrow tissues by fibrous tissue, and the development of anemia. This may occur in some children with rickets.

FOOD SOURCES

The dietary sources of vitamin D are fatty fish, cod-liver oil, eggs, milk, butter, cheese and other foods to which vitamin D has been added.

DEFICIENCY SYMPTOMS AND SIGNS

The clinical picture of vitamin D deficiency depends upon the age of the individual involved. The most striking features relate to changes in the skeleton as a result of a loss of calcium. The major symptoms and signs of both rickets and osteomalacia are:

Rickets (mainly seen in children)

Infants

- excessive sweating
- irritability
- delayed development of movements
- softening of the skull bones
- thickening of the top of the skull
- teeth appear late
- enlargement of the joints where the ribs meet the breastbone
- chest and spinal deformities
- bowed legs

Adolescents

- aching legs
- swelling of the ends of long bones
- knee aches and pains

- impaired immunity with repeated infections
- poor musculature
- poor growth

Osteomalacia (mainly seen in adults)

- bone pain
- bone tenderness
- weakness of certain muscles, particularly of the hip girdle (difficulty in getting out of a chair or climbing stairs)
- deafness
- waddling gait

THOSE WHO MIGHT BEST BENEFIT FROM VITAMIN D

- those who are exposed to little or no sunlight
- the elderly
- those who live in industrial, urban communities
- people living in institutions
- dark-skinned people living in a northern climate
- those who have a dietary deficiency of vitamin D and calcium (e.g. the elderly, vegetarians, Asian immigrants and Rastafarians).
- those who do not absorb vitamin D or calcium
- patients on long-term drugs for epilepsy

DOSAGE AND TOXICITY

The prevention of vitamin D deficiency usually requires the administration of only 400 IUs of vitamin D per day by mouth, though a higher dosage may be necessary in premature infants.

In those with a vitamin D deficiency caused by a dietary deficiency or a lack of sunlight, doses of several thousand IUs of vitamin D per day can be taken, **but only under medical supervision.**

The dosage should be tailored to the individual's response. There should be an improvement in muscle strength and in muscle tone, but there may, for a short while, be an increase in bone pain.

A failure to respond suggests poor absorption of the vitamin from the intestine, a co-existent calcium deficiency or malabsorption, or a disturbance of vitamin D metabolism caused by kidney or liver disease.

In these last two situations, specialized forms of vitamin D may have to be taken.

Too much vitamin D produces marked elevations in blood calcium levels, and symptoms such as feeling generally unwell, drowsiness, abdominal pain, increased thirst, constipation and loss of appetite. In the long term, it can produce soft tissue calcification, kidney damage and kidney stones. This can be treated by stopping the vitamin D supplements and, in severe cases, by taking steroids. **People with a condition called sarcoidosis should not take any supplement containing vitamin D without medical supervision.**

Vitamin E

Vitamin E, along with vitamin C, is one of the most popular vitamin supplements and has, from time to time, been recommended as a treatment for almost every conceivable medical condition. A large proportion of the medical profession has reacted by saying that there are *no* known indications for vitamin E. Both views are extreme and, not surprisingly, the truth lies somewhere between them.

Vitamin E was first discovered in the 1920s and most of the early research was done on animals. By 1959 it was accepted in the USA as an essential dietary agent and by the mid-1960s there were more than 2,000 research papers on vitamin E. It is now recognized that what was originally called vitamin E is actually a family of compounds called tocopherols. The name comes from two Greek words, *tocos* (child birth) and *phero* (to bring forth). It was coined because vitamin E deficient animals were unable to have successful pregnancies.

WHAT IT DOES

The tocopherols are all fat-soluble and their absorption from the intestine depends upon effective fat digestion and fat absorption. So, diseases of the stomach, pancreas and liver can produce a vitamin E deficiency just as they predispose to deficiencies of the other fat-soluble vitamins (A, D and K). Vitamin E is thought to be particularly valuable in that it is an anti-oxidant. Living tissues are particularly sensitive to the damaging effects of oxygen and other oxidizing substances called free radicals (see page 146) which can seriously damage the structure of cell membranes, as well as the contents of living cells; accelerated damage may lead to cell death. Vitamin E helps protect cells from this kind of damage.

FOOD SOURCES

Good sources of vitamin E include most vegetable oils, nuts, seeds, soya and lettuce, and there is some vitamin E in eggs, dairy products, and minimal quantities in animal produce. Many vegetable-derived foods contain polyunsaturated fats. These can easily be oxidized by oxygen in the atmosphere, particularly when also exposed to heat and/or light, and it is this process that turns vegetable and other oils rancid. Vitamin E, because of its anti-oxidant (anti-oxygen) activity, retards this process and vitamin E, in this respect, can be thought of as nature's preservative. In fact, vitamin E can be used as a preservative for processed foods. Unfortunately, and disappointingly, other chemical anti-oxidants are usually used instead.

DIETARY REQUIREMENTS

The requirements for vitamin E depend upon the intake of polyunsaturated fats. The higher the intake, the higher the requirements of the vitamin. However, most dietary polyunsaturates naturally contain adequate quantities of vitamin E. An intake of 8–10 mg of alpha-tocopherol, or its equivalent, is required by most adults per day. Less is required in infancy, and more during pregnancy and lactation.

Premature infants are particularly prone to a deficiency of vitamin E and supplementation may be necessary, usually by injection.

DEFICIENCY SYMPTOMS AND SIGNS

There are no true deficiency symptoms and signs that one can rely upon. The need for vitamin E supplementation is usually made purely as a result of clinical suspicion by a doctor.

THOSE WHO MIGHT BEST BENEFIT FROM VITAMIN E

There are a number of well-defined indications, some rare and some common, for taking vitamin E.

Clearly, vitamin E is most likely to be beneficial in someone who is already deficient in it. A healthy individual who eats a well-balanced diet, and who doesn't have any special need to increase his vitamin E, is most unlikely to benefit from the vitamin.

Patients with coronary artery disease have been given vitamin

E in doses in the region of 300–1,200 IUs per day, but its value is uncertain. Vitamin E has been most studied as a treatment for poor circulation in the legs usually found in smokers. Stopping smoking, regular exercise, and the taking of vitamin E, 300–600 IUs a day, is of proven value when followed for at least six months. This treatment offers a real alternative to major surgery in some people.

Vitamin E can also lower raised cholesterol levels, particularly in young people. Its cholesterol-lowering effect in older people has not been properly investigated.

Those who have suffered a single or a recurrent stroke may, by taking vitamin E (as well as other nutrients), and by making appropriate dietary changes, reduce their risk of having further strokes. Aspirin, which is often used in the treatment of mild recurrent stroke, has effects which in some respects are very similar to vitamin E and the two can be taken together.

Premature infants have especially high needs for vitamin E. They have very low levels in their blood, and a lack of the vitamin means that they are particularly susceptible to potentially damaging effects from oxygen. Often they have to have oxygen administered to them in an incubator, and this additional oxygen may produce lung and eye damage. It appears that these potentially damaging effects from additional oxygen can be reduced by giving vitamin E.

Other conditions for which vitamin E has been successfully given include premenstrual syndrome, premenstrual breast tenderness, period pains, menopausal hot flushes, certain blood diseases, e.g. sickle cell anemia and thalassemia, Dupuytren's contracture (disfiguring and shortening of the tendons in the hand, sometimes associated with diabetes), chronic leg ulcers and osteoarthritis. In some conditions, such as cystic fibrosis and other diseases of the pancreas or liver, specialized forms of vitamin E may be required as absorption of dietary vitamin E is impaired.

DOSAGE AND TOXICITY

For most conditions, vitamin E is given in a dose of 300–600 IUs per day.

People with liver, pancreatic or gastrointestinal disease must take their vitamin E by injection, or in a water-soluble or other specialized form, because their absorption of fat is upset.

Vitamin E can have toxic effects. Minor gastrointestinal upsets can occur, but, more seriously, people taking anticoagulants (blood thinning tablets), particularly if taking large doses of vitamin E, can be prone to excessive bleeding. **No one taking anticoagulant agents for conditions such as thrombosis, or pulmonary embolism, should take vitamin E unless it is *closely* supervised by their medical practitioner.**

There have been occasional reports of diabetics taking vitamin E being able to reduce their insulin requirements; it is certainly possible that diabetics starting on vitamin E could have hypoglycemic attacks.

Vitamin K

Vitamin K is a term used to describe a group of chemical substances, deficiencies of which lead to bleeding disorders.

WHAT IT DOES

The most important function of vitamin K is in the production of blood clotting factors, particularly one called prothrombin.

While the major source of vitamin K is food, some is produced in the intestines. It is estimated that dietary intake accounts for some 300–500 mcg of vitamin K per day. Not all of this is absorbed, but it easily satisfies the normal requirement of approximately 1 mcg per kilogram of body weight per day. As well as this dietary source, some of the vitamin is made by bacteria in the small bowel. Vitamin K produced by bacteria in the large bowel is not absorbed. Excess vitamin K can be stored in the liver. In newborn babies, the requirement for dietary vitamin K is considerably greater, probably because the infant's bacteria-free intestine does not produce any vitamin K.

FOOD SOURCES

These include turnips, greens, broccoli, cabbage, lettuce, liver, green tea and cereals. Vitamin K is found in lower amounts in many other foods.

DEFICIENCY SYMPTOMS AND SIGNS

A deficiency of vitamin K can produce a bleeding disorder, but this rarely occurs except in those who have some pre-existing illness. Deficiency comes about as a result of one of three mechanisms: a lack of dietary intake or production by the small bowel bacteria, poor absorption, or poor utilization by the cells of the body.

The most important clinical situation in which vitamin K deficiency occurs is in hemorrhagic disease of the newborn. Newborn infants have a low vitamin K level because the placenta does not transmit fat-soluble substances easily and the bacteria-free gut of the infant doesn't yet produce any of the vitamin. Inadequate vitamin K levels mean an increased susceptibility to bleeding, particularly in the first few days of life. Premature babies are especially at risk, as are babies of mothers who are taking anti-epilepsy medications. Vitamin K is now often routinely given to newborn infants in the UK, a practice that is well established in the USA. Usually, a dose of 1 mg is given either orally or intramuscularly in the first few hours after birth. Babies born to mothers who are on anti-epileptic drugs should always be given vitamin K.

MINERALS

The minerals, or elements, are a major group of vital substances necessary to normal life.

The essential elements for man can be categorized in different ways. Perhaps the most practical way of thinking of them is to divide them into:

The macrominerals. Calcium, phosphorus, magnesium, sodium, potassium and chlorine—these are the bulk elements that are required in quantities of several hundred milligrams per day. They are involved in structural functions (bones and cells) as well as metabolic ones.

The trace elements. These include iron, zinc, copper, manganese, iodine, chromium, selenium, molybdenum, cobalt and sulphur. These are required in very small quantities (a few milligrams or less per day). They have subtle but vitally important effects on metabolism.

The ultra trace elements. These are now recognized as essential, as the ability to measure them more accurately has been developed.

Research trace elements. This is the final group, and includes a number of different elements that have not yet been proven categorically to be essential for normal human metabolism, but which are present in the body, and which appear to have some influence on its working. The group includes vanadium, nickel, tin, lithium and a few other very rare elements.

In addition to these elements the body also needs hydrogen, nitrogen, oxygen and carbon, but these are not going to be discussed because they are either obtained from the air we breathe (the first three) or are present in all living matter that we eat.

They are basic building blocks of the body that are eventually used in cells once food has been broken down and transported to where it is needed.

As regards which elements are essential and which are not, there is still a lot to learn. But considering that most elements are available, at least in some quantity, in the earth's crust, it would be surprising if such a complicated machine as the human body had not developed some way of taking advantage of whatever elements are present.

So, rather than saying that an element definitely does *not* have an essential or useful function in man, it makes sense to reserve judgment and say rather that its value has not yet been proved.

What Does "Essential" Mean?

The adjective "essential" is only used if the element is present in all healthy tissues; if it has a fairly constant concentration range across species; and if its exclusion from the body causes reproducible physiological abnormalities which are then reversed on giving the element. Such rigid definitions have, to date, restricted the number of essential elements to nineteen. There are currently also some eight "beneficial" elements known. Life is possible without these beneficial elements, but it is a fairly meager form of existence and could not be called healthy. In addition, there are twenty or thirty trace elements which are found in all tissues, but whose concentrations vary and whose physiological roles have not yet been fully worked out. These have been called contaminants, by some experts, until proven otherwise. The dividing line between essential and beneficial, and contaminating and polluting elements, is not fixed and is expected to be redrawn from time to time as diagnostic procedures and scientific instrumentation improve.

The average element composition of a seventy-kilogram man is as follows:

	Milligrams
Oxygen	43,550,000
Carbon	12,590,000
Hydrogen	6,580,000
Nitrogen	1,815,000
Calcium	1,700,000
Phosphorus	680,000
Potassium	250,000
Chlorine	115,000

	Milligrams
Sulphur	100,000
Sodium	70,000
Magnesium	42,000
Iron	6,000
Zinc	2,000–3,000
Fluorine	200–1,000
Copper	50–120

Elements that are present in the body in varying amounts, but usually less than 50 mg, include vanadium, iodine, manganese, selenium, silicon, molybdenum, chromium, cobalt and nickel.

It is clear that the idea of "optimum" nutrition includes the notion of all the nineteen essential nutrients being within the optimum range. As we shall see later, this is not always the case, and less than optimum health occurs all too frequently. The optimum range is wider for some elements than for others, and this is discussed in general terms under each element.

It is also important to realize that there is a substantial interaction between different elements, and between essential elements and toxic elements.

This should be borne in mind when taking mineral supplements as medicines. For example, zinc antagonizes the uptake of copper, and can cause a copper deficiency (see page 72). Zinc deficiency enhances lead toxicity and so on.

It is also important to bear in mind that vitamins and amino acids can influence the mineral status of an individual. For example, histidine is a copper-binding agent and when taken excessively as a supplement can result in excessive copper excretion and thus in a copper deficiency. Vitamin C can also reduce a person's copper status, and can be used in the treatment of copper toxicity.

Interactions between essential minerals and toxic elements are discussed under the relevant sections on toxic metals.

Calcium

Calcium is one of the bulk minerals required by the body.

Of the body's total calcium, ninety-nine percent is required for the bones and teeth. The remaining one percent is in solution and helps biochemical functions of various kinds.

The importance of the right calcium balance for the maintenance of health cannot be overestimated. In this section we will cover the main points of calcium metabolism that are generally overlooked by most doctors.

FOOD SOURCES

Good dietary sources are: milk, cheese, broccoli, legumes, green, leafy vegetables, nuts, seeds, peas, beans and lentils. Because milk products so often cause allergic reactions, be wary of milk and milk products as a source of calcium. There is also insufficient magnesium in milk, and children, especially, who rely on large quantities of milk for their nutrient intake, can end up with a relative magnesium insufficiency.

THINGS THAT AFFECT CALCIUM STATUS

There are a number of different factors that influence calcium status, in addition to dietary intake; e.g. the intake of vitamin D (and the amount of exposure to sunlight), the amount of protein eaten, the level of acid in the stomach, magnesium intake, and the speed at which food passes through the intestine.

Bran

Phytates in bran and unleavened bread (including chapattis) bind calcium and render it unabsorbable. This is one of the potential drawbacks of adding bran to a nutrient-poor diet to increase dietary fiber. Adding bran to a junk-food diet further damages calcium, zinc and magnesium status. For more on the harmful effects of fiber, as well as its beneficial effects, see page 123.

Phosphorus

Although it is an essential nutrient, and sufficient quantities are necessary for calcium to do its job in the body, too much phosphorus can increase calcium requirements which, if not met, can render the individual calcium deficient. A junk-food diet is rich in phosphorus and can produce a relative calcium deficiency and all the problems that this entails. Ideally, the dietary calcium:phosphorus ratio should be approximately 1 or 2:1.

Fat

A high-fat diet reduces the availability of calcium and can produce a net deficiency of this important element.

Vitamin D

Adequate vitamin D is needed for calcium absorption and utilization. It can be synthesized in the skin in response to sunlight (see page 35).

Magnesium

There is also evidence that suggests that calcium metabolism is disrupted if there is too little magnesium in the diet to meet the individual's requirements.

Protein

A high-protein diet increases calcium loss in the urine and can result in higher calcium requirements.

Stomach acidity

For calcium to be absorbed efficiently there needs to be sufficient hydrochloric acid produced by the stomach.

Malabsorption

Poor absorption of food can reduce the absorption of calcium and give rise to either an overt or a hidden calcium deficiency. All kinds of conditions can cause malabsorption, including pancreatic insufficiency, celiac disease, lactase deficiency, cows' milk allergy (and allergies to other foods), intestinal problems (from physical and emotional causes), too little gastric acid (see above) and chronic intestinal infections and infestations, such as worms.

Endocrine status

The hormones that influence calcium status are complex and involved. The main hormone concerned is parathyroid hormone, which increases the activity of vitamin D, increases calcium absorption from food, increases the mobilization of calcium from bones, increases phosphorus excretion via the kidneys, and increases the deposition of calcium in soft tissues of the body (blood vessels, muscles, joint spaces, hair and so on).

Circulating estrogens tend to reduce the sensitivity of bone to the calcium-mobilizing effects of parathyroid hormone. So it is that after menopause, when levels of circulating estrogens fall, bone tends to lose calcium, resulting in osteoporosis, which is a major cause of fractured bones in elderly women. This is discussed in more detail on page 253.

Exercise

Regular exercise seems to increase bone density. Immobilization of the elderly, in bed, causes a reduction of calcium in bone, and can increase the risk of fractures.

Kidney function

Calcium balance also depends on correct kidney function, and in the presence of kidney disease, calcium status can be severely affected even when dietary balance is adequate.

CONDITIONS IN WHICH CALCIUM SUPPLEMENTATION MAY BE USEFUL

It is important to detect calcium insufficiency in adults because prolonged low blood levels of calcium may produce cataracts.

Allergies

In individuals with allergies, calcium insufficiency is often a problem. This may be obvious if the symptoms are clearly related to the gastrointestinal tract, but is less obvious if the problems are asthma, eczema or hay fever.

Post-menopausal women who develop multiple sensitivities, intolerances and allergies are often helped by correcting their calcium status.

Many people on elimination diets for the management of their allergies are on a vitamin D and/or a calcium-deficient diet. This occurs with disturbing frequency in both those whose diets are self-imposed and in patients who have been under medical supervision.

Toxic metal exposure

Calcium and/or vitamin D deficiency predispose to an increased gastrointestinal absorption of lead and aluminum, two elements which are "let in" through the gastrointestinal lining by those mechanisms which also permit the increased intestinal absorption of calcium.

Aluminum is also known to influence parathyroid gland activity, so disrupting calcium status. Both lead and aluminum are known to have widespread detrimental effects on the body, especially on the central nervous system. If someone is exposed to these two elements, calcium supplementation is almost essential.

Mental function

Too much parathyroid hormone can lead to a high blood calcium which is associated with bone pains, psychiatric symptoms, and constipation. This should always be sought as the cause for these symptoms in any psychiatric patient because an excess of parathyroid hormone is easily corrected surgically, with magical results. Conversely, calcium insufficiency is also associated with a wide range of mental disturbances. Defective calcium metabolism is often found in a wide range of psychiatric conditions, many of which respond to calcium supplementation. The most common are depression, anxiety, panic attacks, nervous tics and twitches, insomnia and hyperactivity.

Joint pains and arthritis

Many people with joint pains and arthritis appear to have symptoms attributable to overactivity of the parathyroid gland. This is not a true disease of the parathyroid glands, but is caused by nutritional overactivity as a result of inadequate dietary calcium and/or vitamin D intake, or as a result of a low dietary calcium: phosphorus ratio, or any of the many causes of calcium malabsorption.

Many of these people are improved by calcium supplementation, by stepping up the calcium in the diet, or a reduction of dietary phosphorus or phytates.

DOSAGE AND TOXICITY

When taking calcium it is important to ensure that it is in an absorbable form. This can involve taking a digestive supplement containing hydrochloric acid in the form of betaine hydrochloride or glutamic acid hydrochloride. This is especially important in those who have little or no gastric acid.

Dolomite is relatively unabsorbable and may be contaminated with toxic metals such as lead, arsenic, mercury and aluminum, and therefore should be avoided unless one can be sure that the specific dolomite preparation is free of these contaminants. The same applies to bone meal.

Good sources of absorbable calcium are SandoCal; calcium lactate, gluconate or sulphate; amino-chelated calcium; and calcium orotate. Requirements vary from person to person, but post-menopausal women may need 1000–1500 mg of calcium, and others somewhat less.

Excess calcium

Too much calcium, as a result of metabolic or nutritional disorders, can give rise to kidney failure and a number of other problems. For this reason, it is important to have the condition diagnosed early, even when mild. It can lead to kidney stones, poor muscle tone, constipation, abdominal pains, loss of appetite, nausea, vomiting and deposition of calcium in sites outside bone.

Phosphorus

WHAT IT DOES

Phosphorus is involved, along with calcium, in the formation of bones and teeth, and like calcium, has a number of other functions as well. It is necessary for the working of every cell in the body and is involved in energy production, storage and release. Calcium is the only mineral that we require in greater quantities than phosphorus. Phosphorus is widely available in foods and in the West a deficiency is rare. In fact, many of the problems that we see in our practice are centered around excessive phosphorus in the diet in relation to amounts of calcium and magnesium.

B vitamins are only effective when combined with phosphate in the body. A very important phosphorus-containing compound is adenosine triphosphate (ATP) which is involved in energy production and storage.

The average daily intake of phosphorus in the UK is about 1,200–2,000 mg, and 1,500–1,600 mg in the USA. There is no recommended daily allowance (RDA) in the UK, but the 1980 RDA in the US was 100 mg per day.

FOOD SOURCES

Good food sources of phosphorus include milk and milk products, nuts and wholegrain cereals, poultry, eggs, meats, fish and legumes.

TOO MUCH OR TOO LITTLE?

There are many conditions in which excessive phosphorus could be a contributing factor. A very low dietary calcium:phosphorus or magnesium:phosphorus ratio can bring about a relative insufficiency of calcium or magnesium, simply because the absorption of these two elements is reduced when excessive phosphorus is present. This is discussed in more detail in the section on calcium (see page 44). The ideal calcium:phosphorus ratio is 1:1 or greater.

Soft drinks often contain phosphate and some food additives contain phosphate, so these foods and drinks can upset the calcium:phosphorus and magnesium:phosphorus ratio.

Low blood levels of phosphate can be caused by alcoholism, antacid therapy for gastric ulcers, intravenous glucose, barbiturate therapy, pregnancy, and a vitamin D deficiency. The clinical symptoms of phosphate deficiency are muscle weakness (even to the point where the breathing muscles stop working), and increased susceptibility to infection and anemia. A decreased resistance to infection is related to the poor functioning of white cells that occurs in phosphate deficiency.

PHOSPHORUS SUPPLEMENTATION

We seldom find it necessary to give phosphorus supplements. However, some multi-mineral supplements do contain phosphorus. Post-menopausal women may require phosphorus supplements along with calcium and magnesium to prevent osteoporosis (see page 253). Excessive phosphorus can lead to increased requirements of calcium and magnesium.

Potassium

In the UK, the daily intake of potassium is estimated to be 2,000–4,000 mg daily. The daily intake of sodium is estimated to be 3,000–6,000 mg. There is some evidence to show than "primitive" diets and unprocessed-food diets consumed in non-industrialized nations supply the body with more potassium than sodium. There is increasing evidence that the reversal of the dietary sodium:potassium ratio from a "natural" pattern can contribute to a number of different medical conditions seen in modern Westernized society.

Most of the potassium in our bodies is inside the cells, at a concentration thirty times greater than that in the fluid surrounding the cells. The sodium:potassium ratio is 1:10 inside the cells, and 28:1 outside. The difference in concentration across the cell membrane is actively maintained by what is called the "sodium pump." This is a biochemical mechanism that pumps the sodium out of the cell. The kidney regulates sodium and potassium balance and helps maintain the blood potassium level within a fairly narrow range, despite a wide variation of dietary intake and total body content of potassium. So it is that blood levels of potassium can be normal despite considerable potassium depletion of the body as a whole. A normal blood potassium level is therefore no guarantee of overall potassium adequacy.

WHAT IT DOES

Potassium is important in a wide range of bodily functions and is present in every cell in the body. It is especially essential for the correct working of the heart, the muscles and nervous system, and for the maintenance of normal blood glucose levels.

FOOD SOURCES

Strict vegetarians have a high-potassium, low-salt diet if they do not add salt to their food. This is because fresh fruits, vegetables and whole grains are rich in potassium. On the other hand, meat eaters tend to eat too much sodium in relation to the potassium in their diet.

Mild potassium depletion and its related symptoms can be helped by taking fruit juices or vegetable soups several times a day. Salt substitutes, available in health food shops, have a high potassium chloride content and this can be an inexpensive way of obtaining extra potassium.

There are lots of potassium supplements available on the market, but many of them upset the stomach and are expensive. Potassium gluconate can upset the stomach, but it is cheap and readily available from a pharmacy without prescription. Effervescent potassium chloride is also available, and this is another way of increasing potassium intake.

DEFICIENCY SYMPTOMS AND SIGNS

Potassium deficiency produces muscle fatigue, poor appetite, mental apathy and fatigue, depression, constipation caused by poor muscle tone in the intestines, an irregular heartbeat, and muscle cramps. Weakness, irritability, tissue swelling, headaches, bone and joint pain, and a rapid heartbeat are also sometimes seen.

DIURETICS AND POTASSIUM

Certain diuretics (drugs that increase urine production) are sometimes used in the treatment of high blood pressure and heart failure. There are two groups of diuretics: those that cause the body to retain potassium and those that cause the body to lose it. The potassium-losing diuretics can cause a rise in blood glucose levels. This causes a further loss of potassium. Retention of potassium in the body depends on there being enough magnesium, but the potassium-losing diuretics also tend to cause a loss of magnesium. So, one can become magnesium deficient and potassium deficient, yet taking more potassium does not necessarily cure the symptoms. **Clearly, this needs close medical supervision.**

CAUSES OF POTASSIUM DEFICIENCY

As well as the potassium-losing diuretics mentioned above, chronic diarrhea, excessive salt, intestinal malabsorption, the ingestion of aspirin, prolonged laxative therapy, diabetic acidosis, certain gastrointestinal disorders and steroid therapy are all causes of potassium deficiency.

TOXICITY

Excessive amounts of potassium (for example 18,000 mg per day) can stop the heart beating. Certain illnesses such as kidney failure, severe dehydration and severe adrenal insufficiency can raise blood potassium to toxic levels. **These are medical emergencies and have to be dealt with in the hospital.**

POTASSIUM AND BLOOD PRESSURE

There is evidence to show that a low potassium intake can predispose to high blood pressure. This is discussed in more detail on page 223.

Sodium

The average adult has 70–100 g of sodium in his or her body. It is mainly outside the cells, in contrast to potassium which is mainly inside the cells.

Sodium is intimately related to the maintenance of the body's fluid balance and blood pressure. So the higher the level of blood sodium, the higher the blood pressure, and vice versa.

Daily intake is approximately 4–6 g, but there is evidence to suggest (see page 222) that this is too high.

Most of our dietary sodium is in the form of table salt, but an appreciable amount is derived from sodium nitrate, which is used as a preservative in meats, and monosodium glutamate, a flavor enhancer. In fact, we take in so much sodium that it is difficult to conceive that dietary sodium was once scarce. Nevertheless, sodium is an essential mineral that our bodies regulate and conserve.

Excessive sweating results in a loss of sodium simply because the sodium content of sweat is high (hence its salty taste). Working in hot environments, vigorous exercise, or the excessive use of saunas can cause a considerable sodium loss and a resulting sodium deficiency. The manifestations of sodium deficiency include nausea, vomiting, dizziness, cramps, exhaustion, apathy, and, if extreme, circulatory failure.

Most of these symptoms can be corrected by replacing the water that has been lost along with the salt. However, if sweating has been really considerable, it may be necessary to take finger dabs of salt as well. This should be done very carefully as it can be an excessive shock to the system. Salt tablets or high-salt solutions cause the water to remain in the stomach an unduly long time, and this can lead to problems too. Ideally, you should replace lost salt at the next meal.

SODIUM AND BLOOD PRESSURE

Excessive sodium can increase blood pressure, and a shortage of sodium can produce a low blood pressure.

TOXICITY

It appears that the average intake of salt per person in the Western world is above the minimal nutritional needs of the vast majority of people. Excessive amounts of salt, especially in infant milk formula, can be fatal. It is important to be very wary of giving salty foods to infants.

Magnesium

Magnesium has long been known as a treatment for high blood pressure in pregnancy, and as an anticonvulsant. Its effects on the heart were first described as long ago as 1935. However, magnesium could be considered a forgotten mineral until recently, when more reports of its importance have appeared in the medical literature.

WHAT IT DOES

Magnesium is the second most abundant mineral inside cells after potassium, and its distribution across cell membranes is closely linked with calcium and phosphorus metabolism. The average human adult has 20–30 g of magnesium, seventy percent of which is contained in teeth and bones; the remainder—the physiologically important component—is found mainly in the cells. The average daily intake of a healthy adult should be 400–800 mg, but requirements can increase in certain circumstances, such as with high-protein, high-calcium, high-phosphorus, or high-vitamin D intakes.

A diet high in refined and processed foods is often deficient in magnesium, and this is made more significant if bran is added to such a diet because it binds what little magnesium is present, so rendering it less easily absorbed.

Magnesium is essential for many metabolic processes, especially the cellular "pumps" which maintain the correct distribution of sodium, potassium and calcium across cell membranes. Magnesium deficiency is associated with muscle cramps, or, in extreme cases, tetany—continuous cramps, especially of the hands and feet.

Because magnesium is involved in so many enzyme systems a deficiency has widespread metabolic consequences.

FOOD SOURCES

Sources rich in magnesium include nuts, shrimps, soybeans, whole grains, and green, leafy vegetables (magnesium is a component of chlorophyll, so the greener the vegetables, the more magnesium there is). Tap-water in hard water areas is also an important source of dietary magnesium.

DEFICIENCY SYMPTOMS AND SIGNS

The symptoms of magnesium deficiency center around the neuro-psychiatric end of the spectrum of disorders and include:

- loss of appetite
- nausea
- apathy
- weakness and tiredness
- numbness and tingling
- confusion and disorientation
- learning disability and memory impairment
- vertigo
- convulsions, epilepsy
- muscle cramps, grimaces, jerks, tremors
- tremor and jerks of the tongue
- eyes flick uncontrollably
- muscular incoordination
- insomnia
- hyperactivity
- constipation
- heart rhythm problems
- susceptibility to the toxic effects of digoxin
- hypoglycemia
- difficulty in swallowing
- abnormal ECG
- premenstrual symptoms

Magnesium status should be assessed in anyone with these complaints. Because magnesium is needed for vitamin B1 metabolism, many of the symptoms can be associated with a vitamin B1 or B6 deficiency (see pages 11 and 20) and these should be looked for in anyone complaining of these symptoms.

CONDITIONS IN WHICH MAGNESIUM SUPPLEMENTATION MAY BE USEFUL

Until recently, doctors measured serum magnesium (the amount in the blood), which turns out to be an extremely poor indicator of magnesium status. As a result, doctors' awareness of magnesium deficiency has been low. The medical literature is full of situations where magnesium deficiency is probably of significance. A few of the conditions in which magnesium is of proven value are:

Osteoporosis

Osteoporosis is a condition in which calcium is removed from the bones, and the result is brittle bones that fracture easily. It is common in old people and especially in post-menopausal women. Two hormones, calcitonin (CT) and parathyroid hormone (PTH), regulate the skeletal turnover of calcium. Magnesium suppresses PTH and stimulates CT secretion, thus favoring the deposition of calcium in the bones and the removal of calcium from soft tissues. Furthermore, magnesium enhances calcium absorption from food and its retention in the body, whereas increasing calcium intake suppresses magnesium absorption. So there are sound theoretical grounds for using magnesium supplements in preventing or treating osteoporosis.

Joint problems

When deposition of calcium in soft tissue is increased, by a deficiency of magnesium, muscle and joint aches and pains could result. In our clinical experience, magnesium supplementation can be beneficial, in addition to other therapeutic interventions (see page 247).

Psychiatric symptoms

These include nervousness, anxiety, insomnia, childhood hyperactivity, depression, anorexia, apathy, weakness and tiredness. Many of these are associated with vitamin B1 deficiency, and magnesium is essential for the efficient utilization of vitamin B1 as well as B6. Magnesium deficiency is also associated with increased lactate levels which in turn have been linked to a wide range of psychiatric symptoms. (Vitamin B1 deficiency can result in increased lactate levels.) So, clearly, magnesium deficiency must be considered as a possible cause of, or contributing factor to, a whole range of psychiatric symptoms.

Premenstrual syndrome

Magnesium supplementation, along with vitamin B6, can be of real value in the management of the premenstrual syndrome (PMS). Vitamin B6 alone increases red-cell magnesium levels, which are often low in women suffering from PMS, and magnesium supplementation along with several other nutrients has been shown to increase premenstrual progesterone levels. Also, women in the premenstrual phase are more subject to hypoglycemia and it has been found that hypoglycemia is more marked in magnesium deficiency. Magnesium reduces the extent of reactive hypoglycemia and its symptoms (see page 292).

Heart disease

Spasm of the coronary arteries and increased excitability of the heart muscle, due to magnesium deficiency, can produce abnormal cardiac rhythms and even cause sudden death from a heart attack. People who die from heart attacks have been found to have lower magnesium in their heart muscle than those dying from car-accident injuries.

Magnesium deficiency caused by water tablets

Short-term, vigorous diuretic treatment, or moderate-dosage, long-term treatment can give rise to significant magnesium shortages. This depletion is also often compounded by hospital diets, which are surprisingly low in magnesium, a soft water supply, and, in some people, a high alcohol intake. Research from Dublin has found that the most common symptoms include depression, muscle weakness, and a disorder of heart rhythm which doesn't respond to digoxin treatment. Psychiatric symptoms may also appear as a result of low blood sugar (hypoglycemia) (see page 292) due to magnesium deficiency. It seems that the elderly are most at risk, especially those who have an excessive alcohol intake, a diet low in magnesium, or a soft water supply.

Hypertension

Magnesium deficiency has been recognized as a possible causative factor in hypertension (see page 223).

Kidney stones
Research has shown an abundance of evidence linking too much oxalic acid in the urine and urinary oxalate stones to a variety of nutritional problems, including magnesium deficiency. Supplements of magnesium and vitamin B6 have been found to prevent urinary oxalate stone formation.

Alcohol problems
Magnesium is one of the elements that is depleted in chronic alcoholism, probably as a result of decreased intake, the poor absorption of what is eaten, and poor reabsorption of magnesium by the kidneys. Alcohol acts as a diuretic and promotes the loss of both potassium and magnesium in the increased urine output. It has been found that levels of magnesium in sweat and blood can be low in alcoholics and that this can be partially corrected after three weeks of abstinence.

Diabetes
Diabetes mellitus causes substantial magnesium loss partly because of the large volumes of urine passed. This loss can further be contributed to by the kidney disease so commonly seen as a complication of diabetes.

Epilepsy and convulsions
There is a definite correlation between magnesium deficiency and the incidence of convulsions. This is discussed further in the section on Epilepsy (see page 355). We believe that epileptics should have their magnesium status assessed.

Childhood hyperactivity
It seems from our professional experience that many hyperactive children have poor magnesium status and that their symptoms may very well be due, at least in part, to an existing magnesium deficiency. Hyperactive children and learning-disabled children very often drink a great deal of cows' milk. While many of their symptoms may well be attributable to cows' milk intolerance (see page 129), it is quite feasible that too much cows' milk can predispose to magnesium deficiency as a result of its extremely low magnesium:phosphorus ratio.

MAGNESIUM SUPPLEMENTATION
The cheapest form of magnesium supplement is magnesium oxide, and 100 mg of magnesium oxide provides approximately

60 mg of elemental magnesium. Other forms of magnesium include animo-chelated magnesium, magnesium aspartate, or magnesium orotate. Magnesium gluconate or magnesium chloride can also be used orally, but these are less satisfactory. In the premenstrual syndrome, as much as 200–400 mg daily of magnesium may be necessary; in other conditions, 100–300 mg in adults is usually all that is necessary. Calcium and magnesium supplementation should be in the ratio of one or two parts of calcium to one of magnesium. Excessive magnesium supplementation can cause diarrhea.

Iron

Iron is a constituent part of the proteins hemoglobin and myoglobin which act as oxygen transporters in red blood cells and muscles. It is also a vital component of many of the body's enzyme systems. In a healthy adult male, about two thirds of the total of 4–6 g of iron in the body consists of hemoglobin, which is found in the red blood cells. The second largest amount consists of storage iron which is found mainly in the liver, spleen and bone marrow. A third and much smaller quantity includes compounds such as myoglobin and iron-containing enzymes. Finally, there is a very small amount of iron that is carried around in the blood by the iron-binding protein, transferrin.

FOOD SOURCES

Rich sources of iron are organ meats (liver, kidney and heart), egg yolk, legumes, cocoa, cane molasses, shellfish and parsley. Poor sources include milk and milk products, white sugar, white flour, polished rice, potatoes and most fresh fruits. Intermediate iron-containing foods are muscle meats, fish and poultry, nuts, green vegetables, and wholemeal bread. Over-boiling vegetables can reduce their iron content by as much as twenty percent.

DEFICIENCY SYMPTOMS AND SIGNS

Iron deficiency can cause many symptoms, most of which are linked to the anemia it produces. The symptoms of anemia resulting from iron deficiency include listlessness, fatigue, a very obvious heartbeat on exertion, sometimes a sore tongue, cracks at the corners of the mouth, difficulty with swallowing, and concave nails. In children, poor appetite, poor growth and a decreased resistance to infection are common. Abnormalities of the gastrointestinal tract, including the production of too little stomach acid, have long been observed in iron deficiency anemia. So iron deficiency can cause too little stomach acid and iron malabsorption, as well as being caused by these two situations.

Iron deficiency can exist without any blood changes and without the person being anemic, and this is far more common than is realized. One study in Canada showed that nineteen percent of the population had evidence of deficiency but only two percent were anemic!

HOW COMMON IS IRON DEFICIENCY?

Iron deficiency is very common both in the UK and the USA. Those most at risk are children, pregnant women and those with heavy periods, strict vegetarians and people from low socioeconomic groups who have a poor diet. Others who may be at risk are those with malabsorption problems, those who are on limited exclusion diets for food allergy, and those with very little gastric acid following the removal of part of the stomach in an operation for ulcers. A study of fifteen- to twenty-five-year-old women in England revealed an iron intake of only seventy to seventy-five percent of the officially recommended levels. It has been claimed that worldwide iron deficiency is the most common nutritional disease—much of it totally unrecognized.

HOW DO YOU KNOW IF YOU ARE IRON DEFICIENT?

Your doctor will be able to tell if you are iron deficient if you have any of the aforementioned symptoms; a response to iron supplements can also be an extremely useful confirmation. Often, within a few days, the common symptoms, especially muscle tiredness, respond to iron supplementation.

WHY BOTHER ABOUT IRON DEFICIENCY?

First, because it is so common, and second because doctors often rule it out if they find no evidence of anemia. This means that the various other conditions and diseases get missed and remain untreated, often for years.

For example, people who go to their doctors with clinical features of poor thyroid activity and in whom the laboratory tests for thyroid function appear normal, should be considered as possibly iron deficient because, in animals at least, the conversion of one type of thyroid hormone into another has been shown to be defective in iron deficiency.

Iron deficiency should also be suspected in children with learning and behavior disorders (see page 362) and this is often overlooked. Children who are iron deficient also have a higher than normal ability to absorb lead from their food and this can have a cumulative effect on their behavioral and learning problems (see page 360).

Vegetarians are at risk from iron deficiency because iron absorption is impaired by whole grains, soya and other legumes. However, vitamin C improves the absorption of iron and most vegetarians eat a diet rich in this vitamin.

Vegetarians are further at risk if they also drink tea, as tannin-containing beverages such as tea, taken with meals, can contribute to iron deficiency by inhibiting iron absorption. It therefore seems sensible for vegetarians to avoid tea around mealtimes. This is doubly important during pregnancy when iron requirements increase.

Coffee has also been shown to reduce iron absorption from food. In one study a cup of coffee reduces iron absorption from a hamburger meal by thirty-nine percent as compared to a sixty-four percent decrease with tea. No decrease in iron absorption occurred when the coffee was consumed one hour before the meal, but the same degree of inhibition was seen when coffee was taken one hour later. Also, the stronger the coffee, the greater the reduction in iron absorption.

It makes sense, then, if you are at risk from iron deficiency, not to drink tea or coffee at mealtimes. If you want to drink it, do so at least one hour before a meal or one and a half to two hours afterwards. The harmful effects of coffee are discussed on page 131.

DOSAGE AND TOXICITY

Iron supplementation was routine for pregnant women until quite recently, but as a *British Medical Journal* editorial states: "Surely obstetricians need no longer give all expectant mothers iron in an attempt to prevent appreciable anemia in seven percent." In the light of the increasing evidence that iron deficiency is widespread, this statement is not entirely appropriate, as it only takes into account anemia as a sign of iron deficiency, and not iron deficiency without blood changes.

However, another aspect of iron supplementation during pregnancy needs to be taken into consideration: that iron (and folate) supplementation inhibits the absorption of zinc. While a woman's requirements for iron are undoubtedly increased during pregnancy, the routine supplementation of pregnant women with iron seems to us to be foolhardy; zinc deficiency is associated with a poor pregnancy outcome, including possibly congenital malformations, and zinc adequacy in the average pregnant woman is questionable (see page 66). It is more sensible to ensure that women have adequate levels of iron before becoming pregnant, by eating a proper diet, fairly rich in vitamin C (which promotes iron absorption), and that they avoid tea and coffee at or after meals.

Iron overload can occur for many reasons, including as a result of increased intestinal absorption and over-enthusiastic supplementation. It can cause damage to the liver after many years.

Routine multi-mineral supplements should contain iron and zinc in the approximate ratio of one or two parts of iron to one of zinc, as more iron than this inhibits zinc absorption.

Iron deficiency and bowel symptoms

Reginald was a sixty-six-year-old retired insurance manager who had had indigestion and abdominal problems for over fifteen years. An operation for gallstones had only produced minimal improvement in his abdominal pains, bloating, gas, and tendency to diarrhea. He himself had tried a number of different diets, without any obvious benefit, but noticed that his symptoms became worse when he ate bran. Further investigation, including a barium meal, had not shown any serious abnormality. When I saw him, he really was at his wit's end as to what could be causing his bowel symptoms. Investigations showed that he had a low serum iron, 10.3 micromols/liter, normal range 14.3–36. Iron deficiency can cause poor acid production by the stomach, which can be a cause of indigestion and lead to an accumulation of abnormal or unusual bacteria in the intestines. Reginald also had evidence of these abnormal bacteria, which were probably causing his abdominal bloating. Treatment with iron supplements—ferrous sulphate, 200 mg, one a day—for three months, together with a diet avoiding whole grains, resulted in gradual, but substantial, improvement. His iron level returned to normal and the evidence of abnormal bacteria in the intestines cleared. He was able to tolerate foods, such as wholegrain bread, that had previously caused some abdominal pain and bloating. Nutritional deficiencies may frequently exist in patients who have bowel problems and may not only be caused by underlying bowel disease, but may in turn contribute to it. It is thus important that all patients with a long history of bowel complaints are assessed nutritionally.

Iron can be taken in the form of iron gluconate or iron fumarate. Preparations of iron containing 50–100 mg of iron can cause intestinal upsets, constipation and black stools.

In severe iron deficiency, injections of iron may be necessary. If a dose of 50 mg or more of iron is to be taken, it should be administered several hours away from any zinc supplements.

Zinc

Zinc is fast becoming recognized as a very important nutrient involved in a wide range of metabolic processes which become disturbed in many diseases. Despite the fact that there are many thousands of published papers (two and a half thousand in the last two years alone) indicating the clinical importance of zinc, only a handful of clinicians are applying the knowledge that *is* available.

We now know a lot about the deficiency effects, the role of zinc in enzyme function, dietary requirements and the toxic effects of zinc. However, there's a lot to learn about interactions between zinc and other nutrients, things that affect individual requirements, zinc metabolism and people's tolerance of excesses, not to mention the precise mechanisms by which a deficiency of zinc exerts its observable effects.

A lot of knowledge about zinc deficiency has come from animal studies, but a rare disease in children has also provided many useful clues. This condition is called acrodermatitis enteropathica, and it is caused by an hereditary absorption defect. Features include a loss of hair, skin troubles and diarrhea. Symptoms start early in infancy, but only in formula-fed babies. In the classical, untreated condition, such babies die from zinc deficiency. It was found that giving breast milk cured the condition because of the high levels of zinc it contains. Now, zinc supplements can be given and such babies live and thrive.

FOOD SOURCES

The best dietary sources of zinc are fresh oysters, ginger root, muscle meats such as lamb chops and steak, pecans, split peas, brazil nuts, beef liver, non-fat dry milk, egg yolk, wholewheat, rye, oats, peanuts, lima beans, soy lecithin, almonds, walnuts, chicken, buckwheat, hazelnuts, clams, green peas, shrimps, turnips, parsley, potatoes, garlic, wholewheat bread, carrots, beans, raw milk, pork chops and corn.

DEFICIENCY SYMPTOMS AND SIGNS

- slow growth
- infertility/delayed sexual maturation
- low sperm count
- hair loss
- skin conditions of various kinds
- diarrhea
- immune deficiencies
- behavioral and sleep disturbances
- night blindness
- impaired taste or smell
- impaired wound healing
- white spots on fingernails

The degree to which zinc deficiency contributes to a wide range of common clinical situations has not yet been thoroughly researched and evaluated. However, many physicians who assess the zinc status of their patients on a routine basis are aware of the number of patients whose problems respond well to zinc supplementation.

CONDITIONS WHICH MAY OR CAN BE CAUSED BY ZINC DEFICIENCY

- Frequent and/or severe infections.
- Many skin problems.
- Delayed wound healing and post-operative "complications."
- Congenital malformations.
- Retardation of growth and/or sexual maturation.
- Impotence, infertility and low sperm count, reduced sex drive.
- Behavioral and sleep disturbances.
- Psychiatric problems.
- Dandruff, hair loss.
- Impaired glucose tolerance.
- Impaired taste, smell and dark-adaptation.
- Connective tissue disease.
- Reduced appetite.
- Gastrointestinal problems (diarrhea).

Those who might have an inadequate dietary intake of zinc are:

- Those with anorexia nervosa, those on fad diets, and those on weight-reducing diets.
- Those on exclusion diets for food allergies.
- Strict vegetarians.
- Those on restricted protein diets.
- Those on synthetic diets (for the management of inborn errors of metabolism or malabsorption states).
- People who eat meat substitutes (soya "meat," etc.).
- The elderly.
- Alcoholics.

Some people eat enough but do not absorb it properly. These include:

- People on high-fiber diets (including lots of bran).
- Those taking iron tablets.
- Children with acrodermatitis enteropathica.
- People suffering from celiac disease (see page 208).
- People with achlorhydria and hypochlorhydria.
- Those suffering from alcoholic cirrhosis.
- People with pancreatic insufficiency.
- The elderly.

Some groups of people lose zinc and so need more. These include:

- People suffering from starvation, burns, diabetes mellitus.
- Those taking diuretics.
- Those taking the drug penicillamine.
- Those with chronic blood loss, or on dialysis (chronic renal disease).
- Those with exfoliative dermatitis, excessive sweating.
- Sufferers from inflammatory bowel disease, intestinal parasites and hookworm.
- Alcoholics.
- People with liver disease (including viral hepatitis).

- Those with diarrheal fluid loss and ileostomy fluid loss.
- After surgery or after trauma.

Some people have increased needs for zinc because of the following conditions:

- cancers
- growth spurts and puberty
- pregnancy and lactation
- psoriasis

It has been suggested by many researchers that zinc in the household food supply in the UK and in the USA may well be inadequate. The refining of foods substantially reduces their zinc content and inadequate zinc intake may be much more widespread than is generally appreciated.

ZINC-NUTRIENT INTERACTIONS

The availability of zinc to the body's cells is influenced by other nutrients, including iron, manganese, selenium and copper. Excess zinc inhibits the absorption of copper and can lead to a copper-deficit anemia. Oral iron supplements can interfere with zinc absorption which is especially important in pregnant women (see page 66).

Zinc is essential for the metabolism of vitamin A.

Protein intake influences zinc absorption—the higher the protein intake the higher the zinc requirement.

It has been known since 1934 that zinc is necessary for the growth of animals. Retardation of growth is an early and prominent feature in young animals experimentally deprived of zinc. Zinc is required for optimum growth recovery rates in children with malnutrition, and children with the hereditary zinc deficiency disease acrodermatitis enteropathica have a poor growth-rate. The rate of increase in growth parallels zinc supplementation. Formula-fed infants do not grow as well as breast-fed babies and this has been related to better zinc intake in breast-fed infants. Zinc deficiency during pregnancy is also associated with lower birth weights.

ZINC AND LACTATION

It has now become clear that the availability of zinc from human milk is greater than from cows' milk, soya milk, and combined formulas, and that more attention should be paid to the trace element levels in infant formula.

A woman's zinc requirements increase during pregnancy and lactation and this should be borne in mind because her dietary zinc may be borderline or indeed inadequate at the best of times. One study measured the zinc content of the food that pregnant and lactating women were eating and found that the average daily intake of zinc was only forty-two percent of the recommended daily allowance.

ZINC AND PREGNANCY

For many years it has been known from animal studies that zinc deficiency is associated with decreased fertility, increased rates of miscarriage and increased rates of congenital malformations.

Researchers from the University of California studied mice fed a diet moderately deficient in zinc from day seven of pregnancy until birth. Offspring of these mice showed depressed immune function through to six months of age. Also the second and third generations, all of which were fed the normal control diet, continued to show reduced immune competence, although not to the same degree as in the first generation.

Studies published in the *British Journal of Obstetrics and Gynaecology* failed to show any association between zinc deficiency and problems in pregnancy, but these studies used serum and hair zinc-levels which are very unreliable methods of assessing zinc status.

It appears that zinc deficiency during the last two thirds of pregnancy can alter the basic development of the immune system, and several researchers conclude that adequate dietary zinc is essential during both pregnancy and lactation to ensure the development of an intact immune system in the offspring.

It is clear that zinc is a critically important element which must be available to the developing fetus, in adequate amounts, for normal development. It makes sense for all women of child-bearing age to eat a diet which will provide an adequate amount of zinc. This is especially true for women who have already had one or more problem-pregnancies or babies.

ZINC AND IMMUNITY

Zinc deficient animals and children have an increased susceptibility to infections. It is now clear that zinc has a profound influence on immune responses.

Oral zinc supplementation has been shown to be beneficial on the immune response of old people.

It seems, from the research available, that zinc deficiency could well play a part in the suppression of the immune system which is often observed following bereavement or viral infections such as glandular fever. Long-standing vaginal trichomoniasis responding to oral supplementation with zinc has also been reported.

A recent study has demonstrated that sucking zinc gluconate lozenges (containing 50 mg of zinc) may reduce the duration of the common cold.

Acquired immune deficiency syndrome (AIDS) is another area where investigation of the zinc status of sufferers and the effects of zinc supplementation may turn out to be highly profitable.

ZINC AND THE SPECIAL SENSES

There is a considerable amount of evidence which shows that zinc is an important factor in maintaining the integrity of the special senses.

Vision

It is clear that zinc is essential for maintaining normal vision, and night-blindness that is not due to vitamin A deficiency can respond to zinc supplementation.

Zinc deficiency has also been implicated in congenital fetal abnormalities involving the eye.

Taste

Animal and human studies and clinical observations in humans have shown a definite correlation between zinc deficiency and an impaired or disordered sense of taste, and that zinc supplementation can correct this.

Abnormalities in the sense of taste in patients having regular kidney dialysis have been shown to be reversed by oral zinc supplementation.

Smell

The power of smell has been reported to be diminished in zinc deficiency. Zinc supplementation in those with a loss of the sense of smell has led to mixed findings and it appears that an impairment of this sense is not a condition that consistently responds to zinc supplements.

ZINC AND REPRODUCTIVE FUNCTION

Zinc is necessary for the production of sperms, the development of primary and secondary sexual characteristics, and all phases of the reproductive process in the female from estrus to birth and lactation.

Zinc deficiency has been clearly shown to be a cause of low sperm count and male infertility.

ZINC AND WOUND HEALING

Clinical observations in humans have shown that there is an association between low zinc and chronic ulceration from various causes. Several studies have found that zinc improves the healing rate of surgical wounds.

ZINC AND ACNE

Studies in Sweden and the UK have shown that zinc supplementation can be of benefit in acne.

ZINC AND HAIR LOSS

Zinc is well recognized as being involved in hair growth. Patients with acrodermatitis enteropathica lose their hair and hair loss has also been observed in zinc-deprived animals. Supplementation with a high dose of zinc has been shown to reverse hair loss in those with alopecia, with a rapid restoration of dense, thick hair growth. It may well be worth considering zinc supplementation if you have patchy or total hair loss.

ZINC AND MUSCLE FUNCTION

Recent reports have shown that zinc depletion reduces muscle strength and endurance; this suggests that oral zinc supplementation would increase stamina by prolonging muscle contraction.

Two studies of athletes in training revealed lower levels of serum zinc compared with those of controls. It is possible that increased sweating, increased blood volume, protein-rich diets and increased sweat losses could account for the lower levels. Anyone undergoing rigorous athletic training should be assessed for zinc deficiency and should take supplements where appropriate.

ZINC AND MENTAL FUNCTION

It has long been known that children with acrodermatitis enteropathica are mentally lethargic, have poor concentration and are sullen, schizoid, depressed, miserable, irritable and tearful, never smile or laugh, are difficult to soothe and not soothed by close bodily contact. The restoration of smiling after zinc supplementation is one of the earliest signs that the acrodermatitis is under control. The mechanisms by which these changes are brought about is not understood.

Researchers in England found that patients recently admitted to a psychiatric hospital had low plasma magnesium and zinc when compared with controls.

Mentally retarded children who eat dirt have been shown to have a low hair-zinc and elevated hair-copper when compared to those who do not. Researchers feel that trace-mineral status should be evaluated in such children and that such an evaluation would be a valuable contribution towards better nutritional care of the mentally retarded.

One researcher has reported that babies waking one or more times at night between midnight and 7 A.M. improved their sleep pattern when given 12 mg of elemental zinc and 0.925 mg of manganese. He also noted that the babies had an increased appetite, and a reduction in irritability, diarrhea, skin rashes and pallor.

Anyone of any age who has a mental disturbance or a behavior or sleep disorder should be examined for zinc deficiency and given a therapeutic trial of zinc if necessary.

ZINC AND RHEUMATOID ARTHRITIS

Low serum zinc has been recorded in a number of inflammatory conditions including rheumatoid arthritis. Reseachers in Seattle gave a zinc supplement, three times daily, to some patients with chronic, active rheumatoid arthritis; others were given a placebo. Those on zinc supplementation for twelve weeks did better than did the placebo group and had marked improvement in joint swelling, morning stiffness, walking time, "overall condition" and joint tenderness, when compared with the control group.

ZINC AND INFLAMMATORY BOWEL DISEASE

It is well recognized that zinc is absorbed poorly in various malabsorption syndromes. What is less well known is that zinc deficiency is common in inflammatory bowel disease (Crohn's disease more than ulcerative colitis), caused by impaired absorption, loss from the surface of the intestine, loss of zinc in the urine, poor appetite and poor food selection.

ZINC AND ALCOHOL

Poor nutrition and a diuretic effect which results in more zinc being lost in the urine may both contribute to zinc deficiency in alcoholism. Alcoholics with zinc deficiency can develop an acrodermatitis-like, zinc-responsive skin rash. Anyone who drinks a lot should be suspected of being zinc deficient.

There is a definite relationship between alcohol consumption during pregnancy and fetal abnormalities. There is now considerable evidence for a link between zinc deficiency and alcohol intake in the mothers of these children. It seems likely that zinc deficiency promotes the teratogenic effects of alcohol, resulting in the series of congenital abnormalities that are now so well described in the fetal alcohol syndrome.

ZINC AND DRUGS

Anyone taking drugs should be aware that some of them influence zinc metabolism. Drugs which produce a depletion of zinc include penicillamine, steroids, ethanol, diuretics and excessive tea and coffee. Laxative abuse and fiber supplementation can also reduce zinc absorption. Serum zinc/copper ratios are reduced in women taking combined oral contraceptives. The anticonvulsant medication, valproic acid, has been shown to bind zinc, and its teratogenicity and side-effects (anorexia, hair loss, liver toxicity etc.) could be related to drug-induced zinc deficiency.

As more becomes known about drug-nutrient interactions it is likely that other drugs will be recognized as interfering with normal zinc metabolism. On the other hand, it is likely that as an awareness of the role zinc inadequacy plays in the cause of a range of clinical conditions, zinc supplementation and nutritional handling may complement or even replace some current drug regimes.

Anyone taking long-term steroids, penicillamine or diuretics, and all alcoholics, should have their zinc status regularly monitored and supplementation instituted where appropriate.

ZINC AND TOXIC METALS

Lead and cadmium both inhibit, amongst others, zinc-dependent enzymes. So, clearly, the toxicity of these elements is reduced in the presence of adequate zinc. In fact, zinc and vitamin C have been shown to reduce blood levels of these poisons in workers who make lead batteries. Lead and cadmium exert a more toxic effect in the presence of zinc deficiency. This is highly relevant when assessing the behavioral effects of these elements in children, when zinc supplementation should seriously be considered.

ZINC AND ESSENTIAL FATTY ACIDS

Zinc is necessary for the correct metabolism of essential fatty acids and their conversion to prostaglandins—in fact many of the symptoms of essential fatty acid deficiency are mimicked by zinc deficiency.

ZINC SUPPLEMENTATION

Oral zinc supplementation is relatively safe and nontoxic. Most of the studies have been done using sulphate, but amino-chelated zinc, zinc orotate, or zinc acetate, citrate and picolinate can be used. It is well known that supplementation with zinc can reduce copper absorption and cause copper deficiency in the long term. For this reason, zinc supplements should be taken before or after mealtimes by one hour or more to avoid interaction with dietary elements.

You can see from this chapter that zinc is a very important element in the maintenance of health and in the treatment of a wide range of disorders. The best way to find out if you are zinc deficient is to take zinc and see if you get better.

EFFECTS OF FOOD ON ZINC ABSORPTION

Several foods seem to reduce the absorption of zinc and so should not be eaten at the same time as zinc supplements. These include soya protein isolates, soya-base milk formulas, coffee, cows' milk, cheese, hamburgers, celery, lemon, brown bread, iron supplements, wholewheat bread, high-fiber diet foods, bran.

There is evidence that someone who has a low-zinc diet appears to absorb more efficiently whatever zinc there is in the diet.

Items which have been shown *not* to interfere with dietary zinc absorption include bacon, white toast and human milk. Nutritional supplements with a significant inorganic iron content, such as those often prescribed to pregnant women, can also inhibit the uptake of zinc. There is no convincing evidence to date that zinc absorption is influenced by hormonal factors, but it has been shown that vitamin D enhances the absorption of zinc. There is no evidence that vitamin C influences zinc absorption.

Though zinc may be found in high concentrations in cows' milk and soya-milk infant formulas, it is most easily absorbed from breast milk.

Absorption of zinc is best at night

A sixty-three-year-old lady who had been shown to be zinc deficient on the basis of hair, sweat and serum tests, was put on a zinc supplement. Repeat testing after two months showed that there was really no difference at all in her zinc levels, indicating that absorption of the zinc supplement was not taking place. Knowing that zinc absorption can be interfered with by a number of other different dietary constituents, she was advised to take zinc on an empty stomach last thing at night. At retesting, her zinc levels had shot up well into the normal range and it was evident that she was now absorbing the zinc. Nine months later, when she came back for retesting, her zinc levels had dropped back into the deficient range. On closer questioning, it was learned that she had been taking her nutritional supplements once a day; she found it a bit of a nuisance to take the zinc last thing at night, and so had resumed taking it at breakfast time. She was advised again to take her zinc supplement at bed-time and her zinc levels have remained normal ever since. This is just one example of making use of the fact the zinc absorption is better when it is not interfered with by other dietary constitutents.

Copper

Copper has been known for over 150 years to exist in plants and animal tissues. More than fifty years ago it was shown to be essential for animals. Human copper deficiencies were reported forty years ago and, more recently, copper deficiency states have been discovered.

Copper deficiency produces anemia, skeletal defects, degeneration of the nervous system, reproductive failure, elevated blood cholesterol, cardiovascular problems, impaired immunity, and defects in the pigmentation and the structure of hair.

Copper is one of those elements which can easily be taken in excess, although it is essential for normal metabolism. The average adult has approximately 60–110 mg of copper in the body, one sixth being in the liver, one sixth in the brain, one third in the muscles, and the remaining third dispersed throughout the rest of the body. The liver controls copper storage and any excess is excreted via the bile, though if your copper intake increases, so does the amount retained.

There are a number of copper-containing enzymes that have been isolated, several of which are involved in brain metabolism.

Copper is also involved in the oxidation of vitamin C.

About thirty percent of the copper we eat is absorbed, and a typical daily dietary intake is 2–5 mg of copper. This means that the daily absorption is somewhere between 0.6–1.6 mg.

Factors which reduce the absorption of copper include excessive vitamin C or zinc, raw meat, calcium, molybdenum, mercury, lead and sulphide.

FOOD SOURCES

This very much depends on the copper content of the soil, and the copper content of the water in which the foods are prepared. Because of this, any tables of food-sources of copper should be treated with caution. However, rich food-sources of copper include oysters, kidney, dried legumes, liver and nuts.

COPPER AND HEART DISEASE

There is evidence to show that copper is involved in the regulation of blood cholesterol—a copper deficiency leads to an elevated blood cholesterol. There is also some evidence to suggest that an inadequate copper intake is associated with an increased rate of cardiovascular disease due to atherosclerosis.

There is an interaction between zinc and copper which is not yet fully understood, but relates to cardiovascular disease, atherosclerosis, and serum cholesterol. A US researcher found that an increase in the zinc to copper ratio raised the blood cholesterol levels in rats. He compared coronary heart disease with death rates in forty-seven US cities, and related it to milk intake (because the zinc to copper ratio in milk differs from one area to the next in the US). He discovered a correlation between high zinc to copper ratios and higher death rates from heart disease. He also noted that the copper content of foods today is lower than it was thirty-five years ago, and that in the US many people are eating less than the recommended daily allowance of 2 mg.

COPPER AND ARTHRITIS

Many people swear that wearing a copper bracelet reduces their arthritic pain. There is very little objective scientific evidence that this is so, though one only has to talk with people who find their copper bracelet useful to realize that there may well be some value in it. One Australian study found that thirty-one out of forty arthritic patients felt better when wearing their copper bracelets. The researcher, Dr. Ray Walker, found that the copper bracelets lost an average of 13 mg in weight per month. This was presumably due to the loss of copper from the bracelet into sweat and then its absorption by the skin. Obviously, a little could also be lost into clothing, bath water and so on.

The way in which such bracelets work is not understood, though it may very well be related to the activity of the enzyme superoxide dismutase, which has a copper-containing form. Copper deficiency would limit the production of the enzyme and this would result in a failure to "mop up" those substances in the body that can cause inflammation and pain. Furthermore, John Sorenson, professor of Pharmacy at the University of Arkansas, has noted that copper salicylate (a sort of aspirin containing copper) can be useful in arthritis and in the treatment of ulcers.

It is possible that anti-inflammatory compounds, such as aspirin and phenylbutazone, combine with copper in the tissue of the stomach, the copper then being transported to the site of inflammation. Aspirin is *extremely* potent in its ability to combine with copper.

COPPER AND MENTAL FUNCTION

In view of the fact that copper is involved in the production of a number of brain chemicals, disruptions of copper metabolism can understandably produce mental symptoms.

Dr. Carl Pfeiffer of the Brain Biocenter in Princeton, New Jersey, has long claimed that excessive copper, especially when combined with deficiencies of zinc or manganese, can be involved in the development of schizophrenia.

It has been our experience that a number of people with schizophrenia and/or severe mental disturbances of one sort or another very often have high serum- or hair-copper levels. Reducing these levels with the use of vitamin C, zinc, manganese and B vitamins, results in an improvement in those conditions.

COPPER AND THE CONTRACEPTIVE PILL

As mentioned on page 312, the Pill raises blood copper levels and can reduce the body zinc status. Also, during pregnancy, elevations of copper and decreases of zinc can occur as a result of normal hormonal actions.

Postnatal depression and psychosis, as well as depression while using the Pill, could possibly be linked to the severely reduced zinc to copper ratios that can occur.

COPPER AND DRINKING WATER

The copper content of drinking water depends on the type of piping it flows through (very often copper) and the hardness of water itself. Hard water tends to coat the inside of the pipes and provide a protective barrier between the water and the copper pipes. The copper content in hot water is generally higher than in cold water because of the increased solubility of copper at higher temperatures. It is possible to buy a domestic filter through which all drinking water is passed. This is worth doing because too much copper reduces the availability of zinc to the body and most of us are already rather short of zinc. You should never fill up the kettle, or drink water from the hot-water tap, as it can be very high in copper.

COPPER DEFICIENCY AND ZINC

Excessive zinc supplementation can cause a copper deficiency. However, in an adult, 30–50 mg of zinc per day is unlikely to produce severe copper deficiency, though on this kind of level of supplementation it is important to monitor both zinc and copper status.

Vanadium

Vanadium is probably a trace element for man and may be of value in protecting against heart disease and cancer. Much has yet to be learned about vanadium, whose biochemistry is very complex.

The total amount of vanadium in the average adult body is probably in the range of 17–43 mg. It is involved in growth and fat metabolism.

It has been found that vanadium deficiency results in increased blood cholesterol and triglyceride levels. Animal studies have revealed that vanadium deficiency results in an impaired reproductive performance that does not show up until the fourth generation of animals mated.

It is also possible that an adequate vanadium intake will protect against the development of heart disease. Vanadium has also been recommended for treating atherosclerosis.

FOOD SOURCES

Good sources of vanadium include buckwheat, parsley, soybeans, safflower oil, eggs, sunflower-seed oil, oats, carrots, cabbage, garlic, tomatoes, other vegetable oils, rice, sunflower seeds, corn, green beans, and oysters.

VANADIUM AND MANIC-DEPRESSIVE ILLNESS

Researchers at the University of Dundee showed that elevated levels of vanadium in hair were present in manic patients, and that these elevated levels fell towards normal as the subjects improved. In contrast, they found that depressed patients have raised levels of vanadium which appeared to fall with recovery.

Iodine

Iodine has been known to be an essential trace element for over 150 years. Nevertheless, it is estimated that more than 200 million people throughout the world suffer from iodine deficiency diseases, mainly because they live in iodine-deficient soil areas.

The main iodine deficiency sign is an enlargement of the thyroid gland in the neck (goiter). Giving iodine to such people cures the goiter and adding iodized salt to their diet can prevent it from occurring at all.

Iodine is essential for the production of thyroid hormones which play a fundamental part in controlling metabolism.

Since thyroid hormones are so important in the maintenance of normal metabolic processes in the body, a defect in their production can play havoc with the body's normal functioning.

Eating too much iodine suppresses the thyroid gland. This fact is put to good use in people who have an overactive thyroid gland (thyrotoxicosis) and can bring about a resolution of the overactivity when used in conjunction with low-dose lithium under medical supervision.

Iodine excess can aggravate acne (see page 275), and skin contact with iodine can lead to dermatitis.

FOOD SOURCES

Foods rich in iodine include clams, shrimps, haddock, halibut, oysters, salmon, sardines, beef liver, pineapple, tuna fish, eggs, peanuts, wholewheat bread, cheddar cheese, pork, lettuce, spinach, green peppers, butter, milk, cream, cottage cheese, beef, lamb and raisins. Between eighty and eighty-five percent of our total dietary intake of iodine is derived from dairy products, meat, fish, poultry, grain and cereals.

In 1950, the British Medical Association recommended intakes of 100 mcg of iodine daily for adults, and 150 mcg for children, adolescents and pregnant and lactating women. An intake in adults of 50–1000 mcg of iodine per day is considered to be safe.

However, some experts are concerned that there is too much iodine in our diet. This is because iodine is used in the dairy industry, in coloring dyes and in dough conditioners, and they feel that the iodine should be replaced wherever possible by compounds containing little or no iodine. Too much iodine—as in some tonics—can result in a skin condition similar to acne.

Goiter can also be induced by a high dietary iodine intake, just as by an iodine deficiency. This occurred in Japan, where certain groups of fishermen who ate seaweed consumed 10,000–200,000 mcg of iodine per day.

Silicon

Silicon appears to be an essential element, though we need more information to fulfill the criteria for it to be called truly "essential" (see page 43).

Silicon is very similar to carbon, which in turn is found everywhere in nature. Silicon can form long, complex molecules in the same way that carbon can. However, the bond between silicon atoms is stronger than that between carbon atoms, which makes silicon-containing molecules relatively stable and structurally strong. So, structurally "strong" tissues such as arteries, tendons, skin, connective tissue, cornea and sclera (white of the eye) contain large amounts of silicon, whereas other tissues such as liver, kidney and blood contain very little. Collagen, the tough substance that holds other tissues together, contains a lot of silicon. Silicon is a structural part of collagen and silicon-containing substances are found in all cartilage.

In atherosclerotic arteries there is fourteen times less silicon than in disease-free arteries. There does, therefore, seem to be a link between silicon status and the incidence of arteriosclerosis. Researchers in the USA and in Finland have found that in areas with a high silicon level in the drinking water, there is a reduced incidence of arteriosclerosis.

Molybdenum

The average adult has 8–10 mg of molybdenum, concentrated mostly in the liver, kidney, adrenal glands, bones and skin.

It is possible that molybdenum deficiencies will become recognized as an important aspect of health and disease, since the refining of food reduces its molybdenum content substantially.

It is possible that molybdenum deficiency is linked to an increased risk of cancer of the esophagus, but this has yet to be proven. Molybdenum and copper interact with one another, and a high copper intake increases the rate of molybdenum excretion. There is some evidence that sensitivity to bisulphites which are used as preservatives of salad greens may be in part due to molybdenum deficiency.

Chromium

Chromium is an essential trace element, recently discovered to be necessary for blood sugar control. Because chromium is present in blood in very minute quantities, in the past there have been problems with its accurate measurement. This means that early scientific literature cannot be relied upon to present a true picture. However, with more recent advances in analytical techniques, chromium can now be measured accurately in body tissues.

WHAT IT DOES

Chromium may turn out to be an important factor in the development of a number of chronic degenerative diseases in the Western world. It is evident that not only are some diets deficient in chromium, but that these very same diets increase the excretion of chromium in the urine, so resulting in a depletion of whatever chromium reserves an individual may have.

Refined carbohydrates have had the chromium removed from them during processing and they also tend to increase the rate at which chromium is excreted in the urine, so diets high in refined carbohydrates can produce a chromium deficiency. This may have some bearing on the fact that there is a whole range of different diseases (including diabetes, heart disease and hardening of the arteries), that are more prevalent in the Western world where there is a higher intake of refined carbohydrates. Something else that may be relevant is that refined carbohydrates cause a rapid increase in the blood sugar level, which in turn results in an increased secretion of insulin, to handle the sugar. With increased circulating insulin levels, the demand for chromium increases, as we shall see.

FOOD SOURCES

Good sources of chromium include brewers' yeast, black pepper, calf's liver, wheatgerm, wholewheat bread, and cheese.

CHROMIUM LEVELS: CHANGE AND AGE

Chromium levels are high in newborn infants and children up to ten years old, and levels decrease with age. This probably reflects the development of a chromium deficiency. It seems to parallel the observation that glucose tolerance (the ability to control blood sugar levels) deteriorates with age, while at the same time the incidence of certain of the chronic degenerative diseases increases.

CHROMIUM AND GLUCOSE TOLERANCE

Insulin is essential to control blood sugar levels, and to enable glucose to enter the cells, and glucose is a vital part of the energy production of almost every cell in the body. When the body fails to control blood sugar, and the level increases above the normal range, the condition is known as diabetes mellitus (see page 286). This disease is associated with an increased risk of death from heart attacks, strokes, and damage to blood vessels affecting the function of the eyes, kidneys, and the blood supply to the skin. Another complication of diabetes mellitus is the malfunction of nerve fibers (neuropathy) which produces a whole range of, often diffuse, symptoms. Chromium has now been proved to be essential for the action of insulin and the maintenance of normal blood sugar levels.

The human body can't utilize chromium in the same form that exists in such things as car bumpers. It has to be in the form of a molecule in which the chromium is combined with vitamin B3 (nicotinic acid) and three specific amino acids. This is called the Glucose Tolerance Factor (GTF). The richest known natural source of preformed GTF chromium is brewers' yeast, whose GTF activity is ten times higher than that of any other food.

GTF chromium in food is absorbed much more efficiently and utilized more effectively than is any other form of chromium. However, ordinary chromium salts can be absorbed to a lesser extent by humans and it appears that the ability to convert this inorganic chromium into GTF chromium is important in the resistance against the development of arteriosclerosis and diabetes mellitus.

THE EFFECTS OF CHROMIUM DEFICIENCY

Most of the studies on the effects of chromium deficiency have been done in animals. The following are the effects of chromium deficiency:

- impaired handling of glucose
- reduced effectiveness of insulin
- corneal opacity
- atherosclerosis
- depressed sperm-formation
- elevated blood sugar and hypoglycemia
- loss of sugar in the urine

There have now been many studies on the effect of chromium supplementation on people suspected of being chromium deficient. Studies with inorganic chromium have tended to produce different results from those utilizing GTF chromium-rich yeast or GTF chromium. It seems that supplementation with chromium can produce a range of effects. For example, one study, in New York, looked at the effects of chromium-rich yeast on glucose tolerance and blood fats in elderly people. The results support a thesis that elderly people have a low level of chromium and that an effective source of chromium, such as brewers' yeast, can improve their carbohydrate tolerance and total blood fats.

Studies on laboratory animals have found that supplementation with chromium produces a significant regression of hardening of the arteries.

Several other studies have shown that chromium supplementation, preferably in the form of GTF chromium, improves the body's sensitivity to insulin, reduces blood glucose levels, and improves blood fat levels, suggesting that chromium in this form might have a protective effect against atherosclerosis.

CHROMIUM SUPPLEMENTATION

Adequate chromium intake can be assured by taking several grams of brewers' yeast per day, unless you are yeast sensitive. An inexpensive way of taking chromium is to arrange with your local pharmacist to make up a bottle of trivalent chromium chloride providing 200 mg per day in 5 mls of water. GTF chromium appears to be the chromium supplement of choice. **However, many GTF chromium preparations are yeast-derived, and the same cautions for yeast-sensitive people apply to the GTF chromium as well as to the yeast itself.** There are some companies that state that their GTF chromium is yeast-free, but so far we have no information on the metabolic activity of yeast-free GTF chromium.

Manganese

This is a rather enigmatic, but nevertheless essential, element that is found in bone, soft tissues, pituitary gland, liver, and kidney, in decreasing order of concentration. It is necessary for normal intra-uterine growth, growth generally, normal cartilage, the functioning of nervous tissue and for many of the body's "activator" systems. Manganese is also known to be essential for the metabolism of amino acids and carbohydrates.

Manifestations of manganese deficiency include disc and cartilage problems, glucose intolerance, reduced brain function, middle-ear imbalances, birth defects, reduced fertility, and growth retardation.

A healthy body contains 12–20 mg of manganese. The body loses about 4 mg a day of this element, so to be safe it makes sense to at least replace this amount, whether in food or as supplements.

When taking a supplement, take 10–20 mg a day of manganese chloride or manganese amino-chelate. Leafy, green vegetables and whole grains are the main sources of manganese in the diet and tea is an exceptionally rich source. One cupful contains 1 mg of the element.

Selenium

Selenium deficiency was first described in animals but has now been documented in humans as a result of studies on patients who, because they are very ill and cannot eat, are being totally artificially fed. Selenium deficiency has also been implicated as a cause of heart disease, cancer and a number of other conditions which are dealt with below.

In human beings, the role of selenium is not well understood, though a considerable amount of evidence is emerging to demonstrate that it is essential in man.

WHAT IT DOES

At present the only known function in man for selenium is as a component of an enzyme which protects cells against oxidative damage (see page 146).

FOOD SOURCES

There is no evidence that selenium is essential for plant growth. This means that arable farmers do not get upset when the soil becomes depleted of selenium because their crop yields do not fail. This does not apply to farmers dealing with livestock, as severe selenium depletion results in muscle disease in animals. Good sources of selenium are grains, fish and most wholefoods.

DEFICIENCY SYMPTOMS AND SIGNS

The main situations in which selenium deficiency has been documented are those in which people respond to selenium supplementation after developing symptoms on prolonged, total artificial feeding. According to our own observations, however, there are certain groups that are particularly at risk. We have found that certain groups of patients tend to be low in selenium, for example those with liver disease (primary biliary cirrhosis or alcoholic cirrhosis), cancer patients, those with cardiovascular disease and some older patients with arthritis. It is important to remember that someone with selenium deficiency which occurs as a result of an inability to consume and/or absorb food, or with continual gastrointestinal losses secondary to intestinal disease, is probably deficient in a number of other nutrients also.

CONDITIONS IN WHICH SELENIUM SUPPLEMENTATION MAY BE USEFUL

There is now increasing evidence that ensuring an adequate selenium intake may be a very positive preventive medical step. Here are some situations in which a future for selenium looks hopeful.

Cardiomyopathy (Keshan disease)

Chinese researchers were first to show that selenium deficiency was one of the principal factors responsible for a heart condition that affects mainly children and young women living in rural areas of Keshan, a selenium-deficient area of China.

We think that, in the light of current knowledge, any individual with unexplained cardiomyopathy of this kind should be assessed for selenium adequacy.

Cancer prevention

There have been a number of studies associating selenium deficiency with an increased risk of cancer.

Studies have shown that selenium inhibits tumor formation in spontaneous breast cancers in mice, and the development of other specific tumors in mice. Initial epidemiological studies in man have suggested that regional or national variations of dietary selenium intake could be responsible for the statistical associations between diet and deaths from cancer. Cancer patients have lower levels of selenium in their urine than do any other groups investigated.

It seems, therefore, that selenium deficiency could be an important causative factor in the susceptibility to cancer. Any preventive medical efforts should take this into consideration. It is also important to bear in mind that selenium deficiency can be a direct *result* of certain forms of cancer.

Heart disease

Research in Finland, which has one of the highest national cardiovascular death rates in the world, has shown an association between cardiovascular death, heart attacks and low serum selenium levels.

Cirrhosis and alcoholism

Selenium deficiency has been well documented as occurring in alcoholics. It is most likely that this is due to an insufficiency of selenium in the diet, or altered metabolism involving increased loss of selenium in the urine or feces.

Artificial intravenous feeding

As has been pointed out already, selenium deficiency has been documented in patients who are being fed intravenously. Anyone on long-term intravenous feeding should be monitored for selenium status and, ideally, selenium should be supplied in adequate amounts (up to 200–250 mcg per day in the average adult).

Chemical sensitivity

One researcher theorizes, on the basis of anecdotal reports, that hypersensitivities to chemicals are primarily related to oxidation mechanisms, and that selenium and other dietary anti-oxidants might minimize the ill-effects of such chemical exposure. Certainly, in our experience, nutritional supplementation in such individuals, who are often quite ill, can result in considerable clinical improvement. (See page 180.)

Dandruff and ringworm

Selenium-containing shampoos such as Selsun and Lenium contain considerable amounts of selenium. They are undoubtedly effective as a treatment for dandruff, but no one knows how they work.

Selsun shampoo can be applied to the skin for ringworm on the body and other superficial fungal skin infections.

Mercury toxicity

Selenium can be used in the treatment of mercury toxicity, (see page 98). Acute poisoning with inorganic mercury is very dangerous, and aggressive treatment is required. However, with lesser degrees of mercury toxicity in animals, it has been demonstrated that selenium compounds counteract the toxicity of both inorganic and organic mercury compounds. It seems likely that the protection afforded by selenium also applies to man.

TOXICITY

Though selenium is an essential nutrient, it is possible to have too much. The toxic effects of selenium have been recognized for a long time as a result of observations made on animals and humans living in geographical areas with a high-selenium soil content.

Sources of selenium toxicity

Potentially toxic sources of selenium in the environment are:

- Industrial, such as:
  smelting—copper, lead, zinc; pyrites-roasting; lime and cement (some areas); glass and ceramics; rubber; steel and brass; paint and ink pigments; plastics; photoelectric; chemical.
- Non-industrial:
  selenium-containing shampoos (e.g. Selsun, Lenium); high selenium in the soil in certain areas.

Selenium-containing shampoos, such as Selsun and Lenium, which contain selenium sulphide, can be a source of total body selenium toxicity because they are absorbed through the skin even though selenium sulphide has a very low toxicity in comparison with selenite.

Symptoms of selenium toxicity

The symptoms of selenium toxicity are:

- Hair loss.
- Nail signs—in sequence of events:
  brittle, white spots,
  pale nailbeds,
  breakage of the nails (thumbs always first),
  fluid around the nail,
  loss of nail.
- Tooth decay.

- Nervous system—in sequence of events:
  loss of sensation in hands and feet,
  pins and needles,
  pain in the hands and feet.
- Poor appetite and weight loss.
- Gastrointestinal disturbances.
- Reddish pigmentation of the skin.
- Sour taste in the mouth.
- Garlic-like odor on the breath.
- Dizziness, malaise, pallor.

SELENIUM SUPPLEMENTATION

Since vitamin E and selenium are so closely related in their effect on the body, you should always take vitamin E along with selenium.

There are different forms of selenium supplements and it appears that some are more biologically active than others.

If you are going to take 100–200 mcg per day of selenium in the form of selenomethionine in brewers' yeast, you must bear in mind the apparent frequency with which yeast intolerance or sensitivity occurs. If this happens, it would be sensible to use a sodium salt of selenium (e.g. selenite or selenate) or selenium-enriched kelp.

Nickel

Nickel has recently been found to have a physiological role in both animal and human metabolism. More is known about the effects of nickel in certain animals than in man because it is very difficult to prepare a nickel-free diet for humans. In rabbits and dogs, nickel in tissues outside the intestine intensifies the blood-sugar-lowering effect of insulin, and large doses alter fat metabolism. In humans, it acts as an antidote to the blood-pressure-raising action of adrenalin, which constricts blood vessels and stimulates the heart.

The nutritional requirements for nickel have not yet been established. High levels of nickel in the serum are found after heart attacks, in people with strokes and severe burns, and in women with toxemia of pregnancy or uterine cancer. Low levels occur in people with cirrhosis of the liver or chronic kidney failure.

Exposure to nickel is widespread because it is found in coins, jewelry, kitchen appliances and so on. The most commonly observed ill-effect of nickel is dermatitis in nickel-sensitive people.

Commonly occurring items containing nickel are:

- Personal objects:
  - suspender clasps
  - snap fasteners
  - jewelry clasps
  - clasps of wristwatches (and the watch itself)
  - car keys
  - pocket knives
  - metal eyeglass frames
  - hooks and eyes
  - earrings
  - brassiere clasps
  - cigarette lighters
  - metal studs or buttons on jeans
  - coins
  - zippers
- Household objects:
  - vacuum cleaners
  - needles
  - thimbles
  - telephone dials
  - knitting needles
  - sewing machines
  - scissors
  - drawer handles
  - baby carriages
- Office materials:
  - typewriters
  - staplers
  - paper clips
  - staples, etc.

Dr. John Howard, with whom we work very closely, has noticed that patients who are nickel sensitive (jewelry, watches, etc.) tend to have a higher than normal sweat nickel level. We have noticed that these patients also have an increased tendency to food allergies. When they start to recover from their illness, even without necessarily avoiding nickel, we find that the sweat-nickel level often comes down to the normal range. The precise mechanism by which this occurs has not yet been established.

Lithium

It is probable that lithium is an essential element, though a lot of work has yet to be done in order to clarify its actions. There is no recommended daily allowance as lithium deficiency itself has not yet, to our knowledge, been reported in man.

It has been found that lithium is effective in the treatment of acute mania and depression, and it is now a standard treatment for manic-depressive psychosis, in the form of lithium carbonate, taken in the dose of 400 mg several times a day. However, since lithium is potentially toxic, people on such treatment have to have their lithium levels measured routinely to ensure that they are not being poisoned by it.

Lithium has also been used in the treatment of alcoholics because it produces a taste aversion to alcohol.

Low-dose lithium carbonate (100–300 mg once or twice daily) has also been reported anecdotally as being effective in controlling many of the more unpleasant symptoms of the menopause and premenstrual syndrome. A lithium-based ointment has been effective in the treatment of genital herpes.

TOXICITY

Excess lithium disturbs mineral transport across cell membranes as well as fluid balance. Symptoms include nausea, vomiting, tremors, thirst, excessive urination, thyroid swelling, weight gain, drowsiness, confusion, disorientation, delirium, skin eruptions, and at worst seizures, coma and even death. Irreversible kidney damage has been reported in some people who have been on long-term treatment for manic-depression, **and for this reason people taking lithium should do so only under medical supervision.**

LITHIUM SUPPLEMENTATION

There is no evidence at the moment that lithium supplementation is required in people who do not suffer from manic or ordinary depression.

Lithium supplements, along with iodine, may be of value in overactivity of the thyroid gland, **but these should only be taken under medical supervision.**

Fluoride

Fluoride is present throughout the body and is best known for its ability to reduce tooth decay.

It has never been shown to be essential to life, as far as we know, but it seems important in the maintenance of normal bone and tooth structure. It has been used to curb osteoporosis and to stop the loss of hearing associated with otosclerosis.

In Colorado, in 1916, a dentist noticed that his patients' teeth were mottled, but had few cavities. The city's water supply was analyzed and found to contain two parts per million of fluoride as soluble salts. It now appears that the optimal concentration for good tooth structure is only one part per million.

Fluoride in drinking water definitely protects teeth against decay. However, excessive fluoride intake causes mottled teeth with white patches over the surface of the teeth and yellowy brown staining. In severe cases, the tooth enamel is pitted and the teeth corrode.

Fluoridation of the water supply has reduced dental decay by between forty and seventy percent in the children born after this treatment began.

However, there is considerable opposition to the fluoridation of municipal water supplies, on the ground that we already receive enough fluoride from other sources, and that there are ill-effects from fluoridation.

Tea is very rich in fluoride, and many industries emit fluorine fumes in the processing of minerals. Fluoride in toothpaste directly reduces bacterial growth in the mouth and thereby reduces tooth decay. This works in adults as well as children.

There is a lot of controversy on the subject of fluoride, even though the prevention of dental decay is an obviously desirable goal.

A comparison of cancer rates in the ten largest cities in the USA fluoridated before 1966, with the rates in the ten largest cities during the pre-fluoride period 1944–1950, and not fluoridated as of 1969, demonstrated a significant increase in the incidence of cancer in the areas where the municipal water supply was fluoridated. However, there are other studies which do not support this finding and the question has not yet been resolved.

There is some suspicion that congenital malformation may be associated with a fluoridated water supply.

FOOD SOURCES

Wheat, carrots, beets, squash, sauerkraut, currants, cabbage leaves, potatoes and lettuce, as well as tea.

THE FLUORIDE DEBATE

The fluoride debate continues and we cannot come down on one side or the other. Perhaps the best compromise is to ensure that children have their teeth treated with fluoride by their dentist and use a fluoride toothpaste twice a day, rather than fluoridation of the water supply. We are not convinced that fluoridation of the water supply is an entirely safe procedure for all.

Cobalt

Cobalt is an essential trace element and is usually thought of as being physiologically active only when present as vitamin B12.

Inorganic cobalt, however, is by no means physiologically inert. However, in the past, because cobalt is present in such small quantities, it has been very difficult to clarify its importance in human metabolism other than as a part of the vitamin B12 molecule.

While cobalt excess has been recognized for many years, it is only recently that a researcher in Chicago observed that hair cobalt levels are very low in violent offenders compared with normal people.

TOXICITY

In 1966, a new disease appeared in heavy beer-drinkers in Canada, Belgium and the USA. It was characterized by heart failure caused by a condition called cardiomyopathy. It was believed that this was due to excess cobalt added to the beer to produce a nice frothy "head." The sufferers were drinking between six and thirty bottles of beer per day.

Too much cobalt can also cause too many red blood cells in rats, mice, guinea pigs, ducks, chickens, pigs, dogs and humans. A high-protein diet can give considerable protection against the toxicity of cobalt.

Other Minerals

Other minerals that are important to optimum function of the body include sulphur. Elements which are being researched and which may well turn out to be essential include rubidium, strontium and tin, but in view of the fact that supplements are not generally given, they are not discussed further here.

TOXIC METALS

Ever since man started to extract and use metals, he has been able to take from the earth's crust toxic substances that are normally present in only very small quantities, and to concentrate and disperse them throughout the environment.

We are now confronted with levels of certain toxic metals

(especially lead, cadmium, mercury and aluminum) at concentrations which were not present during our evolution. Although we call them *toxic* metals, there may well be certain biochemical processes that are dependent on very small quantities of these elements. As yet, no deficiency symptoms and signs of these elements have been described in humans. The more usual problem is one of excess. Clearly they represent an adaptive stress and it is, therefore, hardly surprising that toxic signs and symptoms have been clearly described.

This section does not look so much at the *extremes* of toxic exposure to these elements, such as are found in industrial environments. Here, we are more interested in describing the relationships between man and low environmental concentrations of these elements: their sources, their effects, and what we can do to protect ourselves against them.

Lead

For centuries it has been recognized that lead is toxic to humans. "Classic" lead poisoning is well recognized as potentially fatal. But what concerns us more is the recent evidence which shows the more subtle detrimental effects of chronic low-level lead exposure. By low-level, we mean a level insufficient to produce "classical" lead poisoning. There are some factors, primarily, but not exclusively, nutritional, that tend to enhance the toxicity of such low levels of exposure. The main problems caused by low-level exposure to lead are:

- stillbirths
- developmental abnormalities
- learning, behavioral and nervous system problems
- cancer
- heart disease and high blood pressure
- kidney and metabolic disease
- vague symptoms (lethargy, depression, muscle aches and pains, frequent infections, etc.)
- immune dysfunction

THE CURRENT LEVEL OF LEAD POLLUTION

Lead is naturally present in the earth's crust in small concentrations, but for centuries man has been mining it and spreading it throughout his environment. The degree of contamination is now so great that the average Westerner has a total body-lead burden some 500 to 1000 times greater than the background levels encountered by pre-technological man. Studies of the lead content of polar ice and remote oceanic waters suggest that worldwide lead pollution has occurred and is occurring to a degree that represents a threat to the ecological stability of the entire biosphere.

While significant lead pollution in remote areas has been documented, far higher levels are encountered in populated areas. The major sources of lead in an urban environment are:

- atmospheric lead—gasoline exhaust, lead smelters, coal burning, refining lead scrap
- dust and dirt
- leaded house paint
- drinking water and lead plumbing, rainwater, snow
- vegetation growing by roadsides
- some canned foods
- milk from animals grazing on lead-contaminated pastures
- bonemeal, organ meats
- improperly glazed pottery and painted glassware
- putty, solder, lead-shot, car batteries
- cigarette ash, tobacco
- hair blackeners, Indian mascara
- occupational exposure

Lead interferes with the normal function of other trace elements and physiologically important metallic ions. Because lead inhibits zinc-dependent enzymes and there are at least 100 such enzymes known so far, the potential ill-effects are legion. This is doubly important since zinc deficiency is probably widespread in the general population.

THRESHOLD OF TOXICITY

For decades it has been said that there is a threshold of toxicity for lead (as well as for other toxins). Since lead is a potent toxin and is not thought to be essential in mammalian cells, the wisdom of such a view was not questioned. With technological advancement, however, we have the ability to perceive more subtle effects; so, if there is no threshold (as seems likely), the point at which no toxic effect from lead can be observed will inevitably be reduced as more sophisticated studies are conducted.

CHILDHOOD HYPERACTIVITY AND LEARNING AND BEHAVIOR DISORDERS

Increased body lead burdens have been repeatedly found to be associated with learning and behavior disorders in children. Several researchers have found that there is a link between hyperactivity and blood lead levels and have then gone on to show that treatment to reduce lead levels results in an improvement in classroom performance. Others have shown that body lead burdens, as judged by tooth-dentine lead levels, correlate with IQ and functions of classroom performance. Studies using hair lead levels as an indicator of lead exposure have shown an association between hair lead and learning disability, poor learning ability or "minimal brain dysfunction." None of these studies took into consideration nutritional status, and/or diet.

PRECONCEPTIONAL AND ANTENATAL INFLUENCES OF LEAD

Most of the work that has been done on the influence of lead exposure on the mother and father *prior* to conception has been done on animals. Pregnancy and lactation are particularly important times because requirements for protective nutrients, such as vitamin D, iron, zinc and calcium, are known to be increased, and thus the potential for lead toxicity is increased, especially since zinc is so often deficient in the diet.

ADOLESCENCE

Adolescence is a period when hormonal changes occur and when an individual's requirements for calcium and zinc are increased. So the potential for lead toxicity is increased. Lead has been implicated in the development of criminal and delinquent behavior and tends to occur in the lower socioeconomic groups that are more subject to dietary deficiencies of the protective nutrients.

MENTAL DISEASE

Little attention has been given to the role of low-level lead in the development of mental symptoms that require treatment. In view of the vast sums of money spent, in the West, on drugs which act on the brain, the search for common causative factors seems to us to be of paramount importance. Apart from dietary factors, lead fulfills many of the criteria as a significant factor.

CARDIOVASCULAR DISEASE

In the UK, illness and death from cardiovascular disease is most common in areas where the lead content of tap-water is highest, and the concentration of the protective nutrients, calcium and magnesium, lowest.

Chromium has a protective effect against lead toxicity. The association between chromium deficiency and cardiovascular disease has been well documented and chromium supplementation has been shown to have a beneficial effect on glucose tolerance, and on the protective HDL-type of cholesterol. Chromium is deficient in the highly refined carbohydrate diet eaten in the West, which itself is known to be associated with an increased incidence of cardiovascular disease and which is also deficient in other lead-protective nutrients.

A high-animal-fat diet tends to increase dietary requirements for various lead-protective nutrients (calcium, magnesium, zinc), and a high-fat diet itself is known to be linked to an increased incidence of cardiovascular disease.

While all this evidence is circumstantial, it all points in one direction: that lead exposure is an important contributory factor in the production of some cardiovascular diseases, including hardening of the arteries, gout, and high blood pressure.

CANCER

The degree to which lead may contribute to the development of cancer has been looked at but is, as yet, not conclusive.

IMMUNE DYSFUNCTION

Lead is known to harm the immune system and render an individual more susceptible to infection.

VAGUE SYMPTOMS

The degree to which low-level lead exposure contributes to the development of vague symptoms such as lethargy, tiredness, aches and pains, depression and susceptibility to infections, has not been fully assessed clinically, but has been suggested by some researchers.

LEAD EXPOSURE AND NUTRITION

There are now several nutritional protective factors that are known to help reduce the metabolic ill-effects of lead.

These include:

- vitamin C
- zinc
- calcium
- magnesium
- iron
- vitamin D
- protein and amino acids
- chromium
- vitamin E and selenium
- other nutrients

Aluminum

Aluminum is now recognized as a toxic metal and it is widely distributed in the environment. The presence of aluminum in the earth's crust has meant that man has been exposed to it over the centuries. What is new is the fact that we are now exposed to soluble, readily absorbable forms of the metal. Since the development of extraction processes for obtaining metallic aluminum, this metal has been used extensively in the manufacture of cookware, household and industrial utensils, packaging materials, aluminum cans and so on.

Aluminum salts are added to table salt to stop it from attracting water and becoming difficult to pour; we take gallons of aluminum-containing antacids per year; we add aluminum to flour to bleach it; we put it in deodorants and antiperspirants. These are completely different forms from that in which aluminum existed during our evolution. It is no wonder that there are now so many toxic effects from aluminum.

EFFECTS OF ALUMINUM OVERLOAD

The major effects of aluminum overload seem to be on the central nervous system, though it does have effects on the parathyroid gland, influencing the degree to which it responds to low serum calcium by excreting parathyroid hormone. It also seems to have an effect on bone metabolism, possibly directly as well as via the parathyroid gland. Pre-senile dementia (Alzheimer's disease)—a condition in which an individual becomes senile before his time—seems to be associated with aluminum overload. Postmortem brain aluminum measurements reveal a considerably higher level of aluminum in the brains of people with the condition than in those dying from other causes.

People on kidney dialysis machines have, in the past, been shown to have a tendency to develop a brain disease in which there is dementia and in which neurological damage develops. One of the problems with early dialysis machines was that blood phosphorus levels tended to become too high, and calcium and phosphorus problems ensued. Excessive amounts of aluminum hydroxide were then used in an attempt to reduce the degree to which phosphorus is absorbed from the gastrointestinal tract. It has since been shown that the amount of aluminum in tap-water can be a determining factor as to whether or not an individual develops dialysis dementia.

Aluminum can accumulate in the liver, interfering with its working, and its effects on the kidneys include nephritis and degeneration. It has been found that the aluminum content of joint tissues in patients taking aluminum hydroxide can be raised.

As yet, insufficient work has been done to implicate aluminum in a wide range of different conditions, to be able to say quite categorically that it is involved. However, in our clinical experience we have very little doubt that aluminum *is* involved in childhood hyperactivity, Alzheimer's disease, and a small percentage of non-specific "joint problems."

WHAT YOU CAN DO TO AVOID EXPOSURE TO ALUMINUM

We recommend that our patients avoid the use of aluminum cookware, and use, instead, Pyrex or glassware saucepans. Failing that you can use high-quality, enamel cookware, or even stainless steel. However, stainless steel saucepans are a rich source of nickel, and if you are nickel sensitive you should avoid using them.

If it is impossible to replace your aluminum cookware with other pans, then try to keep at least one non-aluminum saucepan in which to cook vegetables or fruit. The acidic nature of these foods increases the degree to which aluminum can be scoured from inside the pan and incorporated in a soluble form into the food. By using an alternative pan for fruit and vegetables you will reduce the amount of aluminum you eat.

Mercury

Mercury is a heavy metal that is a liquid at room temperature. When the weather is warm, mercury vaporizes to some degree so that there is always some in the air, coming from the ground. Probably all living things have contained mercury since the beginning of life, but only in tiny amounts, and fish are no exception. More mercury is found in prehistoric fish than in the bones of present-day fish.

As with so many other metals, man has managed to disseminate this toxic substance into the environment without due caution. Mercury has long been known to be toxic in high quantities, but it is only recently that we have begun to recognize the adverse effects on health resulting from low-level exposure. We are exposed to mercury in the environment at levels much greater than those which occurred during our evolution, and those of us with mercury-amalgam tooth-fillings are exposed to even more (see below).

When we ingest or breathe elemental mercury, it leaves the body fairly quickly (half disappears in five days), unlike lead and cadmium, which remain. It takes quite a lot of mercury every day (about 100 mg) to make us ill.

Methyl and ethyl mercury can permanently damage the brain when the level in food is twenty to forty parts per million. These compounds have been used for twenty years or more as dressings for seeds, to prevent mold. If seed that has been preserved with inorganic mercurial compounds is used to make bread, then this can be *extremely* toxic. Such seeds are intended to be used for sowing rather than milling. We have seen several cases of mercury intoxication as a direct result of organic mercurial compounds used as fungicides. It was an organic mercurial compound that resulted in the Minimata River disaster, in Japan, where local people were eating fish and shellfish polluted by a factory making plastics, discharging methyl mercury sulphide and chloride upstream. These seafoods contained twenty to thirty parts per million, and there are a number of cases where there was death or permanent damage to the central nervous system. Cats, pigs, dogs, crows, sea birds, crabs, fish and shellfish died. Rabbits, horses and cows did not. Women who had no symptoms themselves produced babies with cerebral palsy, small heads, and mental retardation, proving that methyl mercury is more toxic to a growing fetus than to an adult.

Mercury can be methylated in the environment, so a certain amount of natural "background" mercury in nature is in the form of methyl mercury. This methylation is done by bacteria, even by bacteria occurring in the mouth.

The effects of mercury toxicity involve primarily the nervous system. The main ones are mental and neurological symptoms (which can mimic multiple sclerosis). Doctors should check patients with symptoms of multiple sclerosis for mercury toxicity, especially if the diagnosis is in doubt.

MERCURY AND DENTAL FILLINGS

Mercury has long been used mixed with silver for dental fillings. It has always been considered to be safe but there is increasing evidence to suggest that this is not so.

One researcher in the USA has shown that mercury-containing fillings can suppress the white blood cells involved in the immune response.

Electric currents are produced in the mouth ("galvanism") as a result of a mixture of metals (say a gold bridge and a mercury filling) and the degree to which this occurs can depend on the content of the saliva and the types of foods eaten. A salty food will produce a greater current than a non-salty food.

It has been shown that mercury vapor is released from fillings when one chews, and it has also been shown that bacteria in the mouth can actually methylate mercury, producing the more toxic methyl mercury.

The extent to which these phenomena cause health problems in individuals has yet to be fully elucidated, but it is quite possible that it has been underestimated.

In the USA, a number of people have reported the alleviation of chronic symptoms after removal of their mercury amalgam fillings. Under these circumstances, it is important that the dentist uses rubber dam—a sheet of rubber which encircles the teeth—in order to prevent the mercury from the amalgam fillings which are being drilled out from being swallowed. The mercury is sucked out by the assistant and this reduces further exposure of the patient to mercury. We have seen a number of people with elevated hair mercury levels, which caused us to suspect chronic mercury intoxication, whereas in fact it was just the after-effect of having had mercury fillings removed without the rubber-dam procedure. After dental treatment involving the use of mercury amalgam, urinary mercury excretion can be increased for up to a week or more.

Dentists and their staff are at risk from the mental and neurological complications of chronic mercury exposure, and this is probably an underestimated aspect of a dentist's work. Many dentists are still lax about the way in which they treat this extremely toxic element and we feel it is sensible for dentists to have mercury-screening on a regular basis, to ensure that they are not accumulating too much.

Some people with mercury-amalgam fillings have urticaria or eczema-like rashes on the skin, which resolve following the removal of their amalgam fillings and their replacement with other, non-mercury-based filling materials. This should be considered in anyone who has had mercury in their mouth for more than five years. Nickel in dental materials can also cause problems for people with such material in their mouths.

MERCURY EXPOSURE AND NUTRITION

It has long been known that mercury toxicity can be modified by dietary vitamin C.

Mercury exposure seems to reduce vitamin C levels in tissues, and a major protective effect of very high levels of vitamin C (equivalent to 35 g per day for a 70 kg man!) has been demonstrated in guinea pigs. This does not, however, necessarily mean that you should take large amounts of vitamin C if you are exposed to mercury. In fact, the reverse may be true. Animal studies have shown that a high dietary vitamin C intake increases the tissue levels of orally administered mercury, but not of injected mercury. It is possible that vitamin C helps in the absorption of mercury via the digestive tract.

Vitamin E has been shown to have a protective role in minimizing the neuro-toxic effects of methyl and ethyl mercury in animals. Several researchers have noted that certain people who had raised levels of mercury compounds in either their blood or hair, did not display any signs of mercury toxicity, although adverse effects would normally have been expected, and that this might relate to their vitamin E intake.

Supplementation with selenium seems to increase the apparent protective effect of vitamin E.

Cadmium

Doctors have long known that cadmium can be poisonous in excess.

At the turn of the century, and up to the Second World War, cadmium had been rejected as a proposed coating for food cans on the grounds of its toxicity.

In spite of its toxicity, after the Second World War, cadmium was used to coat ice-trays in electric refrigerators. It is extremely effective as an anti-corrosive agent and is replacing zinc as the plating on metal.

Cadmium is found in sources of zinc, even in its purest form. The zinc used for galvanizing iron (roofs, pails, water-storage tanks, etc.) is generally the cheapest grade of zinc, and contains up to two percent cadmium.

Whenever a slightly acid liquid comes into contact with galvanized metal, it dissolves some zinc and cadmium. Rain water is slightly acid from the dissolved carbon dioxide and pollutants in the air. Falling on a tin roof, collected in a gutter, stored in a galvanized-iron cistern, rain water will contain zinc and cadmium. Soft water also dissolves zinc and cadmium. Ideally, you should flush the water pipes out first thing in the morning, before drawing water for breakfast drinks.

In Westerners, the body contains approximately 30 mg of cadmium, and as little as 10 mg or less in certain African populations. The Japanese sometimes have as much as 50 to 60 mg.

Cadmium, once in the body, probably stays for the whole of a person's life in the kidneys, liver and blood vessels. As little as 2 mcg a day, absorbed and retained, results in a body burden of 30 mg over forty years.

Cadmium exerts its toxic effects primarily by displacing zinc from important enzyme systems so rendering them inactive.

The human kidney contains eight to ten times as much cadmium as do the kidneys of any other mammal, except those pets who are exposed in the same way as we are.

When we swallow cadmium, only a small amount is absorbed from the digestive system—perhaps ten percent—most of which is put out in the urine.

When we breathe cadmium, we retain about half of it, absorbing it from the lungs. Cigarettes are a very concentrated source of cadmium, containing 16–24 mcg per cigarette. Thus, a smoker can contaminate a whole roomful of people, and the blood and sweat levels of cadmium in smokers can be two or three times higher than those in non-smokers.

Other sources of cadmium include rubber tires, plastics, pigments, plated-ware, alloys, insecticides, and solders. Some foods have a lot of cadmium, especially oysters, foods contaminated during processing, some instant coffees and teas, some canned foods, kidneys of pigs given cadmium as a worm-killer, gelatin, fish dried on chicken-wire, and some cola drinks.

Some red and yellow pigments contain cadmium, and in fact one of us has seen a child poisoned by cadmium, as the family lived in a house which was a converted pottery that had an extremely high cadmium level in the soil in which they grew the family vegetables.

Cadmium is everywhere in our society, so it is difficult to avoid it. But what are its effects on human health?

TOXICITY

The earliest sign of subtle cadmium toxicity is a rise in blood pressure. When we look at human kidneys, we find that people who die from high blood pressure have either more cadmium or less zinc in their kidneys than people who die of other causes. Cadmium displaces the zinc, and poisons some of the zinc-dependent systems that control blood pressure.

There is good reason to believe that smokers should have their cadmium levels monitored on a yearly or two-yearly basis if they persist with their toxic habit.

METHODS OF TREATING CADMIUM OVERLOAD

If, on the basis of a hair mineral analysis and other tests, there is evidence of excessive cadmium accumulation, it is important to remove the source of cadmium.

It has been shown that vitamin C, iron, and zinc all protect against cadmium toxicity. Iron adequacy seems to reduce the absorption of cadmium from the digestive tract, and also possibly reduces the toxic effects of cadmium on the kidneys.

Cigarette smokers are known to have reduced levels of vitamin C, while at the same time having an excessive exposure to cadmium. So it seems only sensible for cadmium-toxic individuals to take regular supplements of vitamin C, especially if they are smokers, and to ensure that they are not iron deficient. Vitamin B6 may also increase cadmium toxicity.

How to Minimize the Effects of Toxic Metals

- Avoid exposure to them at home and at work. Especially avoid tobacco smoke, exhaust fumes and cooking in unsuitable pots.
- Eat plenty of fiber and nutrient-rich vegetables and fruits.
- Do not buy fruit and vegetables from displays on stalls or outside greengrocers' shops where they may have been exposed to leaded exhaust fumes.
- Correct any nutritional deficiencies you have by improving your diet. Some people may also need to take a multivitamin and multi-mineral supplement.
- **For those with proven toxic metal overload medical treatment will be essential.**

PROTEINS AND AMINO ACIDS

Proteins are one of the essential food ingredients and there is a minimum quantity that we have to eat if we are to remain healthy. This minimum daily intake depends on body size, rate of growth and the presence or absence of disease.

Unlike fats and carbohydrates, you cannot reduce your protein intake without producing adverse short- and long-term effects on your health.

Proteins are composed of long chains of building blocks called amino acids. The sequence of amino acids is characteristic to a particular protein and determines its character and function. There are some twenty or more amino acids, some of which are essential and some non-essential. We normally think of dietary proteins being broken down into their constituent amino acids by digestive enzymes. There is now considerable evidence to show that chains of amino acids that have been incompletely digested can be absorbed into the bloodstream and cause a whole range of symptoms from low or high blood sugar or even have drug-like actions on the brain. This is one mechanism of food intolerance.

Essential and Non-essential Amino Acids

The essential amino acids are those that cannot be formed in the body but yet are required for normal health. They therefore have to be obtained from the diet. Non-essential amino acids can be synthesized in the body but may also be obtained from the diet.

The essential amino acids are leucine, isoleucine, lysine, methionine (and its related compound cystine), phenylalanine, threonine, tryptophan and valine. In infants, histidine is also essential.

The non-essential amino acids are alanine, aspartic acid, glutamic acid, glycine, serine and tyrosine.

Protein is often divided into first and second classes on the following basis. First-class protein contains significant quantities of all the essential amino acids, so if one consumes enough one will obtain all the essential amino acids. Examples of first-class proteins include animal meat, fish, eggs and dairy products.

Second-class protein contains some of the essential amino acids but not all, and the missing essential amino acids will have to be made up either by eating some first-class protein or another second-class protein which contains the missing amino acids. Vegetable proteins are second-class proteins, so it is important that a vegetarian diet should be balanced to provide a healthy intake of all the essential amino acids. Combinations such as five parts of rice to one of beans will provide all the essential amino acids.

The body's requirements for protein increase during periods of growth, such as in infancy, during pregnancy and breast-feeding, during recovery from weight loss or in the healing of tissues or recovery from burns. On the whole, we in the West consume considerably more protein than we actually need. Biologically speaking, to make animal protein, a lot of vegetable protein has to be sacrificed. This makes it sensible to eat first-class protein (much of which comes from meat in our culture) only during periods of growth or repair. Normally we do not need to eat much animal-derived protein—we can remain perfectly well on vegetable protein. This also makes sense from a conservationist point of view. An acre of land can grow a considerable amount of vegetable protein, many times more than the amount of animal protein that can be produced by an animal grazing on that same area of land.

What Amino Acids Do

Amino acids are the building blocks for protein, which in turn are often the building blocks of the body. Proteins can be roughly divided into two types: those that are structural and those that have a specific, sometimes metabolic, function. Structural proteins are found in muscle, bone, connective tissue, and to a much lesser extent in the walls of cells. Functional proteins include hormones such as insulin, digestive enzymes and antibodies. Amino acids themselves may be needed not only in the formation of proteins, but in the formation of essential functional molecules such as neurotransmitters (chemicals that transmit electrical nerve impulses in the brain to influence mood and behavior). Hormones, such as thyroid hormone, require the presence of one or more essential amino acids for their formation.

Protein and Amino Acid Metabolism

Dietary protein must, like all the foods we eat, first be digested.

Once the constituent amino acids are formed, they are then absorbed by the small intestine and transported to the liver where they are used to re-form new proteins. This appears, at first, to be a considerable waste of biological effort, in that this long chain of amino acids is broken down, and then a new protein, with a different sequence, formed. Unfortunately, it is necessary because we cannot use the protein molecules of another species of plant or animal. If we were to, we would take on the biochemical and physical characteristics of the foods that we ate. Occasionally, small fragments of amino acids, three or four in number, are absorbed intact, and function as mini-hormones interfering with normal hormonal metabolism. This is occasionally a problem clinically.

Once amino acids arrive at the liver, some are used intact, and others are chemically rearranged. The enzymes that convert them are known as amino acid transferases. They all require vitamin B6. Thus, vitamin B6 requirements are very dependent upon protein intake and many processed foods have a relatively low level of vitamin B6 compared with their protein content.

Excessive amounts of protein in the diet are metabolized but, unlike fats, cannot be stored. Protein breakdown products are mainly carbohydrate-like molecules which are further metabolized to water, carbon dioxide, energy, and urea, which carries the residual nitrogen components of a protein. The urea is formed in the liver and excreted by the kidney into the urine.

Nutritional Losses of Amino Acids

Little attention has been given to the effects of cooking and processing upon the amino acids in foods. We take for granted that a dish containing meat will contain the basic constituents of that meat. However, the processes of heating and preserving can produce chemical changes. The amino acid lysine, for example, can be reduced in amount by heating a protein with sugar. This could, in theory, produce a relative lysine deficiency. This interaction between simple sugars and amino acids can occur in the oven at home as well as in the laboratory. Another example is the preservative sulphur dioxide, which can have adverse effects on the amino acid methionine.

Not all cooking is bad. Many plant proteins, particularly those in beans and peas, contain substances that prevent pancreatic digestive enzymes from breaking down protein. High concentrations of such a compound are particularly found in soybeans, and are destroyed by cooking. Failure to cook some beans adequately can have unpleasant consequences (such as diarrhea), because agents that inhibit digestion and other normal biochemical processes are still present in significant concentrations in either the uncooked or partially cooked food.

Protein Requirements

Protein requirements vary throughout life. They also vary from country to country, which could in part be due to differences in body size. The World Health Organization recommendations of 1974 suggest a protein intake of up to 37 g per day for a moderately active adult man, and 29 g for a woman. This rises to 39 g per day during the latter half of pregnancy and 46 g per day during breast feeding. In the USA, recommendations are some ten to fifteen percent higher. Protein requirements increase in the elderly and in vegetarians.

In practical terms, the recommended daily allowance of protein could be provided by as little as half a pint of milk, one egg, two ounces of meat, and two or three ounces of wholegrain cereals a day. Some people, with a healthy appetite, satisfy their protein requirements at breakfast alone. Most of us could halve our protein intake and still easily satisfy our needs.

Conditions in which Protein Restriction May Be Necessary

There are a few conditions in which protein restriction may be advisable. Obviously, individuals with rare disorders of amino acid metabolism need specialized diets, often for life. People with liver disease may, particularly if there is an element of liver failure, have to restrict their protein intake. In those with kidney failure, the kidney is unable to excrete all the nitrogen-containing urea produced by the liver, and the blood urea level rises. This, and other waste compounds, accumulate, resulting in ill-health.

Some types of kidney stones have been linked to a high-animal-protein diet, and a reduction in animal protein with the substitution of vegetable protein is sometimes advisable. If someone eats a lot of animal protein, the kidneys produce a relatively acidic urine, and too much calcium, which may lead, in some cases, to osteoporosis—a thinning of the bones. Again, a limitation of animal protein is recommended.

Therapeutic Uses of Amino Acids

We tend to think of vitamins, minerals and, more recently, essential fatty acid supplements as being the major nutritional supplements today. But a new concept in nutritional therapeutics has arrived with the use of amino acids as therapeutic agents. In certain diseases there may be increased demands for certain types of proteins, and if these proteins are high in one particular amino acid, then the demand for that amino acid may well be increased and perhaps not satisfied by the diet. In other diseases there is a disruption or disturbance in the metabolism of a particular amino acid. Lastly, it is possible that individual requirements for any given amino acid vary considerably. So it might be possible to influence the outcome of certain diseases by using specific amino acids. Indeed, certain drugs, such as anti-inflammatory agents used in the treatment of arthritis, may actually work by affecting amino acid metabolism (in this case, tryptophan). Doubtless, over the coming years there will be a considerable increase in interest in, and research into, the use of amino acids for specific clinical problems.

Here are just a few examples of some therapeutic uses of amino acids.

ARGININE

Shown to improve sperm count and sperm motility in some men with poor sperm counts and infertility.

CYSTEINE AND CYSTINE

Used as mucolytic agents to help bring up phlegm and sticky mucus in people with conditions such as chronic bronchitis, cystic fibrosis, and bronchiectasis.

ISOLEUCINE, LEUCINE AND VALINE

Low levels of these three amino acids are found in those seriously ill with liver disease, and their intravenous administration may be of some value for those in coma as a result of liver abnormalities.

PHENYLALANINE

Used in the treatment of pain both as the form D-phenylalanine and the mixture D-L-phenylalanine (DLPA). Effective pain relief has also been obtained with D-leucine. These amino acids may well work in the same way as opium and heroin but without the same risks of addiction. DLPA has also been used in depression.

METHIONINE

Used in the treatment of paracetamol overdose, it helps to protect the liver against the toxic effects of this painkiller. It has also been used to increase the urinary excretion of toxic overloads of lead and calcium.

HISTIDINE

Of value in rheumatoid arthritis. Low levels of histidine are found in the blood of those with rheumatoid arthritis.

LYSINE

Used particularly for recurrent cold sores and herpes infections.

TAURINE

Taurine has been shown to be useful in conjunction with zinc and B12 in the treatment of senile dementia (Alzheimer's type).

TRYPTOPHAN

This amino acid is one of the most studied in this group. First, there appears to be an association between tryptophan and arthritis. Many non-steroidal anti-inflammatory drugs are effective in relieving the pain of arthritis, though they do not slow down or prevent the disease process. There is a correlation between the degree of pain relief and the level of tryptophan in the blood. High levels of tryptophan are also found in those with jaundice and women who are pregnant, and arthritis often gets better in both conditions.

Tryptophan has also been used in the treatment of depression, particularly if insomnia is a feature. Some studies have shown that tryptophan is as effective as conventional antidepressants, but others have failed to confirm this. One side-effect of tryptophan is sleepiness, which is, of course, useful in those suffering from insomnia. However, it is worth bearing in mind that anyone taking tryptophan may well be drowsy the following morning.

It appears that certain things interfere with normal tryptophan metabolism, particularly estrogen-containing oral contraceptives. This may be because of their effect on vitamin B6 which is essential for the conversion of tryptophan to serotonin. Some women become depressed when on the Pill and this may be a result of its adverse effects on vitamin B6, which in turn harms tryptophan metabolism.

Recent reports, which at the time of writing needed to be confirmed, indicate a negative effect of high-dose tryptophan supplementation involving muscle pains and an increase in the number of a type of white blood cell called eosinophils. It seems possible that this observation, reported in the United States but nowhere else as yet, may be due to contamination and not to the tryptophan itself, it being an essential dietary constituent. Anyone wishing to take tryptophan should discuss the situation with his or her own doctor.

TYROSINE

Tyrosine, like tryptophan and D-L-phenylalanine, has been found to be useful in depression. This amino acid is essential for the synthesis of substances called catecholamines, which include dopamine, and noradrenaline. Some depressed people have low levels of these compounds as a pathological feature of their depressive state. Giving tyrosine is thought to enhance their production and may alleviate the depression.

Diets and Amino Acids

It seems likely that more and more uses for individual amino acids will become apparent as research progresses. A much more complex approach is the question as to whether various diets that have a preponderance of one or other of various amino acids could be of value in the treatment or prevention of certain diseases. For example, it is well known that vegetarian diets reduce some of the risk factors associated with atherosclerosis. This could come about for a number of reasons, including their high content of dietary fiber, their lower refined carbohydrate and animal fat content, their higher mineral content and so on. But the difference in amino acid content of vegetarian proteins as compared with animal proteins might also be a significant factor. One study looked at this and found that in a group of seventy-three patients fed a lacto-vegetarian diet, who had only one serving of milk per day, there were significant changes in the blood amino acid profiles.

ESSENTIAL FATTY ACIDS

One of the essential groups of foods that we need to eat to remain healthy is fat in various forms. Fats give the body its characteristic contours, act as heat insulation and also as a store of readily available energy if food supplies fail. But their most important function is that they produce highly active biological substances that are vital for the normal working of the body. They also form the major structural part of the cell wall in every single cell in the body.

Dietary fats include not only obvious "visible" fats on foods, but also many invisible ones in milk, nuts, lean meat and so on. All fats are made up of substances called triglycerides and each triglyceride is a combination of three fatty acids with a unit of glycerol. The differences between fats occur as a result of the different fatty acids in each.

There are literally dozens of fatty acids in nature, but they break down into two groups which are known as saturated and polyunsaturated. Saturated fatty acids are mainly found in hard fats such as lard, meat and cocoa butter, while the polyunsaturated fatty acids are liquid or soft at room temperature and include the vegetable oils.

Linoleic and linolenic acids are called "essential fatty acids" because they are vital for health, yet can't be made by the body. They therefore have to be eaten in food.

Essential Fatty Acids (EFAs) and Polyunsaturated Fatty Acids (PUFAs)

PUFAs are so-called because of their chemical structure. Not all PUFAs are essential, though the essential fatty acids themselves are all PUFAs. This is important to bear in mind because some processed vegetable oils contain PUFAs which are not only *not* essential, but actually tend to *block* the metabolic pathways of the essential fatty acids. As such, they could really be termed "toxins."

Signs of EFA Deficiency

The following conditions have been found in people who are short of essential fatty acids:

- hair falls out, dandruff
- eczema-like skin lesions
- dry skin
- wounds fail to heal normally
- all body membranes become permeable to water (sweating for no apparent reason)
- excessive thirst (often with concentrated urine due to skin water-loss)
- reproductive failure (especially in males)
- kidneys enlarge, blood in the urine, kidney failure
- liver undergoes fatty degeneration
- salivary, tear and pancreas glands wither
- depigmentation of skin
- impaired cholesterol transport
- capillaries become more fragile
- impaired growth
- loss of muscle tone
- mental disturbances
- poor vision
- heart abnormalities
- diarrhea

- bronchial disorders
- phrynoderma (gooseflesh-like pimples on upper arms, thighs, buttocks)

Omega-6 and Omega-3 EFAs

These two groups of dietary constituents are named on the basis of the number of carbon atoms in a particular part of their chemical structure. An important EFA in the omega-6 series is arachidonic acid, which is not truly essential as it can be synthesized from linoleic acid. Nevertheless, it constitutes a significant proportion of the fatty acid intake in our diet. The most common dietary source of the omega-6 series is linoleic acid, which is found in a wide range of foods, especially vegetables and grains. The other major group of EFAs belongs to the omega-3 series, derived from alpha-linolenic acid, which is present to some degree in wheat, beans and spinach. A further dietary component of the omega-3 series is eicosapentanoic acid (EPA) and docosahexanoic acid (DHAO) which are primarily found in seafoods.

Prostaglandins

Prostaglandins are so called because they were first isolated from the prostate gland of bulls and the name has remained despite the fact that subsequent research has shown that they are produced, at times, in all cells of the body.

The prostaglandins have turned out to be an extremely active group of substances with a wide range of influences on cellular biochemistry.

More than fifty prostaglandins have been identified so far, with a range of differing activities. They are made by the body from essential fatty acids.

Cis-linoleic (LA) is obtained from the diet and is converted into gamma-linolenic acid (GLA). The next step is its conversion into dihomogamma-linolenic acid (DGLA). DGLA is not usually present in the diet, and yet is present in human milk in substantial quantities. It is also present in the evening primrose plant, borage and blackcurrants. The seeds of the evening primrose oil plant contain ten percent GLA in relation to their total fatty acid content. We shall see the significance of this later.

DGLA can then go one of three ways:

1. It can move into fatty membranes all over the body and be stored there.

2. It can be acted upon by the enzyme cyclo-oxygenase to form prostaglandin E_1 (PGE_1). PGE_1 is an extremely active substance with a whole range of properties. Among others, it:

    - prevents platelets sticking together
    - is a vasodilator (i.e. improves circulation by enlarging the blood vessels)
    - inhibits inflammatory reactions
    - lowers arterial blood pressure
    - inhibits excessive cholesterol production
    - stimulates underactive brown fat—the fat that helps "burn off" rather than store excess calories
    - enhances the effects of insulin
    - activates T-lymphocytes in the immune system
    - inhibits abnormal cell proliferation
    - appears to have neurotransmitter effects

    PGE_1 is low in allergic individuals, diabetics, depressives, alcoholics, people with atherosclerosis (hardening of the arteries).

3. It can be converted into arachidonic acid, which in turn can produce either a group of substances called leukotrienes, which tend to promote inflammation, or can go into the body's fat stores, or be acted upon by an enzyme to produce the substances called thromboxanes, a second series of prostaglandins and prostacyclins.

The 2-series thromboxanes, the most significant of which is termed TXA_2, make smooth muscle contract and promote platelet stickiness, so increasing the likelihood of clots forming in blood vessels. This might seem strange, but it is important to remember that when we cut ourselves we have to have a system that makes the blood clot or we would lose it all. Natural body chemicals therefore act on the blood to clot it in these circumstances and others have the reverse effect, so that the blood does not clot in our blood vessels. The balance between these two mechanisms is critical.

The 2-series prostaglandins produce a reddening of the skin, and tissue swelling, and are important in the pain-producing properties of bradykinin and histamine. Prostacyclin produces a widening of blood vessels and inhibits platelet stickiness.

Because of the natural controls on this complex system, the balance between PGE_1-series and 2-series is easily influenced.

There is a constant interplay of the anti-inflammatory PGE_1 and the pro-inflammatory PGE_2. It is now evident that a number of conditions can result from the excessive production of 2-series prostaglandins and their associated byproducts. The ways in which the relative production of the 1-series and 2-series prostaglandins can be influenced are critically influenced by the nature of the food we eat.

The omega-3 series of fatty acids have come into the limelight over recent years because it now appears that they are essential for optimum health in a significant proportion of people. They form the series-3 prostaglandins (PGH_3), prostacyclins (PGI_3), and thromboxanes (TXB_3). The series-3 prostacyclin (PGI_3) appears to be more strongly anti-clot-forming than does PGI_2. This is one of the reasons why, on an extremely high-fish diet, people (e.g. Eskimos) bleed easily and have poor clot formation, but a very infrequent incidence of heart disease.

Nutrition and the Prostaglandins

As we have just seen, essential fatty acids are metabolized into potent, biologically active materials. We know that in the West the major causes of death are the result of chronic degenerative diseases, the two major ones being cardiovascular disease and cancer. Aside from these, a great deal of human suffering centers around psychiatric problems, arthritic-type problems, diabetes, auto-immune problems, skin problems, allergy, obesity, childhood learning or behavior problems, premenstrual problems in women, gastrointestinal problems and recurring infections—all of which involve prostaglandin metabolism. These groups of diseases form the bulk of the work of any general practitioner and most of what is dealt with by a whole range of medical specialists. There is now considerable and growing evidence which implicates the faulty metabolism of essential fatty acids in the cause of many chronic health problems.

ACTIONS OF PROSTAGLANDIN E_1 (PGE_1)

The direct actions of PGE_1 are listed on page 110.

As arachidonic acid in the diet comes mainly from meat, there is probably more arachidonic acid available to meat eaters than to vegetarians. So, if a diet is high in arachidonic acid and low in cis-linoleic acid, the body will naturally produce increased amounts of series-2 prostaglandins and reduced amounts of PGE_1. In view of the fact that many of the series-2 prostaglandins favor inflammation and blood clot formation, people who rely heavily on animal protein could run into cardiovascular problems that are related to blood clots (such as strokes and heart attacks).

INHIBITORS OF PRODUCTION OF PGE_1

The enzyme delta-6-desaturase, which converts dietary cis-linoleic acid into gamma-linoleic acid, is dependent on zinc and magnesium being present. Thus, dietary insufficiency of these two essential minerals, which is very common, results in a reduction of PGE_1 synthesis and its consequences. There are other factors which reduce the activity of this important enzyme: excessive dietary animal fats, cholesterol, alcohol, diabetes, ageing, and viral infections. Vitamin B (pyridoxine) deficiency, which is also common, reduces the conversion of GLA to DGLA and thus reduces PGE_1 production. Zinc, niacin (vitamin B3) and vitamin C are necessary for the production of PGE_1 from DGLA. Thus, dietary insufficiencies of any or all of the above nutrients can reduce PGE_1 synthesis and promote adverse health effects.

LEUKOTRIENE SYNTHESIS

Leukotrienes are extremely potent biological substances, intimately involved in the inflammatory response. When excessive leukotriene synthesis occurs, inappropriate inflammation follows. When there is a lot of arachidonic acid present, there is an increased tendency for leukotriene to be synthesized. The enzyme that promotes this reaction is inhibited by vitamin E. It is possible to measure the existence of leukotrienes produced in inflammatory skin responses. It has, for example, been shown that people with psoriasis have increased levels of leukotrienes in the affected skin. It has been observed that benoxaprofen (an anti-prostaglandin drug) improves psoriasis. Unfortunately, the side effects of this particular anti-prostaglandin drug were so severe that it had to be removed from the market, but other safe ones are available.

Aspirin is the oldest medication known to prevent prostaglandin production and it is probably via this action that it has so many valuable effects in the body. Today, many new anti-prostaglandin drugs have been developed. One example, ibuprofen, is used for arthritis and menstrual pains. It was found that the menstrual fluid of women with severe period pains contained lots of prostaglandins. Giving an anti-prostaglandin drug, such as ibuprofen, cures the pains in under an hour by reducing the level of prostaglandins present in the uterus. It could, of course, be that certain women are susceptible to producing these excessively high levels of prostaglandins because of a faulty diet that is too rich in animal proteins and saturated fatty acids, and deficient in certain vitamins and minerals (see below).

Conditions in which Essential Fatty Acid Supplements May Be Helpful

- eczema
- hyperactivity in children
- dry skin and dandruff
- brittle nails
- frequent infections
- easy bruising
- high blood fats
- schizophrenia
- inflammatory conditions, e.g. rheumatoid and other forms of arthritis
- some kidney diseases
- certain problems with blood clotting
- angina
- multiple sclerosis
- premenstrual syndrome
- benign breast disease
- diabetes
- obesity
- dry eyes (Sjogren's Syndrome)
- Raynaud's Phenomenon

Those people with serious conditions should be under medical supervision.

Nutrients that assist normalization of essential fatty acid metabolism (adult dosage only)

- zinc 10–20mg
- magnesium 100–200mg
- vitamin C 100–500mg
- vitamin E 200–400 IUs
- selenium 50–200mcg
- vitamin B3, B6 5–25mg
- biotin 200–400mcg

Ways of Taking Essential Fatty Acids

If you have a condition that might respond to supplements of essential fatty acids, it is important to ensure first that you are already eating a basic, healthy diet (see Appendix, page 398). Reduce your consumption of animal fats, using good quality polyunsaturated oils and margarine instead, and eat plenty of vegetables, salads, nuts and seeds. Avoid alcohol, smoking and refined carbohydrates.

The two main essential fatty acid supplements are evening primrose oil—which contains gamma-linoleic acid—and fish oil which contains docosahexanoic and eicosapentanoic acids. Some supplements contain a mixture of these. Evening primrose oil is marketed under a variety of names, of which Efamol (250 or 500 mg capsules), is the best known. The most widely available fish oil preparation is MaxEPA. The dosage is 1–4 g of Efamol per day and 4–8 capsules of MaxEPA per day. The smaller doses should be given to children. These supplements are probably best accompanied by a multivitamin and mineral supplement containing vitamin B complex, vitamin C, vitamin E, zinc and magnesium.

People with any form of epilepsy should not take evening primrose oil without medical supervision as there is some evidence that the condition can worsen. Also, those with blood disorders or bleeding problems should only take MaxEPA (purified fish oil) under medical supervision.

Those people, especially children, who cannot take oil capsules can rub the contents of them into the thin skin on the inner side of the forearm or thigh from where it is well absorbed into the bloodstream.

SUGARS AND CARBOHYDRATES

Carbohydrate is the main source of calories in almost all diets, worldwide. The term carbohydrate includes a variety of dietary compounds varying from simple sugars at one end to complex structures composed of many interlinked sugar molecules, such as are found in starch, at the other.

Simple carbohydrates are referred to as sugars. A single sugar is known as monosaccharide. Often two sugars are joined together to form a disaccharide and when many are joined together, they are known as a polysaccharide. A polysaccharide, such as starch, is composed of several chains of single sugars interlinked one with another. In the gastrointestinal tract digestive enzymes break down these polysaccharides into their constituent monosaccharides, which are then absorbed.

What They Do

The most important carbohydrate is a monosaccharide called glucose. The body's metabolism and energy systems have a high demand for glucose. For example, it is the only source of energy usable by the brain, and a low level of glucose in the blood results in a disturbance in brain function, even to the point of coma. When a doctor measures your blood sugar level he is actually measuring the level of blood glucose. Ordinary table sugar is called sucrose and is a disaccharide—a combination of glucose and fructose. Fructose is the major component of fruit, and is also known as fruit sugar. It, like glucose, is a monosaccharide. Disaccharides cannot be directly used by the body, but fructose, like glucose, can.

In the diet, starch, a polysaccharide, comprises about fifty percent of carbohydrate intake. Sucrose (glucose and fructose combined) comprises about thirty percent of carbohydrate intake; lactose (milk sugar) comprises about ten percent, and other less important sugars form the remaining ten percent. Historically, our ancestors consumed considerably more complex carbohydrates and it is only since the middle of the nineteenth century that our intake of refined carbohydrates, particularly sucrose, has been significant.

The metabolism of carbohydrates is geared to the digestion of complex carbohydrates in the gastrointestinal tract. Digestive enzymes in saliva and pancreatic secretions break down complex polysaccharides into their component mono- and disaccharides. The disaccharides are further digested by enzymes present in the lining of the small bowel. In this way, monosaccharides are formed which are easily absorbed into the bloodstream, from which they pass to the liver.

Certain hormones are involved in the control of carbohydrate metabolism—in particular, insulin, adrenalin and glucagon. These all work together to maintain a steady blood glucose level. The major function of glucose in the body is to produce energy, though some is involved in the metabolism of cholesterol, amino acids and fat. When there is an excess of glucose in the diet the extra is converted into glycogen, a polysaccharide which is stored in the liver. If someone starves, this store lasts for twenty-four to forty-eight hours, and after this further glucose must be produced from the body's fat.

If glucose is to be used, it has to cross the cell membranes into the cell substance itself. To do this, insulin and potassium are required. Diabetics who have no insulin, or in whom the body's cells are unresponsive to the actions of insulin, have a high blood glucose level as a result. When excess insulin is injected, the blood glucose level falls dramatically, producing a temporary clouding of consciousness or even a complete loss of consciousness. This is correctible by giving glucose rapidly either by mouth or intravenously.

So, insulin helps lower blood glucose levels, while the other two hormones, adrenalin and glucagon, help raise them.

Popular understanding and food advertising clearly stress the value of glucose and sucrose (table sugar) in helping to maintain energy. However, neither glucose nor sucrose is an essential constituent of the diet. Carbohydrates are, however, essential nutrients and occur in the form of fruits, vegetables, pulses and grains. The intestine is able to digest these down to their component monosaccharides. In the West, man's digestive system has been bypassed, to a large degree, by the food industry, which provides refined carbohydrates—in effect, predigested complex carbohydrates.

Amost everyone is able to digest carbohydrates satisfactorily, but, occasionally, the enzymes necessary for the digestion of disaccharides are absent. When this occurs, eating specific sugars, such as lactose (milk sugar) can produce abdominal bloating, flatulence and diarrhea, sometimes in a dramatic fashion. Lactose (milk sugar) intolerance is by far the most common, and occurs particularly in Mediterranean, Middle-Eastern and Far-Eastern peoples who normally have low intakes of dairy products in their diet. Sometimes it can follow an acute episode of gastroenteritis. If this is the case the person should go on a milk-free diet for at least two weeks (see Appendix 3).

Complex Carbohydrates

Complex carbohydrates can be divided into two sorts: those that are digestible such as starch, and those that are not digestible. These indigestible, complex carbohydrates are referred to as the "fiber" in food. There are many different types of fiber, but they are all derived from the cell walls of plants and include such things as cellulose, hemicellulose, pectins, mucilages and lignin. Though they are not digested in the gastrointestinal tract, they are far from inert, as they bind water and increase the bulk of the stool.

A characteristic of the Western diet is its low content of dietary fiber, and many doctors feel that this is responsible for the high incidence of many modern diseases (see page 123). Sometimes, indigestible carbohydrates can have adverse effects. Some, for example, bind with important minerals such as calcium and zinc, preventing their absorption. Such a compound is phytic acid which is found in unleavened bread.

Certainly, though, the benefits of a high-fiber diet greatly outweigh the negative effects, if any, of having a diet rich in refined carbohydrates such as glucose and sucrose.

Sugar

Table sugar is more accurately known as sucrose. It is a refined carbohydrate and consists of two simple sugars, glucose and fructose (fruit sugar) that are naturally joined together. Sucrose occurs in a number of fruits including cane-sugar, beetroot, dates, figs and maple syrup. Most sucrose consumed in the West comes from cane-sugar.

Sucrose consumption was minimal until the mid-nineteenth century. Up until this time there was a considerable tax on sugar and production costs were relatively high. The removal of the tax and development of efficient production methods produced a massive rise in sucrose consumption. Men consume more than women, and the highest consumption is amongst teenagers. So, male adolescents are particularly prone to high sucrose consumption, often in the form of sweets, cakes, chocolates and soft drinks. Considerable amounts of hidden sugar are consumed as a part of many processed foods. Sucrose has beneficial qualities from a food manufacturer's point of view, in that it acts as a preservative, is a good binding agent and increases the palatability of many foods.

Sucrose is made from sugar-cane and sugar beet. The raw materials are washed with water, and the sucrose extracted by first crushing and chopping the raw material, then dissolving it in water, filtering and purifying, and finally crystallizing it. When processing cane-sugar, various less "pure," but relatively mineral-rich extracts, such as molasses, are formed as by-products. The final product, white or brown sugar, is almost devoid of the vitamins and minerals present in the original plant material.

Sucrose as a food has come in for considerable criticism recently. This is an area of some controversy in which sugar manufacturers have tried to preserve the "good name" of their product.

With the current move among doctors to recommend high-complex-carbohydrate diets, there is an inevitable reduction in the use of refined carbohydrates, and especially sugar. Sugar consumption has fallen by some twenty percent in the last twenty years, and as increasing scientific evidence demonstrates the association between sucrose consumption and various medical conditions, this figure is likely to fall yet further.

BENEFICIAL EFFECTS OF SUCROSE

Perhaps it is surprising that a book like this should include such a list. However, there are a number of clearcut clinical situations in which sucrose is of value. These include:

- *Hypoglycemia, low blood sugar.* This can occur in diabetics who have taken too much insulin. It should, however, be strictly avoided in the management of reactive hypoglycemia (see page 292).
- *Intravenous feeding.* People who are severely ill and are unable to take food by mouth can be maintained for a few days on a sugar, salt and water solution, given intravenously. Chronically ill patients can be maintained for months or years on carefully planned programs of intravenous feeding, which usually include glucose derived from sucrose, fatty acids, amino acids, vitamins and minerals.
- *Hiccups.* These often respond to a sugar and water solution taken by mouth.
- *Wound healing.* Reports suggest that the local application of honey or sugar helps in some cases of poorly healing wounds, and in some severe infections that occur after chest surgery.

ADVERSE EFFECTS OF SUGAR (SUCROSE)

The following conditions are caused by, or can be strongly associated with, significant sucrose consumption. Some on occasion, but not all, benefit from a reduction in sucrose consumption.

- obesity
- cardiovascular disease: hypertension, raised blood fats, increased platelet stickiness, atherosclerosis, vitamin B1 deficiency heart failure
- diabetes mellitus (adult type)
- gastrointestinal disease: indigestion, inflammatory bowel disease, diverticular disease, irritable bowel syndrome, diarrhea
- gallstones
- tooth decay

- kidney stones and kidney failure
- increased susceptibility to infection
- reactive hypoglycemia—low blood sugar
- depression and anxiety, hyperactivity in children, certain forms of criminal behavior
- seborrheic dermatitis, dandruff, eczema
- allergies

Obesity

Obesity is not caused by the consumption of any single food, but comes about as the result of an over-consumption of food in general. So an excess of any carbohydrate, proteins or fats can produce obesity. Having said that, sugar consumption is highest amongst male teenagers, who are frequently very slim; conversely, a plump, middle-aged woman may have a relatively low calorie intake yet is only able to lose weight slowly and it should not be assumed that because she is fat she eats too much. Almost any well-balanced, calorie-controlled diet will make minimal or no use of sucrose. This is not because it causes obesity, but because the consumption of sucrose does not provide any vitamins or minerals. Those countries that have a high intake of sucrose, as well as animal fats, have a higher incidence of obesity and other diseases such as cardiovascular disease, while those less developed countries which have a low intake of refined foods have a very much lower incidence. Sucrose cannot be recommended as forming a substantial part of any weight-reducing program.

Sugar is also very easy to consume in large amounts. Sugary foods are packed with calories which provide energy and nothing else (hence the term "empty calories"). As most of us in the West are not short of energy, these calories simply get made into fat and can produce obesity. It would be very difficult indeed to consume this same number of calories of complex carbohydrate because the sheer bulk of the food would be so great. This is obviously nature's way of helping us control our appetites.

Cardiovascular disease

Sucrose is not the cause of cardiovascular disease and, when compared to smoking, plays a relatively small part. However, it does have a significant effect in the following situations:

- *Obesity.* As sucrose consumption is associated with obesity, and obesity in turn is associated with increased cardiovascular risk, the reduction of sucrose intake in those with cardiovascular disease seems sensible.

- *Hypertension*. In some individuals, a high sucrose intake produces an increased blood pressure.
- *Elevation of blood fats*. Sucrose ingestion, like that of alcohol, markedly raises levels of certain blood fats, particularly the triglycerides. Its effect upon cholesterol is less clear, but it can elevate it in some people. Sucrose should be avoided by those with elevated triglycerides and cholesterol levels.
- *Platelet stickiness*. Certain conditions are characterized by an increased stickiness of blood platelets. These tiny cells are necessary for the clotting of blood but, if overactive, result in an increased liability to blood clotting which can cause a stroke or impaired circulation in the legs. Smokers are particularly at risk. Taking sucrose has been found to increase blood platelet stickiness both in healthy volunteers and in those with peripheral arterial disease.
- *Atherosclerosis and chromium deficiency.* Another effect of sucrose is that it increases losses in the urine of the essential trace mineral chromium. Low levels of chromium are associated with increased atherosclerosis (hardening of the arteries), coronary artery disease, elevated blood cholesterol levels and diabetes. Sucrose consumption has, to some extent, been linked to all of these, and part of its effect may be due to the production of a relative chromium deficiency. It is interesting that practically all the chromium found in sugar-cane is removed in the refining process.
- *Vitamin B1 deficiency.* Vitamin B1 is essential for the metabolism of glucose and a relative deficiency can occur if there is a high dietary intake of glucose or sucrose. This can lead to heart failure.

Diabetes mellitus **(see also page 286)**

Diabetes is not simply caused by eating too much sucrose. The incidence of diabetes in any country is more closely related to an excess calorie intake from both carbohydrates and fats. There will inevitably be a higher sucrose consumption in those countries where there is a higher incidence of diabetes, but there is no clear causal link. However, for diabetics maintained either by diet or insulin, sucrose is now not recommended in any significant quantity.

Current dietary advice to diabetics urges an increased intake of complex carbohydrates, high in fiber, from such sources as whole grains, lentils, beans, nuts and seeds, rather than the intake of glucose and sucrose. Glucose and sucrose can be helpful for diabetics who are experiencing a hypoglycemic episode which can occur in both those on insulin and those receiving oral antidiabetic drugs.

Gastrointestinal disease

Professor John Yudkin has been at the forefront of the anti-sugar lobby for nearly thirty years, and at a time when it was certainly not fashionable to do so. He described a group of patients with indigestion, over fifty percent of whom had a significant reduction in their symptoms after avoiding sucrose in their diet.

People with Crohn's disease have been found to have a higher sucrose intake than their healthy counterparts. Some researchers have suggested that there might also be a link between refined carbohydrate intake and colitis. As the nutritional state of people with colitis and Crohn's disease is often impaired or borderline, it seems sensible to avoid a food that provides a low intake of essential vitamins and minerals and may also be a possible causative factor.

Low-sugar, high-fiber diets have been recommended in the treatment of diverticular disease and, with the use of unprocessed bran, have been found to be highly effective.

Occasionally, people are intolerant of sucrose. This is because they lack the enzymes necessary to digest it. They have to avoid not only table sugar, but certain fruits in which sucrose and related sugars are found. The ingestion of sucrose in such individuals results in abdominal bloating and diarrhea within an hour or two. An abnormality of digestion like this is usually lifelong and sufferers are only too familiar with what causes their diarrhea. The condition occurs in as many as 1 in 1,000 of the population and is easily underdiagnosed.

Gallstones

Cholesterol-containing gallstones are linked to obesity, and a high sugar consumption is linked to being overweight. Researchers at Bristol Royal Infirmary have shown that a diet providing the average amount of sucrose consumed in the UK produces an increased concentration of cholesterol in bile and therefore an increased risk of gallstones. They concluded: "The risk of gallstones might be reduced by avoidance of refined carbohydrate foods."

Tooth decay

It is widely accepted that a high-sucrose diet is linked to an increased risk of dental decay. Those people and nations who have a low intake of sucrose have a much lower incidence of dental caries.

It appears that it is not just the amount of sugar eaten, but the frequency and type. The consumption of foods in which sugar is sticky or caramelized (and thus easily adheres to the teeth) is more likely to cause dental problems. The bacteria in the mouth require sugar to grow and multiply. In so doing, they release harmful acids that dissolve the dental enamel and lead to dental decay. The avoidance of refined carbohydrates is an important part of the control of dental decay.

Kidney disease

Some people appear to retain salt (and water along with it) when consuming a diet high in sucrose. In a weight-reduction program in which the intake of refined carbohydrates is cut dramatically, there is often a marked reduction in weight as a result of a loss of body fluid. The changes in metabolism that occur when avoiding sucrose and other refined carbohydrates cause an increased loss of salt and water in the urine. High sucrose consumption appears to have an adverse effect upon the metabolism of people who have kidney stones (see page 266).

Resistance to infection

Sucrose has a rapid and dramatic adverse effect upon the ability of white blood cells to fight infection. Researchers at the University of Alabama looked at what happened when healthy dental students were given twenty-four ounces of a sucrose-containing soft drink. There was a rapid rise in blood sugar within forty-five minutes, at which time the ability of certain types of white blood cells to ingest and destroy foreign germs was significantly impaired. It is interesting that diabetics, who have impaired glucose tolerance, are especially likely to get infections. People who have recurrent infections, or infections which are resistant to standard treatments, should certainly consider avoiding sucrose altogether.

Hypoglycemia (see page 292)

Behavior and mood changes

A deficiency of vitamin B1 can occur in people who eat a diet high in refined carbohydrates. Vitamin B1 deficiency can be a cause of, or aggravate, existing depression and anxiety. Vitamin B1 demands are increased by diets high in refined carbohydrates, and sugars such as sucrose contain none of the B vitamins that are necessary for their metabolism. The aim is to correct the deficiency and to avoid sucrose.

Opinion is divided as to the part played by diet in relation to childhood behavior. Some children experience adverse reactions to sucrose in food (see page 361).

Skin diseases

Many people who have poor skin, or are susceptible to blemishes and pimples, improve by cutting out sugar and refined carbohydrates (including ice cream, sweets and chocolate) from their diet and following a good, basic, healthy diet (see page 398).

Conclusion

As we have seen, sugar consumption is associated with poor health. While some people can tolerate quite large amounts without any apparent immediate ill-effects, the long-term liabilities of consuming sugar are such that we recommend everyone to reduce sugar consumption to a minimum.

DIETARY FIBER

Over the last twenty years there has been considerable interest in the importance of fiber in the diet, to the point that we call it "fiber fever." While the importance of dietary fiber is beyond doubt, there are some liabilities, as we shall see later. Before this there had been a general view that indigestible plant residues were of little or no nutritional value. However, their effect on intestinal movement and the absorption of nutrients, and the association of a low-fiber diet with certain Western diseases have been the subject of considerable interest over the last decade.

Fiber comes almost entirely from plants, and plant fibers differ with the type of plant as well as with its age. Fiber is, in fact, a family of substances, not just one. The members of the family include cellulose, hemicelluloses, lignins, pectins, gums and mucilages. All of these form the walls of plant cells, except for some of the mucilages, which are found in algae and seaweed.

Fiber's main property is that it binds water in various ways. This produces a considerable increase in bulk of the stools. So it is that the volume and physical properties of the stools of people who go on a high-fiber diet changes. Fiber also binds various minerals and other things such as bile salts, toxins and drugs.

Some types of fiber are digested but others remain undigested, even by the bacteria in the large bowel. This is particularly true of wheat fiber; some vegetable fibers may be partially digested by the large-bowel bacteria.

Dietary intakes of fiber in Western societies vary considerably. The average intake is around 20 g a day and should be about 30 g.

Despite the considerable research on the importance of fiber in the diet and the effects of adding different types of fiber to the diet, very few researchers have considered the effects of other nutrients present in high-fiber foods, and what benefits could be obtained from their non-fiber constituents by eating more high-fiber foods. We think this is of considerable practical importance. Though much of the epidemiological work has been done in Third World countries, the result has been a recommendation to use substantial quantities of a type of fiber, bran, which was not the subject of study in the epidemiological work and is not the type of dietary fiber consumed in many Third World or "primitive" communities. High intakes of fruit, vegetables, and different types of cereals are usually much more commonplace. Green, leafy vegetables, while being a reasonable source of fiber, and probably the type that our ancestors would have eaten historically, are also an excellent source of vitamin C, beta-carotene, magnesium and folate. A number of studies have stressed the importance of these factors in the prevention of cancer.

Benefits of Dietary Fiber

It does seem from the studies so far that an increase in dietary fiber may be of particular importance and benefit in certain conditions. The main ones are:

- *Obesity.* Ensuring a high intake of fiber may be beneficial for those on weight-reducing programs by preventing constipation and perhaps also by improving blood sugar control, which may be of help in appetite stimulation. Fiber also makes foods very filling and so discourages the over-consumption of other foods which are rich in calories and thus very fattening. However, increasing dietary fiber intake alone is not likely to increase weight reduction, even though it is fair to say that those who eat complex carbohydrates (as opposed to refined ones) all their lives, tend to be slimmer.

- *Gallstones*. There is evidence that the ingestion of wheat-bran may favorably alter bile salt composition so as to reduce the likelihood of gallstone formation.
- *Constipation*. It is now standard practice for most people with constipation to be put onto a high-fiber diet unless there is a serious medical reason not to. The importance of dietary fiber in speeding the passage of food through the intestine and bowel has been well studied and the softer stool of a high-fiber diet is usually a lot easier to pass.
- *Diverticulosis*. Epidemiological studies suggest that diverticular disease goes hand in hand with a low-fiber diet and there is now little doubt that most of those with diverticular disease gain some relief from their symptoms when on a high-fiber diet and that many are cured completely. The underlying bowel abnormality remains, of course, but it does not cause the problems it did.
- *Irritable bowel syndrome*. This has a variety of potential causes, the most important of which may well be food intolerance, particularly to wheat. However, a lack of fiber may play a part, particularly if constipation is a feature. Some sufferers are improved by increasing their fiber intake, but some are made worse, particularly if bran is used (see page 212).
- *Cancer of the large bowel*. High-fiber diets are associated with a lower incidence, worldwide, of cancer of the large bowel, and increasing the fiber intake in the diet might be of benefit in reducing the incidence of the disease in Western countries. Usually, an increase in dietary fiber goes hand in hand with a reduction in dietary fat, particularly animal fat. Certain types of fiber have the ability to absorb particular toxins, including potential cancer-forming ones (carcinogens) formed by bacterial fermentation in the large bowel. The increased intestinal movement of low-fiber diets allows greater fermentation by gastrointestinal bacteria, with increased opportunity of carcinogen formation at this much lower propulsion rate. The exact link between cancer of the bowel and dietary fibers is, however, still not clear.
- *Other cancers*. It is possible that the frequency of other cancers might be influenced by a lack of dietary fiber because of the potential risk of formation and absorption of potential carcinogenic agents from the bowel in people on low-fiber

diets. In one study from Holland, diets containing less than 37 g of fiber a day were associated with an increased risk (approximately threefold) of cancer in general.

- *Coronary heart disease*. Though there are links between a low fiber intake and coronary heart disease, it is too early to say whether increasing fiber alone will reduce the occurrence of this, the most common cause of death in Western countries. The effect of fiber on fat metabolism has been studied in some detail. It does not appear that bran fiber lowers cholesterol levels—exercise and other types of fiber may be more important in this respect.
- *Diabetes*. Over the last few years there have been substantial changes in the dietary recommendations for diabetics. Now, high-complex-carbohydrate, high-fiber diets are recommended. This advice goes along with the avoidance of glucose and sucrose sugars, a reduction in animal fat and salt intake, moderation in alcohol intake and advice to lose weight if the person is obese. Interest has centered on the use of specific types of fiber such as guar gum, a type of vegetable gum, the fiber content of which reduces the rate of carbohydrate absorption. A lot of research in this field has been done in Oxford and in Canada and the results from both centers are similar. It appears that a diet high in vegetable fiber reduces the high swings in blood sugar that can follow certain carbohydrate-rich meals, particularly if they are low in fiber or contain high quantities of simple sugars, and leads to a reduction in total cholesterol both in diabetics who are insulin-dependent and in those who are not.

Adverse Effects of Fiber

The Royal College of Physicians' report, *Medical Aspects of Dietary Fiber,* rightly draws attention to the potential nutritional drawbacks of certain types of dietary fiber. They include:

- *Intestinal obstruction, partial or complete*. A high-fiber diet should not be taken by anyone who has a colon cancer or bowel stricture.
- *Irritable bowel syndrome*—caused by wheat or other grain sensitivity.
- *Celiac disease*.
- *Osteomalacia or rickets caused by calcium malabsorption*. Asian immigrants, particularly in urban communities, are at risk from osteomalacia in adults and rickets in young children,

due to vitamin D deficiency. Both conditions are more likely to occur in winter and spring when there is low sunlight exposure (sunlight stimulates vitamin D synthesis in the skin). The inclusion of chapatis in the diet also means that there is a high intake of phytates. Phytates (especially phytanic acid) are part of the fiber content of wheat. They are known to inhibit calcium, iron, zinc and probably magnesium absorption because of the formation of insoluble phytate salts. They get broken down in the leavening process when bread is made and do not then affect mineral metabolism. However, because no leavening is used to make chapatis, they can cause problems. Rickets and osteomalacia can both be reversed by taking vitamin D, and by avoiding chapatis in the diet. Elderly white people, too, are at risk if they take too much bran.

- *Iron deficiency.* Groups at risk include children under the age of two, menstruating women, and those who eat little meat, particularly if they drink tea. Vegetarian diets are notoriously low in iron, and iron absorption from vegetable sources is further reduced by tea.

  Cereal fiber, because it contains phytate, may also reduce iron absorption. Again, unleavened bread, bran and bran-based foods should not be consumed by those at risk. The iron-binding effect of dietary fiber present in wheat and maize can be reduced by taking vitamin C and fruit juice.
- *Zinc deficiency.* Zinc absorption is blocked by phytates in unleavened bread.
- *Reduced absorption of other minerals*. It is quite probable that magnesium absorption is also reduced by phytate. However, depending on the type of fiber, degradation of the fiber by bacteria in the colon may release some fiber-bound minerals.

Fiber Fever

As has been discussed above, fiber has good and bad effects. The current vogue for adding bran to a junk-food diet is, we consider, a negative piece of health advice. A junk-food diet is deficient in a range of essential nutrients. Adding bran further compromises the absorption of those nutrients that are present. The best way to increase fiber intake is to concentrate on cutting down on refined carbohydrates, eating plenty of fresh fruit and vegetables, whole grains, beans and lentils, and following the basic healthy diet (see Appendix 1, page 398).

WHEAT, COWS' MILK AND EGGS

We have given these foods a separate section because they are those that modern Western society relies heavily upon for its nutrient intake. However, wheat, cows' milk and eggs came late during man's evolution, with the advent of farming. This change occurred approximately 30,000 years ago, which is very recent compared with man's evolution from the apes about four million years ago.

The arrival of farming meant that the proportion of meat in the diet fell drastically, while vegetable foods came to make up as much as ninety percent of the diet. It is interesting to note that with the coming of agriculture, man became an average six inches shorter than his ancestors who did not rely on farming for their nutritional supply. Whether or not this has any significance in terms of health and disease has not yet been decided. However, suffice it to say that we have changed our environment substantially in the last 30,000 years, and it is only reasonable to assume that there is a certain proportion of the population that will have failed to adapt adequately to wheat, cows' milk, eggs, and perhaps to other foods. Conversely, we can assume that there is a percentage of people who manage perfectly well on a high intake of these foods.

Wheat

The benefits and disadvantages of wheat fiber are discussed in more detail elsewhere (see section on Fiber), but we should emphasize here that dietary fiber is essential for optimum bowel function, which can have a wide range of beneficial metabolic effects, including a lowering of serum cholesterol. Nevertheless, there are also disadvantages as regards the absorption of essential nutrients, as well as problems with wheat intolerance.

Certain individuals develop an intolerance to wheat and its products. The most classical form of this is celiac disease, in which the toxic element, gluten, produces a partial destruction of the lining of the small bowel, resulting in diarrhea, bloating of the abdomen, and malabsorption of essential nutrients. Gluten is also present in rye, oats and barley.

Irritable bowel syndrome (abdominal bloating, flatulence, diarrhea and/or constipation) is often caused by an intolerance to wheat and wheat products. Having said this, we must emphasize that there are many other causes for the irritable bowel syndrome. In our practice we have also seen rheumatoid arthritis, tissue swelling, premenstrual syndrome, fatigue, thought disorders, severe mental disturbances, joint and muscle aches and pains and a host of other problems clear up when wheat is excluded from the diet. Some people are able to tolerate white bread but are unable to tolerate brown. This might be because of wheat intolerance (there is more wheat and fiber in brown bread) or because there is usually more yeast in brown bread than white, and such people could be yeast sensitive. Recently, it was found that nearly four out of 1000 blood donors had laboratory evidence of an allergy to gluten in wheat.

It is possible that as a result of aggressive farming policies which depend on insecticides, pesticides and herbicides, the soil becomes depleted of certain essential nutrients. So there is no guarantee that wholegrain wheat, grown on chemically supported farms, is necessarily adequate in essential nutrients.

Cows' Milk

Cows' milk is very often introduced at an early stage in our lives (as is wheat, but milk is usually first), and yet nature designed it for the nourishment of calves, not humans. The substitution of cows' milk for human breast milk is not a sensible idea, since the nutrient content is very different and does not meet all the requirements of a growing infant.

Introducing cows' milk to our children at such an early age produces an aggressive adaptive stress on the system, and a certain percentage of babies are unable to tolerate it. The degree to which the general population can cope with milk has not been clearly defined, but we believe that some sixty to eighty percent of the population could be experiencing detrimental effects from the over consumption of cows' milk and cows' milk products. There is almost no way of actually proving this at the moment, but on the basis of our clinical experience, and the scientific literature that has been published to date, it seems an entirely reasonable figure.

A significant percentage of the world's population has a deficiency in the intestinal tract of the enzyme lactase, which normally splits the sugar lactose which is present in significant quantities in cows' milk. In fact, about fifty percent of the world's population is unable biochemically to tolerate cows' milk. Lactose intolerance is considered in more detail elsewhere (see page 210).

There is a lot of evidence to support the contention that those countries that have a high consumption of cows' milk and cows' milk products also have a very high incidence of cardiovascular disease, and death through heart attack, stroke, and so on. In Ayurvedic medicine, cows' milk is recognized as producing catarrh and mucus. In our experience, this is true in a substantial proportion of those who suffer from these problems. Excluding milk can sometimes cure all such symptoms.

Other conditions which can be associated with milk ingestion are food intolerance and its associated hyperactivity, asthma, rhinitis, recurrent infections, joint aches and pains, kidney disease and a blood disease called idiopathic thrombocytopenic purpura.

Another fact that is now well recognized amongst informed pediatricians is that cows' milk can cause or precipitate eczema in children. Any child with eczema should be considered to be intolerant of cows' milk and eggs until proven otherwise. Some of these children can tolerate cheese, but this is the exception rather than the rule, and a certain percentage can tolerate canned evaporated milk. But some may even have to exclude beef.

Raw unpasteurized milk tends to be more likely to cause a reaction than heavily pasteurized or evaporated milk.

Crib death may be an atypical reaction to cows' milk. Studies on guinea pigs, which involved giving them an injection of cows' milk, found that they died of allergic shock. The researcher then went on to study the effect of introducing cows' milk into the bronchial tubes of guinea pigs, and these animals also suffered from allergic shock. The changes at post-mortem were identical to those found in sudden infant death syndrome (crib death). This may only be part of the story, but it is interesting to observe that the majority of children who suffer crib deaths are bottle-fed on cows' milk. It is well known that dietary substances get into breast milk, and therefore if milk is the culprit, it may be that a mother who drinks cows' milk passes on cows' milk proteins to her baby in her breast milk and sensitizes him or her in the same way.

Because of this, we invariably advise any of our pregnant patients who have a strong family or personal history of milk intolerance, to give up milk completely, both while they are pregnant and breast-feeding.

Anyone with an allergic family history should avoid milk during these times and should not give cows' milk to the baby during the first six months of life.

In fact, in our experience any long-standing illness in childhood, even if there is a formal medical diagnosis, should alert a physician or the child's mother to the possibility of cows' milk intolerance, so common is the problem in childhood.

As well as these problems with allergy, there are other detrimental effects of milk. There is a very low magnesium: phosphorus ratio in cows' milk, and it is quite possible that the large number of magnesium-deficient children we see have a relative magnesium deficiency produced by drinking too much milk.

Alternatives to cows' milk include soya-milk formula, goats'-milk formula, and sheep's-milk formula. However, it is important to bear in mind that some individuals who are cows' milk intolerant will also be unable to tolerate goats' milk. Sheep's milk is now more readily available and may be a useful alternative.

Eggs

Chickens' eggs also form a significant part of the Western diet, particularly in infancy and childhood, as they are very nutritious and are easy to prepare in a number of different ways.

Eggs have been implicated as possibly being a cause of high blood cholesterol and arteriosclerosis, but this is not necessarily true on the basis of the cholesterol content of eggs.

Current wisdom has it that the number of eggs you eat does not much affect blood cholesterol levels, so it is not worth restricting egg intake from this point of view.

Eggs are, however, a common offending food in a wide range of childhood disorders, including childhood eczema, hyperactivity, sleep disturbances, learning and behavioral disorders. Because of this you should bear in mind the possibility of egg intolerance in any problem during childhood. Some people may be sensitive to the yolk but not the white of the egg. Also, eggs cooked in a food—a cake, for example—may not produce an allergic reaction in an egg-sensitive person.

TEA AND COFFEE

Caffeine is one of a number of biochemically active compounds found in tea and coffee. Smaller but substantial quantities may also be found in chocolate, cola-based drinks and a number of medicinal preparations, particularly painkillers. Caffeine has a number of important actions, both on the cardiovascular and the central nervous systems.

Consumption of tea and coffee in the UK, Europe and USA

has been increasing considerably over the last few years. An average cup of strong tea contains 50 mg, and that of coffee 100 mg, of caffeine, but variations are considerable. Pharmacological effects can be experienced from 50 mg upwards, and doses exceeding 250 mg are likely to produce significant effects. The decaffeination of coffee removes practically all of the caffeine, but some biologically active agents remain. Because of the biological activities of caffeine and related compounds, excess tea and coffee consumption may have a number of adverse effects. Obviously, tea and coffee may also be useful as a minor stimulant, and this has been known for quite some time.

Adverse Effects of Tea and Coffee

- *Psychiatric symptoms:* anxiety and nervousness, depression, insomnia and aggravation of pre-existing psychiatric states.
- *Physical symptoms:* passing of excessive amounts of urine, diarrhea, flatulence and gastric stomach, dyspepsia, shakiness and tremor, migraine and withdrawal headache, abnormal heart rhythms, rapid heartbeat, high blood pressure, restless legs at night and high blood cholesterol (approximately eleven percent increase). Painful or lumpy breasts may improve on stopping consumption of tea, coffee and chocolate, as well as stopping smoking.

Consumption of tea or coffee at mealtimes can reduce the amount of iron absorbed from vegetables to one third. This is particularly important for women of childbearing age who are vegetarian or semi-vegetarian, and who consume anything other than minimal quantities of tea or coffee, as they may run the risk of becoming iron deficient.

Tea and coffee also inhibit zinc absorption.

An interesting syndrome of restless or jumpy legs was described as long ago as the seventeenth century. The sufferer complains of an uncomfortable kicking sensation, felt mainly in the lower legs. It only appears at rest, and usually is troublesome at night, and may complicate caffeine-induced insomnia. It often responds to the withdrawal of tea and coffee.

Caffeine is also a potent stimulator of gastric acid secretion, but decaffeinated coffee is even more active in this respect.

Some Actual or Potential Beneficial Effects of Tea and Coffee

- *Asthma*. The stimulant effects of caffeine can have a beneficial effect in asthma. Caffeine is chemically similar to theophylline, a potent medicine used in treating asthma.
- *Pain relief*. Caffeine appears to be effective in improving the efficacy of minor painkillers.
- *Nutritional value*. Tea in particular can be a good source of certain minerals, especially manganese and fluoride.

ALCOHOL, SMOKING AND TRANQUILIZERS

Over the last twenty to forty years, there has been a marked increase in the use of medicinal and non-medicinal drugs. Many socially acceptable drugs, such as alcohol, tea and coffee, are used as minor stimulants or antidepressants. However, the excessive use of alcohol, and the use of legal or illegal drugs, can have devastating effects upon health. Heavy cigarette consumption, too, has an adverse effect on nutrition.

Many people who consume large quantities of alcohol or cigarettes, or who use legal drugs, would like to be able to do without them if they could. A combination of nutritional supplements and appropriate dietary advice may be helpful to them.

Alcohol

Alcohol is probably the most acceptable "social poison" after tea and coffee. The pure alcohol content of various beverages varies. On average, beer is four percent, spirits forty percent, and wine sixteen percent pure alcohol. On average, each man, woman and child consumes ten liters of pure alcohol per annum, equivalent to about two bottles of wine per week. In 1951 it was nearly half this.

Considerable concern has arisen because of this rapid increase in consumption. The adverse effects of alcohol are many.

First of all, it should be remembered that alcohol is a food. It provides calories in the form of carbohydrate. This, in many people, is converted straight to fat. One pint of beer provides

200–250 calories. Hence, many heavy beer-drinkers are often overweight. A certain amount of minerals and B vitamins are provided by beer, but these are inconsequential in that all forms of alcohol have an adverse effect upon the body's nutritional state. Recent advice from the National Advisory Committee on Nutrition Education has urged us to reduce alcohol consumption.

Alcohol has adverse effects on almost every vitamin and on many minerals. In particular, vitamin B1 (thiamin), vitamins B2 (riboflavin), B3 (nicotinamide), B6 (pyridoxine), folic acid, calcium, magnesium and zinc are depleted in the body in those who consume excessive quantities of alcohol, and deficiencies of these nutrients affect one's general health, and one's mental health in particular. As we have learned previously alcohol also interferes with the metabolism of the essential cis-linoleic acid. Researchers in Scotland have shown that essential fatty acid metabolism is severely disrupted in alcoholics and that alcoholics benefit from supplements of evening primrose oil. An "excessive" quantity may be as little as two or three drinks per day (one drink = 8 oz of beer = one glass of wine = one small glass of sherry = one single measure of spirits).

The effect of long-term consumption of alcohol on the body can be devastating. Most of us already know that liver damage can occur as a result of the excess consumption of alcohol over many years, but it is not often appreciated that damage to the nervous system, brain, and heart can also occur and be equally serious. The effects of damage to the nervous system can be partially reversed with high doses of B vitamins, which often have to be given intravenously, rather than by mouth. Alcoholic heart damage may also respond to vitamin B, but damage to the liver is a more serious and long-standing problem, for which alcohol withdrawal is the only effective treatment.

Too much alcohol also has adverse effects upon both the body's metabolism and nutritional state. Obesity is common, especially in younger beer drinkers. Damage to the esophagus, stomach and pancreas, an increased risk of gout, a worsening of diabetes, and raised blood levels of fat, are just some of the metabolic disturbances that can follow a high alcohol intake. Even an occasional drink can have a profound effect. For example, missing lunch and having a couple of drinks instead can result in poor blood sugar control, with low blood sugar and low energy levels in the afternoon. How many office workers find it difficult to concentrate after their liquid lunch?

Also, the risk of certain types of cancer is increased as a result of alcohol consumption. The risk of developing cancer of the liver, esophagus, larynx and mouth are all increased in alcohol consumers.

Women who drink in the weeks just before and during their pregnancy may be putting the child seriously at risk. Children born of mothers who consume substantial amounts of alcohol during pregnancy may suffer characteristic facial deformities, and be mentally retarded. We advise that no woman who is pregnant, or who is trying to become pregnant, drinks alcohol. There may be no "safe limit," however low. Ensuring that your diet is good is of paramount importance.

Finally, some people are allergic to alcohol. This could be an allergy to either the grape or grain used in the production of the alcohol, to the yeast, or to an additive, such as metabisulphite, which is particularly added to wine. This latter can result in an exacerbation of asthma.

Anyone who drinks a lot is well advised to cut down. This is not always easily done.

COMING OFF ALCOHOL

People who have a high intake of alcohol, and who suddenly cut it down or stop altogether, often develop severe withdrawal symptoms. Nervousness, anxiety, insomnia and shaking occur, and may settle down after two or three days. In more severe cases a condition known as delirium tremens starts. This usually develops in the long-standing alcoholic who is suddenly deprived of alcohol, for example, because he or she suffers a car accident or has a heart attack and is admitted to a hospital where the intake of alcohol is abruptly curtailed. They may not admit that they are alcoholic, or may not be able to do so because they are unconscious. The addiction may go unnoticed until one or two days later, when symptoms of delirium tremens develop. These include mental confusion, impairment of memory, hallucinations, agitation, restlessness and insomnia. The hands shake, there is sweating, fever, raised blood pressure and a fast pulse. Though the individual often recovers spontaneously after three or four days, in severe cases the illness can result in death, and the condition should not be treated lightly. Such people may require intravenous administration of vitamins, minerals and water to correct some of the biochemical disturbances that occur. Sedative drugs are also needed.

In the majority of alcoholics, though, severe reactions like these are not common. Lots of people consume anything from four to ten drinks regularly a day and such people may have been advised by their doctor to reduce their alcohol consumption, or may have decided to do so themselves. It appears that eating a good diet and taking various nutritional supplements may be of value. In alcoholics on one rehabilitation program, a "sober rate" after six months' therapy was 37.8 percent. When nutrition education and nutritional supplements were added in, this rose to 81.3 percent.

One particular study, from Inverness in Scotland, suggested that evening primrose oil may have a promising effect in reducing the symptoms of alcohol withdrawal. Alcohol interferes with the metabolism of essential fatty acids, and supplementation with evening primrose oil, which contains a specialized form, gammalinolenic acid, may bypass some of these effects.

Giving this oil to a group of alcoholics reduced some of the symptoms of withdrawal. It is probable that the correction of coexistent nutritional deficiencies, particularly of the B vitamins, vitamin C, zinc and other minerals would produce additional benefits.

The cause of alcoholism and drug addiction is unknown. Obviously stress and psychological factors are important, but biochemical reasons may be of importance too. Underlying physical illness, nutritional deficiencies and even food allergies are well worth considering. Going onto an exclusion diet can be a good time to stop drinking alcohol and smoking.

SOME TIPS FOR CUTTING DOWN ON ALCOHOL

- Follow a basic healthy diet—see Appendix 1, page 398.
- Eat regularly.
- Correct nutritional deficiencies by use of appropriate supplements, e.g. a good, strong multivitamin and mineral supplement and a supplement of evening primrose oil, 500 mg four to eight capsules a day.
- If necessary, avoid situations in which you regularly drink, or where drinking is encouraged, for example, parties, business lunches, and so on.
- Set a target for your alcohol consumption for the day. Some people find it simpler to give up completely rather than to try to reduce their alcohol consumption slowly.
- Keep busy and active. There is a lot of truth in the old saying "the devil makes work for idle hands." Boredom, frustration, and failure are likely to increase the desire to drown your sorrows or lift your spirits with alcohol.

- Take up a hobby or activities that you enjoy, and use them as alternative diversions instead of consuming alcohol. For example, replace evenings at the bar or club with hobbies, interests or a sport.

For most people, reducing alcohol consumption to two or three drinks a day will remove the adverse effects of alcohol, especially if their diet is well-balanced. Some people feel that they have to give up completely, or run the risk of their alcohol consumption slowly rising to its former high levels.

Organizations such as Alcoholics Anonymous are very supportive if you are trying to give up.

Alcoholism and cough mixture

Edward was a sixty-five-year-old retired businessman who had been alcoholic for more than twenty years, sometimes drinking more than a bottle of Scotch a day. He had been off alcohol for six months when first assessed nutritionally. He was still low in magnesium, zinc and vitamins B1 and B2, a common finding in alcoholics. A multivitamin and mineral supplement, including 200 mg of magnesium, 30 mg of zinc, and 50 mg each of vitamins B1, B2, B3 and B6 produced a remarkable resurgence in well-being. At a follow-up visit, however, he complained of a return of his alcoholic craving for the first time in five and a half months. On closer questioning it emerged that he was currently taking antibiotics for a chest infection and was taking cough medicine too. On telephoning the manufacturers of the cough mixture, it was discovered that the preparation contained five percent alcohol, though it was not marked on the label. The alcohol craving returned within one hour of the first dose of cough mixture and gradually became worse over the subsequent twenty-four hours, during which he had taken several doses of cough mixture. The small amount of alcohol in the cough mixture had provoked a return of the alcohol craving. On acquiring alcohol-free cough mixture the craving once again disappeared. This illustrates that reformed alcoholics should beware of consuming even small amounts of alcohol.

Smoking

Cigarette smoking has a powerful anti-vitamin C effect. Smokers have lower than normal levels of vitamin C in their blood and it may take several hundred milligrams of vitamin C a day to correct this deficiency. The effect of smoking upon other nutrients is uncertain, but it may have an adverse effect on B vitamins. Smoking definitely inhibits the workings of the pancreas, a gland that is essential in the digestion of food, and there is little doubt that chronic or intermittent smokers often have poor digestion. Many individuals who are underweight and cannot gain weight will not do so until they stop smoking.

STOPPING SMOKING

Giving up smoking is no easy task, but many have successfully done so and it may be useful to read some tips on how to stop.

- *You* must have decided *yourself* to stop smoking, whether this be for health reasons, financial reasons, or social reasons. Whatever the reason, no matter how trivial, it must be *your* reason. There is no point trying to give up because someone else has told you to. If you are not certain whether you should give up for health reasons, then remember that statistically every cigarette smoked reduces your life expectancy by approximately five and a half minutes.
- Look and see under what circumstances you smoke. Is it when drinking, when relaxing, after meals, when speaking on the telephone, or in relation to other work activities? Being aware of the circumstances under which you smoke may give you clues as to how you could reduce your consumption.
- Reduce the level of stress in your life if your smoking is stress-related. Very often, high levels of cigarette consumption are related to stress, and if you are using cigarettes as a socially acceptable crutch, it is important to recognize this.
- If you are a heavy tea or coffee consumer, try cutting down on these first. Smokers tend to consume a lot of tea and coffee and some of the adverse effects of tea and coffee may increase your desire for cigarettes.
- Follow a basic, healthy diet and eat regularly (see page 398). This may help reduce the craving for cigarettes. Many smokers, particularly heavy ones, have no breakfast in the

morning and rely upon a cup of tea and half a dozen cigarettes to start their day. It is healthier to stimulate your metabolism with a decent breakfast.

- If your diet is questionable, or if you are a heavy smoker, try taking a multivitamin supplement, especially one high in vitamin C, providing about 500–1000 mg or more per day. The relative vitamin C deficiency induced by smoking may produce apathy and depression, which will not help your willpower when trying to give up.
- Occupy your mind. Don't leave yourself idle in the company of cigarettes or where it is easy to obtain them. Maintain your interests and physical and mental activities.
- Oral gratification. Substitution with chewing gum (even nicotine-containing chewing gum) may be helpful. Avoid consuming sweets, chocolates and more food as this will only lead to a marked gain in weight.
- Enlist the support of others. It is much easier to give up if your spouse, friends and work colleagues are non-smokers. When you are ready to give up, tell everyone that you are doing so, so that you will receive their encouragement and support. Remember that many of them may be ex-smokers.
- Save the money you spend on cigarettes. Financial inducement can be a strong incentive. Someone who spends money on one or two packs a day could easily pay for a good vacation each year, save for a luxury car within ten or twenty years, or contribute a significant amount to a pension fund, hobby or interest. Encourage yourself by placing the money you would have spent into a collecting jar, and after four or six weeks count it penny by penny and see just how much you saved.
- Do not give up. If you fail, remember, you can always try again. It may be particularly useful to place yourself on a healthy diet, take some physical exercise and take appropriate nutritional supplements while reducing stress levels at work, in the home, and elsewhere. You can do this while continuing to smoke for several weeks and then when you are ready for it, try again to reduce your cigarette consumption. Some people find it better to stop suddenly, others to reduce their consumption by a cigarette a day over a period of a month or so.

For those who truly cannot or do not wish to give up, but have a serious smoking-related condition, a reduction rather than actually stopping cigarette consumption may provide some benefit.

Reducing your level to approximately five cigarettes per day, particularly if combined with a good diet, may reduce the risks of smoking to practically zero.

Drug Addiction and Drug Abuse

There is increasing concern throughout the Western world about the rise in notified and unnotified drug addicts. It is possible to be addicted to many drugs, both medical and non-medical. Hundreds of thousands of people take medical sedatives every day. It is now widely accepted that many become physically and psychologically addicted to such drugs. They are unable to live without them and their withdrawal produces both physical and psychological symptoms. Organizations have been set up to help people come off sedatives, tranquilizers and sleeping tablets. The medical profession has, unfortunately, been slow to recognize and respond to the problem.

SOME TIPS FOR COMING OFF TRANQUILIZERS

Dependence on tranquilizers is much more common among women than among men. People with anxiety, depression or agoraphobia, insomniacs and those who have been on sedatives for the last twenty or more years form the majority of this group. It is debatable whether such tranquilizers have done more harm than good overall. Certainly, the current situation is nothing that the medical profession can feel proud about, and replacing one sedative or tranquilizer with another is rarely much of a solution. However, short-acting, milder sedatives can usually be substituted for some of the older, longer-acting ones. Such an approach may reduce the morning-after drowsiness that occurs. The following suggestions may be of some help:

- Eat a basic, healthy diet (see Appendix, page 398).
- Come off tea, coffee, cigarettes and alcohol first, before reducing your tranquilizers and sedatives. Do this over several weeks, very slowly, reducing one thing at a time.
- If insomnia is a problem, supplements of calcium and magnesium at night may help. Take more physical exercise: an evening walk of forty minutes to one hour can help you relax. Some people benefit from alternative approaches such as homeopathic or herbal remedies.
- Try to settle the underlying problem causing your anxiety. If anxiety, depression, premenstrual syndrome or agoraphobia are your problems, consider using nutritional supplements, partic-

ularly a vitamin and mineral supplement containing substantial quantities of vitamin C—approximately 1 g per day—and the B vitamins—approximately 50 mg of B1, B2 and B6.

- When you have been on this program for several months, gradually decrease your intake of tranquilizers and sleeping tablets. Your general practitioner can guide you on how best to do this. **Do not stop them suddenly unless the dosage is very small, or you have been on them for only a short while.**

Addiction to non-medical, illegal drugs, such as LSD, cannabis, cocaine, amphetamines, phencyclidine (PCP—angel dust) and heroin, presents an enormous and growing social problem worldwide. The actual effects of such drugs upon nutrient metabolism are unknown, but those consuming illegal drugs, particularly on a regular basis, often eat badly too. Money that would otherwise be spent on food is used to fund the high cost of the drugs and addicts whose incomes are borderline are at real risk from the development of nutritional deficiencies. Their poor nutritional status is likely to impair their physical and mental reserves and so reduce their chances of withdrawing from the drug successfully.

Very often, it is not the drug addict, but his friends or relatives who seek advice or help on his behalf. An essential prerequisite is that the individual himself wants, at least in some way, to "kick the habit." It is pointless trying to treat someone who does not have at least some degree of motivation.

Here are some hints on giving up:

- Get away from the "drug environment."
- Put yourself in the hands of experts who know what they are doing, possibly in a special unit.
- Have a thorough medical examination for any underlying physical illness or nutritional deficiencies. These are surprisingly common.
- Go on a good basic diet (see Appendix 1, page 398), eat regular meals, including snacks.
- If you are physically up to it, get exercise every day.
- Get plenty of sleep and rest. Try to get emotional support, either from a good friend or relative, or from someone who has had experience with drug detoxification.
- Take appropriate nutritional supplements including a good multivitamin supplement.

DRUG-NUTRIENT INTERACTIONS

The last forty years or so have seen a significant escalation in the use of medicines in the Western world. This growing, and in some cases, excessive, use of drugs and medications has brought with it its own diseases, and this, together with the importance of interactions between drugs, is something of which most doctors are becoming increasingly aware.

What is less well known, but just as important, is the interaction between drugs and individual nutrients. Drugs are powerful metabolic agents and it is hardly surprising that they interact with nutrients. It is increasingly being recognized that certain sections of the population, particularly the elderly, have a very borderline nutritional state, particularly for the B vitamins and vitamin C. If they then take a drug which is an anti-nutrient, it may be enough to tip them into a significant and recognizable deficiency state. Conversely, the metabolism of a particular drug can be influenced by a person's nutritional state.

How Drug-Nutrient Interactions Occur

The most common picture is that of a drug acting as an anti-nutrient, and so inducing a deficiency. However, four situations can exist:

- A drug can act as an anti-nutrient (e.g. some anti-epileptic drugs produce a folate deficiency).
- A drug can enhance a nutrient (e.g. estrogens affect calcium uptake and balance).
- A nutrient can act as an anti-drug (e.g. vitamin B6 is antagonistic to the effects of L-dopa, a drug used in Parkinson's disease).
- A nutrient can enhance a drug (e.g. vitamin C increases the effects of the estrogens in the Pill).

The situation can also be further influenced by an individual's own biochemical state, which is determined genetically, and by the presence of a disease which may influence his or her nutritional state.

We think that with all of these complexities doctors should keep their wits about them and be on the lookout for drug-nutrient interactions.

There are essentially three ways in which a drug can act as an anti-nutrient: it can reduce the absorption of the nutrient, it can alter its metabolism in the body, or it can alter the way the body gets rid of it.

Here are some of the more commonly used drugs and their effects on nutrients.

ANTI-RHEUMATIC AGENTS

Many anti-inflammatory agents are commonly used for all types of arthritis. Aspirin can deplete vitamin C levels and it is possible, though by no means proven, that other non-steroidal, anti-inflammatory drugs might have a similar effect.

The anti-arthritis agent D-penicillamine has important interactions with vitamin B6, zinc and other trace minerals. Vitamin B6 activity is reduced in some patients on D-penicillamine, and this can be corrected by the administration of 50 mg per day of B6. Some experts advise routine vitamin B6 supplementation.

Penicillamine has important interactions with trace minerals. It can be used as a chelating agent (a substance that latches onto a mineral and alters the properties and biochemical behavior of that mineral). It has been used therapeutically to reduce copper levels in a condition called Wilson's disease. It is also useful in the treatment of lead toxicity. Copper deficiency can be induced by penicillamine, as may a zinc deficiency.

ANTACIDS

Several antacids have adverse nutritional effects. The long-term use of antacids, particularly those containing calcium in conjunction with a high dietary calcium intake, can lead to too much calcium in the blood and eventually to kidney stones. Antacids containing aluminum can cause aluminum overload and phosphate deficiency can occur.

OTHER DRUGS FOR PEPTIC ULCERS

H-2 antagonist drugs, such as Cimetidine (Tagamet), are powerful suppressors of gastric acid secretion and are used to cure duodenal and stomach ulcers. They may also interfere with vitamin B12 absorption. These drugs are widely prescribed, sometimes on a long-term basis, yet their effects on intestinal function are not yet fully understood. Normal gastric acid production is also important for iron, calcium and magnesium absorption.

DIURETICS

The use of modern diuretics has been one of the major advances in therapeutics. However, excessive potassium loss can easily occur as a result of long-term thiazide diuretics. Diuretics can also cause losses of other important minerals including magnesium, zinc and possibly chromium. A magnesium deficiency may be coexistent with a potassium deficiency and aggravate it. Symptoms of magnesium deficiency, such as nausea, apathy, tiredness and muscle cramps, might easily be dismissed or written off as commonplace, particularly amongst the elderly, and their true cause might not be appreciated. More seriously, digitalis toxicity is provoked not only by potassium but also by magnesium deficiency.

Impaired glucose tolerance can be a feature of long-term diuretic treatment, and this can be reversed by adequate potassium supplementation.

ANTIBIOTICS

Antibiotics are mostly used in short-term courses, so problems of malabsorption or significant drug-nutrient interactions rarely occur. However, the long-term administration of neomycin, particularly to those with liver disease, can produce malabsorption of fat- and water-soluble vitamins. Tetracycline, often used to treat acne, is known to interact with certain minerals, including calcium and iron, though significant deficiencies have not been described in long-term usage. If you are on tetracycline, do not consume calcium-rich foods—at least, not at the same time. It is possible that other more finely balanced trace minerals, such as zinc and copper, may be adversely affected by antibiotics.

Some doctors prescribe multivitamins along with antibiotics to correct any depletion of B vitamins caused by antibiotic treatment. Conversely it appears that the activity of the antibiotics tetracycline and lincomycin can be significantly diminished by the presence of riboflavin (vitamin B2). Nystatin, used to treat yeast infection (thrush), inhibits the activity of vitamins B2 and B6. The adverse effect of riboflavin on nystatin may be enhanced by vitamin C.

If someone on antibiotics needs vitamin B supplementation, then this should be taken at a separate time from the antibiotics.

HIGH BLOOD PRESSURE DRUGS

One drug, Hydralazine, sometimes prescribed by doctors for high blood pressure, is a potent vitamin B6 antagonist.

ANTI-TUBERCULAR DRUGS

Many anti-tubercular drugs may produce B vitamin deficiency. Particularly well recognized is the antagonistic effect of isoniazid on vitamin B6, which can produce nerve damage.

Other anti-tubercular drugs, such as cycloserine, pyrazinamide and ethionamide, can all have adverse effects upon B6 metabolism.

ANTI-PARKINSONIAN DRUGS

Perhaps one of the most widely recognized drug-nutrient interactions is that of the anti-Parkinsonian drug L-dopa with vitamin B6. The therapeutic effects of L-dopa depend upon its conversion to dopamine within the central nervous system, not in the general circulation. L-dopa crosses the blood-brain barrier, but dopamine itself does not. Vitamin B6 enhances the change of dopa to form dopamine in the circulation, thus reducing the amount of dopa available to cross the blood-brain barrier. Vitamin B6 administration abolishes the therapeutic effects of L-dopa. L-dopa can also interact with the dietary amino acid L-phenylalanine. This is why a high protein intake can have an inhibitory effect upon the effectiveness of L-dopa. It may therefore be advisable to avoid taking preparations containing L-dopa after a high-protein meal.

ANTI-METABOLITES

Some chemotherapeutic agents used in the treatment of cancer are themselves anti-nutrients. A good example is that of methotrexate which interferes with folic acid metabolism. Folic acid is important in cell growth, and it is because of this that methotrexate has its anti-tumor activity. It is also the reason it has side-effects.

ORAL CONTRACEPTIVES

Oral contraceptives are known to have adverse effects upon many nutrients, particularly the B vitamins, and routine supplementation with B vitamins should be seriously considered by women taking estrogen-based oral contraceptives for a long time. For more on this, see page 308.

It is impractical and impossible to list all the actual or potential drug-nutrient interactions that could and do occur. Drug-nutrient interactions are more likely to occur in those who are on multiple medications and those who have borderline dietary intakes. As a result, the elderly are particularly at risk. Anyone with poor gastrointestinal function will also be at risk and drug-induced diarrhea will adversely affect nutritional status, particularly for water-soluble nutrients and for those nutrients of which there are not substantial body stores, such as zinc.

The full effect of many medications on a person's nutritional state is not always appreciated. **If you are taking any of the above drugs on a long-term basis, consult your doctor if you suspect that you may be deficient in the relevant nutrient.**

FREE RADICALS AND LIPID PEROXIDATION

Oxygen is essential for basic cell-function in humans and most animals. However, research is showing that this is a mixed blessing. Although it gives us an evolutionary energy advantage over those life forms that do not need oxygen, it is simultaneously a threat to our survival. Oxygen can produce toxic substances, such as peroxide, superoxide, hydroxyl radicals, and "excited state oxygen."

These highly reactive substances combine with other molecules in the body in a destructive fashion. They form "free radicals" which are high-energy chemical substances looking for something to combine with.

It is now becoming evident that free-radical reactions in mammalian systems are probably responsible for such diverse physiological processes as inflammation, aging, drug-induced damage, degenerative arthritis, alterations in immunity, cancer, and cardiovascular disease.

It is now thought that this alteration in cellular material as a result of the release of free radicals is the basis of many disease processes. Also, once they are diseased, tissues undergo peroxidation much more quickly than do healthy ones. This is where nutrition comes to bear on the situation.

Since the utilization of oxygen-breathing organisms has a potentially destructive side to it, it is hardly surprising to learn that nature has provided a method of protecting cells against such oxidative processes. These protective components are called anti-oxidants, and include beta-carotene, vitamin A, vitamin E, vitamin C, selenium-containing amino acids (such as cystine), and enzymes such as glutathione reductase, catalase and peroxidase and superoxide dismutase.

Trace Elements and Free Radicals

While excessive iron is a source of free radicals, there are other minerals that are important for the maintenance of the anti-oxidant activity of a number of enzymes. For example, glutathione peroxidase requires selenium for its activity, and superoxide dismutase requires copper, manganese and zinc. Deficiencies of selenium, copper, manganese and zinc can result in increased susceptibility to free-radical damage of the fat part of cell membranes. Excessive copper can also be a cause of this free-radical peroxidation.

The nutrients mentioned above are all dealt with elsewhere in this book and symptoms and signs of deficiency of these nutrients can, in part, be ascribed to an increased tendency to lipid peroxidation.

The importance of lipid peroxidation is difficult to overestimate. White cells, in the process of inflammation, kill bacteria by releasing hydrogen peroxide, which initiates lipid peroxidation and damages bacteria and viruses. In disease conditions where there is "inappropriate" activity of white cells, such as in rheumatoid arthritis, the destruction of the joint comes about as a result of the release of hydrogen peroxide from the white cells.

So, in inflammatory processes, an adequate supply of the anti-oxidant nutrients mentioned above is essential. It is also worth noting that in disease conditions, requirements for these essential nutrients are often increased.

The whole subject is still in its infancy from the therapeutic point of view, but there are some conditions where it could be beneficial to take appropriate nutritional supplements to reduce free-radical damage.

If we are exposed to excessive oxidation, then our anti-oxidant defense system is activated.

Our ability to supply the appropriate anti-oxidants to meet requirements is a fundamental function of health or disease.

When the oxidative stress becomes too much for our anti-oxidant defense system, damage to tissues starts to occur. If this persists over a prolonged period of time, we get chronic degenerative disease. Our environment provides us with oxidative stress: free radicals could be derived from circulating adrenalin or noradrenalin, which are increased under chronic stress. Photochemical smog is a major external source of oxidative stress, because it produces potent oxidants such as ozone, nitrogen dioxide, peroxyacyl nitrates and numerous hydrocarbon-derived free-radical substances. Cigarette smoke also subjects the lungs and other organs to chronic oxidative stress. Environmental pollutant chemicals and drugs can also be a source of oxidative stress.

In our laboratory we measure our patients' anti-oxidant defenses by looking at the degree to which their red and white cells break up when subjected to a particular dilution of hydrogen peroxide. We also measure the activity of red cell glutathione peroxidase, and if this is low we know that their oxidative stress is high. Then we can say that a particular individual is failing to meet his or her oxidative stress with sufficient anti-oxidant defense. We also measure selenium, manganese, copper, and zinc levels, as well as those of vitamin C, vitamin A, vitamin E, and beta-carotene.

Aging, which is inevitable, may in part be due to the long-term effects of not quite meeting oxidative stresses sufficiently.

Ensuring that your anti-oxidant defenses are good involves eating a healthy diet and also ensuring that your status is adequate as regards zinc, copper, manganese, selenium, vitamins E, A and C and beta-carotene.

ENVIRONMENTAL POISONS

In the twentieth century we live in a very toxic environment. We spray our environment with insecticides, pesticides and herbicides; add artificial substances such as preservatives, taste-enhancers and colorings to our foods; process foods to take out many of the useful nutrients; load the air we breathe and water that we drink with industrial effluent, and so on. This appears to be the price that we have to pay for modern civilization.

Even the household can be a very toxic environment: gas appliances with possible gas leaks, fumes from burnt gas, organic solvents from spray polishes and air fresheners, bleaches, detergents, oils from the garage or car port, etc. These can be detrimental to health and indoor pollution should be kept to a minimum when trying to improve one's level of health.

There are, nevertheless, certain nutritional steps that can be taken to try to enhance our survival potential in this fairly hostile environment. The main thing we can do is to ensure that we consume enough of certain nutrients that help protect our bodies from being too poisoned by all these substances. This is one reason for taking nutritional supplements on a routine basis. The idea that a good, healthy diet is all that one needs just does not stand up any more. A good, healthy diet may have suited a greater number of people before industrialization, but in the presence of so many toxins in the environment, the biochemistry of the body is being assaulted by substances that were not present in our environment during our evolution, and many people simply have not adapted to cope with them.

Substances such as vitamin C, selenium, vitamin E, beta-carotene, zinc and manganese, which may be in short supply, do have a protective effect by enhancing various enzyme activities, as well as increasing, in some instances, the rate of excretion of toxic substances from the body.

PART TWO

Allergies

INTRODUCTION

Over the last few years there has been increasing awareness of the number of diseases and complaints that can be caused, or contributed to, by the presence of allergies.

Though this is a book about nutrition, we cannot confine ourselves to just the subject of food allergies. In the assessment of anyone with an allergic problem we find we often cannot simply consider food allergy or intolerance in isolation, but must also think of other potential causes for a patient's symptoms. It may well be possible to modify allergic processes by paying attention to certain nutritional factors too.

Allergies are enormously common. Conservative estimates are that twenty percent of the population is allergic to something, but when one considers minor allergies such as mild hay fever, wheezy bronchitis in children, minor degrees of eczema and food intolerance, the true incidence of allergy and/or intolerance to one or more environmental agents may well be much higher. This calls for an explanation, because it seems so strange that so many people should be allergic to things in their environment. We believe that changes in the Western diet over the last 100 to 200 years—in particular the refining of food, the use of food additives and the increased consumption of animal produce—and the presence of environmental pollution, have contributed substantially to the prevalence of all forms of allergic disease. The correction or avoidance of these can produce substantial improvements and even cures in some people.

What Is an Allergy

The word allergy is derived from two Greek words meaning "altered reaction" and an allergic individual usually suffers physical symptoms (e.g. headache, vomiting, rashes, migraine, asthma) when he or she is exposed to contact with substances to which he or she is sensitive, though mental symptoms can also occur, as we shall see. The substance which provokes this reaction is called the allergen, and can be house dust, dog or cat fur, a food, a chemical, or a bacterium, to name but a few.

In this part of the book we deal with the three most common sources of allergic reaction—food, chemicals and inhaled allergens.

FOOD ALLERGY

In recent years food allergy has become recognized as a significant contributing cause to a whole range of different medical conditions. As things stand today, anyone denying the existence of food allergy, and its importance in a whole range of physical conditions, could well be accused of burying his head in the sand, because the academic, laboratory and clinical proof of its existence is now incontrovertible.

Where the controversy lies is in the extent to which food allergy plays a part in a number of conditions. There are many myths relating to food allergy which we hope this section of the book will help defuse.

Development of Food Sensitivities and Masking

Adverse reactions to foods were known to the early Greeks, such as Hippocrates, and many a grandmother down the ages knew that certain children and adults reacted adversely to specific foods, and so took steps to avoid them.

Generally speaking, many foods that we have been eating since infancy, once or twice every day, or even more frequently, we continue to eat into adulthood. Examples are wheat, milk, corn and sugar (see page 128).

When solid foods are first introduced, a baby may have an "allergic" reaction to wheat, for example, and develop diarrhea, abdominal colic, crankiness, a runny nose, or even a middle ear infection, asthma or eczema. The cause of these symptoms is generally not recognized and may even be treated as a transient infection if the problem is a runny nose or ear pain.

The offending food continues to be given and the infant usually recovers from the acute symptoms, though there may be persistent, relatively minor symptoms.

Hours, days, months or years later, either following periods of infection or stress, or just due to a gradual failure to remain healthy, symptoms develop.

If the food is withdrawn, the symptoms usually clear within three to five days, though sometimes, especially in children, this can take as long as three weeks. There may be quite marked withdrawal symptoms which usually improve eventually or clear totally. If the person is challenged with the food within the next two weeks or so, during the period of maximum sensitivity, then symptoms will once more appear. The symptoms may be the same as the ones that were present prior to withdrawal and subsequent challenge, or they may be slightly different. The length of time during which sensitivity to an offending food can last is very variable, but in general terms, the longer one avoids the food, the more likely one is able to tolerate it subsequently. Some individuals are particularly sensitive to a given food and may never be able to eat it without producing symptoms. More commonly though, after a period of some weeks or months, the individual can tolerate the offending food in small quantities either on a regular basis or once every four to seven days. This is the basis of what is called the "rotation diet" which is discussed below (see page 169).

Infants in particular, and to a lesser extent, young children, should not have foods withdrawn and then re-challenged without medical supervision. This is particularly true of milk in infancy, which has been implicated in severe allergic reactions even to the point of being life-threatening. **Such challenges should only be done in a hospital under the supervision of a pediatrician who is thoroughly familiar with the hazards of food challenges in infants.**

Masked Allergies

Chronic food allergies are not usually obvious, thus they are often referred to as masked allergies. Unmasking can be brought about by withdrawal of the offending food. There may be withdrawal symptoms for a few days before symptoms then resolve or improve. The person is then in the unmasked state and further consumption of the offending food will produce symptoms again, which are more easily noticed. The most sensitive period is in the three weeks or so following withdrawal of the food from the diet, though sensitivity can remain for months or even years. It is our impression that judicious use of nutritional supplements and methods of coping with stress can reduce this period of sensitivity and improve a person's tolerance to a given food.

Combined Allergy

Sometimes symptoms such as hay fever, running nose, or recurrent infections, are caused by a combination of allergies to inhalants, foods and/or chemicals. This makes things very complex. So the exclusion of a given food may not produce a *total resolution* of symptoms, rather an improvement, as the individual is still subject to reactions caused by inhalants or chemicals. Nevertheless, this is very often a considerable improvement and the individual may be better able to tolerate the inhalant(s) or chemical(s) to which they are still exposed and to which they are sensitive.

Components of Food Allergy

It may be more than just the food itself which can cause an allergic reaction in an individual. Any food is a complex combination of thousands of molecules and it may be one or several of these naturally occurring molecules that produce the reaction.

Also, there is a whole range of other items which can reach the plate that are not necessarily present in a food in its natural state. Food additives include colorings, preservatives, anti-oxidants, and flavorings. Agricultural chemicals such as pesticides and herbicides are added to crops and can contribute to the chemical overload of an individual, making him or her more susceptible to symptoms from the food he or she eats. Antibiotics and hormones, too, are used in animals being prepared for slaughter, or are added to animal fodder. Fungi and yeasts grow on foods,

Warning

If you have any of the symptoms or conditions listed on pages 157 and 158, be sure to see your own doctor for a thorough physical examination, including blood tests if he considers them appropriate. The fact is that though these symptoms can be caused by a food allergy, they can also be due to a whole range of other physical causes with effective medical treatments, which may not be responsive to food allergy approaches. If you delay seeing your doctor because you are conducting food allergy investigations yourself, you may do yourself harm.

especially grains, and these can be a source of clinical symptoms in susceptible individuals. Some people find that they can, for example, tolerate chicken (or the eggs of a chicken) that has been fed on one type of grain, but not on another. So a person may react to a component of the food which was fed to the chickens, rather than to the chicken meat itself.

Signs of Food Allergy and Intolerance

The manifestations of food intolerance are legion and can mimic a whole range of different clinical conditions. They can also play a part in the *cause* of well-recognized and diagnosable clinical conditions such as irritable bowel syndrome, rheumatoid arthritis or migraine.

SOME CONDITIONS WHICH ARE INFLUENCED OR CAUSED BY FOOD INTOLERANCE

- inflammatory arthritis (e.g. rheumatoid)
- migraine and other headaches
- childhood hyperactivity, sleep disturbances, learning disability
- asthma
- rhinitis
- sinusitis
- recurrent infections (e.g. tonsillitis)
- infantile colic and infantile colitis
- mouth ulcers
- eczema and other skin rashes
- urticaria (hives)
- angio-edema
- premenstrual symptoms
- fluid retention
- irritable bowel syndrome (constipation and/or diarrhea, bloating, abdominal pain, gas)
- peptic ulcers and gastritis
- Crohn's disease and ulcerative colitis
- fatigue and excessive sleepiness
- depression

- anxiety
- schizophrenia and other mental conditions
- epilepsy
- hypoglycemia
- aggravation of diabetes
- some kidney diseases
- gall bladder symptoms
- facial flushing
- some types of palpitations
- weight problems
- celiac disease

KEY FEATURES OF FOOD ALLERGY/INTOLERANCE

There are a number of different features which should make you suspect that food intolerance might be an underlying factor in your symptoms. The main ones are discussed below.

In this section we are not going to look at fixed food allergies, such as are found in response to shellfish, strawberries, etc. These allergies tend to last for a lifetime. Here, we are thinking about the subject of "masked" food allergies as it is more difficult to diagnose these and to identify the offending food. Clearly, if a food upsets you very obviously you simply do not eat it.

Fluctuating symptoms that come and go, and do not seem to be related to any particular environmental factor, may very well be caused by eating a particular food of which you are intolerant. The fact that the symptoms may be there one day and not the next, and yet the offending food has been eaten on both days, is no reason to assume that the condition is not due to eating that particular food. All this means is that the individual is oscillating back and forth across the "symptom threshold."

Fatigue. People who are food intolerant are often excessively tired—with a tiredness that is unrelieved by rest. They often feel ghastly in the morning, and gradually perk up during the day (or vice versa), though not to the level that they would consider ideal. Sometimes this fatigue can be so severe that they have to go to bed during the day. It is usually possible to track down a time in their life when the fatigue started to occur—for example, after flu, glandular fever, an operation, stress, pregnancy, etc.

Fatigue and food allergy

Alison suffered from the "tired housewife syndrome" for which there are many causes. In this instance, Alison was put on an elimination diet and it was found that within five days of being on the "modified exclusion diet for adults" (see Appendix 3) she felt less fatigued and less depressed than she had in many years. Reintroduction of food revealed that wheat was the offending food item, and exclusion of this item from her diet resulted in her being able to conduct her life along normal lines. She experienced great relief because she had been told on numerous occasions that she was neurotic, and inadequate as a mother.

Mental and psychological symptoms are another common manifestation of food allergy. Many of those who have spent years on antidepressants and other mind-altering drugs have irritability, depression, anxiety and tension that are directly a result of food intolerance.

Fluid retention may well be a result of food intolerance. Perhaps the most common offenders in this respect are wheat and other grains, though any foods can produce it in susceptible individuals. Many women are put on to diuretics for years in an attempt to reduce their tendency to retain fluid. As we discuss in the section on elimination diets, fluid loss occurs when the offending food is excluded from the diet, with a resultant reduction in weight and passing of large quantities of urine. Fluid retention can also be caused by excessive salt intake and this should be borne in mind too.

Weight fluctuations are very often associated with fluid retention problems. In fact marked weight fluctuation (maybe several pounds within twenty-four hours) can be directly caused by food intolerance. We have had several patients who can eat a diet based on excluding an offending food and who may then eat as little as half a slice of brown bread (for example), and retain as much as four or five pounds or more in weight (all fluid) in a twenty-four hour period. Weight problems themselves can very often be indicators of food intolerance either directly or perhaps as a result of the metabolic effects of the ingestion of the offending food, or because allergic "food addiction" can occur, resulting in bingeing on excessive amounts of carbohydrate. Weight problems are discussed in more detail on page 298.

Muscle and joint aches and pains are a common complaint in food intolerant individuals, and although this can be associated with nutrient deficiencies (magnesium or vitamin B6 for example) they often respond to the exclusion of offending foods. Inflammatory arthritis, including rheumatoid arthritis, is sometimes associated with food intolerance, especially to wheat or milk in younger women and children.

Bouts of racing or bounding pulse, and even abnormal heart rhythms, can be associated with food intolerance as well as deficiencies of certain vitamins and minerals (e.g. B1, B6, magnesium, potassium and copper).

A low blood sugar (reactive hypoglycemia, see page 292). The blood sugar can drop to a point where fatigue, anxiety, lethargy, palpitation, cold sweats, faintness, dizziness, headaches, hunger, aggression, irritability, etc. (not necessarily all together) occur. This is often related to food allergy.

Intestinal symptoms such as diarrhea and/or constipation, typically found in the irritable bowel syndrome (see page 209), are very often caused by food intolerance. Sometimes severe and longstanding constipation in adults or children can be caused by allergy to foods such as wheat, other grains and cows' milk.

Food craving and/or addiction can be part of the food intolerance picture, and one phenomenon that is sometimes seen is that the withdrawal symptoms caused by an allergic addiction can result in a decreased sense of well-being, or other symptoms which can be "made better" by eating the offending food or drink, especially alcohol.

Headaches and migraines (see page 355) are very often features of food allergic conditions.

Facial flushings and sweating. Some individuals with food intolerance notice sweating or facial or body flushing for no apparent reason.

Alcohol intolerance (see page 133). This is an almost certain indicator that someone has developed clinical manifestations of food intolerance.

Classically allergic people are especially at risk. If you have a history of obvious allergies such as hay fever, migraine, urticaria, rashes, asthma or rhinitis, then you should consider intolerance a prime suspect if ever you have any unusual symptoms.

OTHER INDICATORS OF FOOD ALLERGY

There are many other symptoms which can be attributed to food allergy. In childhood (see page 360), they include hyperactivity, learning disorders, clumsiness, excessive thirst, frequent infections (including sore throats and recurrent ear and sinus infections), food fussiness, aching legs, headaches, poor sleep patterns, abdominal bloating, constant stuffy nose, dry patchy facial skin, dry cheeks, ruddy ears, repetitive motions such as rocking and banging, reactions to drugs such as cough medicines and antibiotics, and a history of cows' milk intolerance during infancy.

Stress and Food Intolerance

In our experience, and that of many other doctors, though it has yet to be proved scientifically, when someone is under emotional or psychological stress, they are more likely to develop a food intolerance. A person who is under stress may become inward-looking, so making them much more susceptible to even the slightest of symptoms. Pastimes and therapies such as autogenic training, stress counseling, meditation, yoga and biofeedback, as well as actually trying to resolve the stressful situation, can reduce stress symptoms and so decrease the susceptibility to food and chemical intolerance.

Unfortunately, many long-term food allergy sufferers are dismissed as neurotic or hypochondriac, and many are reluctant even to consider that there might be psychological or emotional factors that contribute to their condition. This calls for very careful and sensitive handling by the doctor concerned, and courage and honesty on the part of the sufferer. In chronic severe food allergies there is often a significant underlying emotional problem.

Making the Diagnosis

The cornerstone of diagnosing food allergies or intolerances is the exclusion of the offending food(s), which produces an alleviation of symptoms, and reintroduction of the food(s), which causes a return of the symptoms.

The main problem is "what food should I exclude?"

If someone eats shellfish and half an hour to an hour later comes out in an itchy rash, or starts wheezing, then one doesn't have to be an expert on food allergies to be able to identify the offending food.

However, when reactions are delayed or symptoms are persistent, the identification of the offending food becomes a rather more skilled matter.

POINTERS IN THE HISTORY

Symptoms. If an individual suffers from food craving, addiction or fluctuating symptoms, food allergy should be suspected.

Onset of symptoms. The date of onset of symptoms can sometimes provide a clue as to whether or not an individual is food allergic. For example, sometimes breast-fed babies can be intolerant to foods in the mother's diet that appear in the breast milk. This is discussed in more detail in the section on Eczema (page 269). Symptoms developing during infancy (such as colic, sleep disturbances, diarrhea), following the introduction of solid foods, can be a good indicator that someone is food allergic. This applies not only to dealing with problems in infancy, but also those in adults. Finding out whether or not an infant spent a lot of time crying or with bowel disturbances and bloating after weaning, is a very good clue to make one suspect that the adult is now suffering from food intolerant problems, since the chances are that those symptoms in infancy were due to an inability to tolerate the foods introduced at that time. The fact that the symptoms resolve during infancy or childhood with no obvious clinical problem does not argue against a diagnosis of food allergy. It could just be that the individual has since learned to adapt to that particular food, either completely or partially, so that there are now no obvious symptoms. At a later point in life, following an infection, stress, or simply with the passage of time, the individual's ability to adapt may have deteriorated, with a re-emergence of the food intolerance symptoms. The symptoms that evolve later on in childhood, teens, adolescence, adulthood or even old age do not necessarily bear any resemblance to the initial symptoms that occurred during infancy.

Major changes in eating habits (diets, etc.) resulting either in a worsening or an improvement of symptoms, also provide a clue to which foods might be a problem. For example, Weight Watchers is a slimming diet that contains milk, wheat and yeast —three very commonly offending foods. Individuals who have trouble losing weight with Weight Watchers may very well be intolerant to the foods that appear in the diet. (See Obesity, page 298.)

Similarly, the Beverly Hills Diet, devised by Judy Mazell, is another diet that can provide a clue. The first part of the diet excludes dairy products and grains, and individuals who do reasonably well on the first part of the diet, and then subsequently "crash," may well be sensitive to either wheat or milk which have been introduced into the diet.

The Atkins Diet involves excluding grain and dairy products, and those who do well on it may actually do so because of exclusion of foods to which they are intolerant.

We quite frequently see patients whose symptoms have become worse when starting on a wholefood diet. The onset of the deterioration may not start exactly at the changeover point because it may take a considerable time for the individual's failure to adapt to the new diet to emerge. In such situations it may be that the individual is sensitive to wheat or some component of the wholefood diet that is being eaten in greater quantities. We have seen rheumatoid arthritis, migraine, asthma and joint pains developing in people within a few weeks or months of going over to a wholefood or high-fiber diet and their symptoms resolving after exclusion of wheat from their diet.

Another type of dietary change that is increasingly common today is when a person becomes a vegetarian (see page 401). If symptoms develop after this, then one should suspect that the individual is eating more of the offending food than they were eating prior to going onto the vegetarian diet. We have seen several cases of people who are sensitive to eggs, dairy products or grains, and whose symptoms either began or became worse on starting a vegetarian diet and resolved when the offending food was excluded.

Other things which may be associated with a change in diet are moving from one country to another, going on vacation, being away at boarding school, staying with relatives, seasonal changes, and so on. Any of these can provide the clue.

The use of the contraceptive pill is not infrequently associated with a deterioration in health, and while this may come about as a result of vitamin and mineral deficiencies, (see page 308), there is also evidence that some women become more food-allergic after going on the Pill. The first step is to come off the Pill, and if the symptoms do not resolve after three months of nutritional supplementation (see page 314), it is well worth embarking upon the full diagnostic routine for food intolerance.

Drugs. If symptoms persist or are worsened after starting a course of drugs such as tranquilizers or sedatives then one should bear in mind the strong possibility of food intolerance.

Infections such as flu, hepatitis or pneumonia, or the use of antibiotics, can sometimes precipitate a range of different symptoms, and while these are easily attributable to the infection itself, there are often food allergic components that can, when treated, result in an improvement in, or resolution of, the symptoms.

Alcohol. A further clue to the diagnosis of food intolerance is the development of an intolerance to alcohol (though this can also be the result of nutrient insufficiencies and disorders of essential fatty acid metabolism). Quite commonly, people who are chronically unwell notice that they can no longer tolerate the same amount of alcohol, or indeed any alcohol at all, whereas previously they were able to consume a reasonable amount without untoward effects. The type of alcohol can be a clue, to some degree, to the suspect food, in that beer, sherry and wines are very rich in yeast, and intolerance to these drinks can be an indicator of yeast intolerance. Whiskey and beer contain grains, and it may be that intolerance to these forms of alcohol is a result of an intolerance to one or more of the constituent grains (see Appendix, page 435). Some wines contain the additive metabisulphite, which can precipitate asthma.

The development of an addiction to alcohol, followed by intolerance of it, is a key diagnostic clue in food allergy which should not be ignored.

PAST MEDICAL HISTORY

A person's past medical history can also give vital clues. Individuals with a history of hay fever, asthma, eczema, urticaria, or immediate food hypersensitivity (such as to shellfish) are more likely to be food intolerant. However, the absence of a history of such allergic conditions does *not* exclude a diagnosis of food intolerance. An individual with celiac disease (gluten sensitivity —see page 208) is also more likely to be intolerant of other foods.

A history of rheumatoid arthritis, or indeed of any persistent joint pains, is also very strongly suggestive of food allergy, though, having said this, we have had a number of failures in trying to cure rheumatoid arthritis using food intolerance methods alone. Inflammatory bowel disease such as Crohn's disease, and ulcerative colitis, may very well have a significant food intolerance component which should be treated if one is to produce a remission in the main condition.

Migraine is a really "hot" sign of food intolerance, and anyone with migraine should be assumed to have some form of intolerance until proved otherwise. Early graying of the hair, around the age of twenty or thirty, is very often an indicator of autoimmune disease and can sometimes be associated with an increased likelihood of food intolerance.

FAMILY HISTORY

Allergies tend to run in families and the stronger the family history of food intolerance or any of the conditions listed on pages 157–158, the more likely the individual is to have food intolerance problems.

TYPES OF SYMPTOMS

Specific foods do not necessarily cause the same symptoms in different people. What is more, the same food can precipitate a range of different symptoms at different times in the *same* individual.

A child with eczema may very well be allergic to eggs or milk, and this should be assumed to be the case until proven otherwise. However, other substances such as citrus fruits and yeast, or a zinc deficiency, can be significant contributing factors to the development of eczema.

Migraine can often be precipitated by dairy products, wheat, coffee, chocolate, and tyramine-rich foods (such as cheese and red wines), but it can also be caused by just about any other food in susceptible individuals.

Women who suffer from fluid retention in the seven to ten days before their periods very often have a wheat or grain intolerance, a yeast intolerance, or an intolerance to dairy products. Premenstrual fluid retention is often made worse by salt, even in small quantities.

LABORATORY TESTS

Skin tests and blood tests can be used by doctors to detect allergy and to identify the specific allergens. However, many of these tests have not been fully validated and can give false results, or are expensive and not generally available.

THE PULSE TEST

This involves taking the pulse before and after eating a food. While the reports of the Royal College of Physicians and the American Academy of Allergy and Immunology disregard it as a valid method of testing, they do not provide any evidence to prove that it is valueless. We, and many other doctors, have found it extremely useful as a guideline to assessing whether or not an individual might be intolerant to a given food.

It is done as follows. Sit in a comfortable resting position; take your pulse before eating, then repeat the pulse-taking at 10,

20, 40 and 60 minutes after eating the suspect food. An increase, *or decrease,* of pulse rate greater than 10 per minute on testing should cause you to suspect the food, even in the absence of any other specific symptoms. Very often symptoms will not occur on the basis of a single ingestion, yet a distinct change in pulse rate occurs. Sometimes, however, symptoms occur without a change in pulse rate, in which case, too, the food should be put on the suspect list and tested subsequently. It is important to exclude other causes of increased pulse rate such as anxiety, emotion, physical activity and so on. For this reason the test should be done resting quietly in a calm and relaxed environment.

DIETARY EXCLUSION

Dietary exclusion and a resulting disappearance of symptoms is the main foundation upon which a diagnosis of food allergy is made.

There are a number of different diets which can be tried. They are discussed below. However, it should be borne in mind that some people may not benefit from an exclusion diet if they are still on certain types of medications, the Pill, alcohol, or cigarettes, or if they have substantial nutritional deficiencies. Nor will they get any benefit if they are in fact not food intolerant. On the other hand, some people who are excessively exposed to chemicals, inhalants, pollens, stress or lack of sleep, may have too high a total burden of environmental stressors to obtain meaningful benefit from an exclusion diet, even if they *are* food allergic. **Certain drugs should not be discontinued suddenly, and certainly not without medical supervision.** Also, if you are being treated for high blood pressure, for example, going onto an exclusion diet may produce a reduction in blood pressure if it involves the exclusion of a food that was contributing to the high blood pressure. So you should really only go on such a diet if you are under medical supervision.

The length of time you need to stay off a given food or foods before a marked improvement of symptoms occurs is very variable. Some children, when they have food colorings removed from their diet, show a dramatic response within seventy-two hours or less. On the other hand, the exclusion of milk and grains can take up to three weeks before demonstrable effects are apparent. So, in certain cases, if the food is not excluded for as long as three weeks, it is easy to draw the wrong conclusion that the individual is not food intolerant or, at least, not intolerant to the foods that have been excluded.

WITHDRAWAL SYMPTOMS

Withdrawal symptoms such as headaches in the first three to five days are a common feature of exclusion diets (even just giving up tea and coffee can cause withdrawal headaches). If these occur, it is a positive sign that you are on the right track. The length of time during which withdrawal symptoms can occur can be reduced by taking a course of Epsom salts at the beginning of the exclusion diet to clear any residual foods from the gastro-intestinal tract so that there is no possibility that substances to which the individual is intolerant are still being absorbed once the food has been excluded from the diet. Some sufferers from migraine have the worst migraines of their life during this withdrawal phase. It may be necessary, in extreme circumstances, for the family doctor to be on standby to give an injection of a major painkiller.

Symptoms diminish on withdrawal of the offending food, but if a rechallenge with the offending food is tried shortly after that, the symptoms can be more severe than they were prior to the withdrawal of the food originally. Maximum sensitivity tends to occur for about three weeks after withdrawal of the food, and it is during this time that the reintroduction of foods should be tried. If foods have been excluded for a prolonged period, their reintroduction may well result in no worsening or development of symptoms. This can lead to the false conclusion that the individual is not sensitive to that particular food. The way to get around this is to reintroduce the food and eat it regularly for a whole week to see if the cumulative effect causes any recurrence of symptoms. However, eating the same food on a daily basis is not a particularly good idea for somebody who is particularly prone to the development of food intolerances, as he or she can actually develop a *new* food intolerance as a result of eating the same food item every day.

Some people, and it is difficult to predict which, may have to avoid a given food for a very long time. These are the minority, though, and most people with masked food intolerances can, after two or three months of avoidance, get away with one or two meals containing the offending food once every four to seven days.

Certain foods tend to top the list of offending foods. The main offenders are:

- wheat, rye, oats, maize (corn)
- milk products and beef

- hens' eggs and chicken meat
- chocolate, tea, coffee
- cane and beet sugar
- colorings and preservatives
- yeast
- pork
- peanuts
- citrus fruit
- alcohol

EXTREMELY SIMPLE TEST DIETS

The modified exclusion diet for adults

A so-called hypo-allergenic diet, or modified exclusion diet (see page 429), is the most appropriate diet for a large majority of food intolerant people, and works quite well. However, there is a subgroup of people who are quite severely allergic and need a more rigorous diet such as the lamb and pears diet (see below). It is vital that the instructions on how to follow an exclusion diet, given in the Appendix on page 425, are read and understood before starting, and are followed during the diet period. Exclusion diets are best done *once* and *well*. Several half-hearted attempts will serve no purpose.

Lamb and pears diet

Clinical experience shows that a diet of glass-bottled mineral water, lamb or turkey, and pears, for a period of five days after a bowel cleansing program using Epsom salts, can be very useful. It is a very "primitive" diet and is highly unlikely to cause allergies. The regime for this diet can be found on page 429. This is then followed by reintroduction of foods, either one a day, or one at each meal, three times a day, assessing the response according to the principles outlined in the section entitled "Reintroduction of Foods" below.

Juice fast

Some individuals find that a juice fast for a period of five or six days produces an alleviation of symptoms. We do not use this as there is a significant number of individuals who are sensitive to one or more of the juices (such as orange or apple) that are commonly used on juice fasts.

Water-only five-day fast

We have considerable experience of putting patients on this program, and it is sometimes highly beneficial. If they have failed on a modified exclusion diet or a lamb and pears diet, then putting them on a five-day water diet provides reasonably conclusive proof that they are, or are not, food intolerant. However, there are certain metabolic changes that take place on a water-only fast, including changes in thyroid hormone function and an increase in hormones from the adrenal cortex (which have an anti-inflammatory action). It is just possible that some of the symptoms alleviated by a five-day water fast are sometimes in fact alleviated not by the fast itself but by the secondary effect of increasing the secretion of cortisone-like hormones. Such a drastic fast as this can rebound on the individual in that every food as it is reintroduced seems to cause a reaction. **Thus reintroduction should really be done under medical supervision.**

Rotated diet

In this diet, foods of the same family are eaten only once in every four days. If symptoms occur on only one of the four days, this provides a clue as to which foods of that or the previous day might be contributing to the symptoms. This diet can also be used in the treatment (not just the diagnosis) of food allergies.

REINTRODUCTION OF FOODS

The reintroduction of foods should ideally be done during the unmasked period if you are going to base the presence or absence of an intolerance to a specific food on the basis of only one meal. If you have avoided the food over a longer period of time (three or four weeks or more), then you should not introduce more than one food every few days, as you may require a build-up of food challenges in order to precipitate symptoms. It is also worth mentioning here that wheat, and possibly also rye, oats, barley and corn, should be tested for a two-day period, as very often the reactions are delayed by twenty-four hours or more. If you don't do this, you can become confused as to which specific food might be causing the symptoms. For example, you might test wheat on one day, and then eggs on a subsequent day, and then develop symptoms. It would be tempting to assign the precipitation of symptoms to the eggs, whereas, in fact, they may well be due to the wheat. This delayed reaction occurs mostly with wheat, rye and corn, though it can occur with other foods in certain people, and this should be borne in mind when trying to interpret the significance of the development of symptoms after the reintroduction of foods on a daily basis. If in doubt, you should omit the food and then retest it subsequently.

Symptom scoring and sheet

It is quite useful to have a "run-in" period before you start an exclusion diet, during which you record your symptoms on a sheet of paper and score them subjectively (0 = no symptoms, 1 = mild, 2 = moderate, 3 = severe). Then, when you are on the exclusion diet, it is easier to list the severity of any particular symptom as you proceed through the diet. This provides a useful reference to go back to help identify possible offending foods.

Weight reduction

If you lose more than five pounds in the first five or seven days on an exclusion diet, it suggests that you have lost primarily fluid, rather than fat. The off-loading of this retained fluid is an excellent sign that the fluid retention was allergic. Even if your symptoms have not improved over the first few days, weight loss of this order shows that you are on the right track and should persist with the diet.

Reasons for failure of an exclusion diet

Some patients do not do well on exclusion diets, and the reasons are many. First, the person may not be food intolerant at all—the symptoms may be caused by some other condition or illness. Many hormone conditions, chronic infections, intestinal infestations, nutrient deficiencies, vertebral misalignments, and other physical conditions can mimic the symptoms of food intolerance. If all the other reasons for the failure of the diet have been excluded, then it *is* worth going back and taking a look at the original diagnosis and treatment—perhaps something has been missed out, maybe the headaches are due to stress or a misaligned vertebra; tiredness due to a thyroid deficiency or anemia; irritable bowel syndrome or diarrhea due to some intestinal parasite in the bowel; and depression/anxiety/sleep disturbances due to magnesium or vitamin B1 or B6 deficiencies, for example.

A common reason for failure is that the diet has not been done properly, and the offending foods which should have been excluded, have not been—either accidentally, or in a deliberate attempt to thwart the efficacy of the diet, as some people do not really want to lose their symptoms for some psychological reason (see pages 176–177).

Some people don't get better on an exclusion diet because they continue to be exposed to some other environmental factor to which they are allergic—a chemical, an inhalant such as a pollen, grass or mold, a food additive, cigarette smoke or whatever.

Another reason for failure is that the diet itself contains a food item to which the individual is intolerant. A more restricted diet may then need to be followed.

If a person is under severe stress, not sleeping well, being continuously criticized by someone in his or her immediate environment, or is afraid to let people know that he or she is on an elimination diet, this can be too much of a strain to allow obvious responses to occur. Ideally, an exclusion diet should be done when the individual is not under stress, and when the diet itself can be done properly. It may be a good idea either to take time off from work or to go away from home in order to follow the diet carefully.

DRAWBACKS AND DANGERS OF EXCLUSION DIETS

There are a number of different drawbacks to following the exclusion diet route.

The main problem to be borne in mind (and this is especially relevant to growing children and pregnant or breast-feeding women) is that going on a stringent diet involving the exclusion of certain foods can actually result in a compromise of nutrient intake causing true malnutrition. Some of the worst cases of malnutrition that we see are in patients who have been put on severely restricted diets either on their own initiative, or on the advice of their doctor. **So if you are putting a child on an elimination diet for anything more than two or three weeks, professional dietary advice should be sought on how to ensure an adequate intake of nutrients to provide him or her with the necessary nutrients to continue to grow and develop normally.**

Being on an exclusion diet can be difficult socially because it makes going out to people's homes for dinner or eating in restaurants difficult. When on an exclusion diet for diagnostic purposes you may simply have to turn down dinner invitations for the first two or three weeks in order to establish the diagnosis of food intolerance. Once you have actually made the diagnosis and are reintroducing foods, it may be possible to go out to dinner and simply "take the consequences." It is worthwhile making a note of what foods you eat, then if an untoward reaction occurs that night or the following day or two, it is sensible to phone the person who prepared the meal to ask them the specific contents of sauces, etc.

The Treatment of Food Allergy

We have looked at food allergy in some detail but so far have not yet seen what to do if an individual is allergic or intolerant to a specific food. Clearly the ideal solution is to avoid the offending foods. This is the most sensible approach. It may involve some hardship for the individual, but more often than not, if the symptoms go, the social and gastronomic drawbacks of excluding a given food are usually considered well worth while.

After avoiding a food for eight to twelve weeks, it is well worth trying it again (in small quantities), to see if the symptoms come back. Many people can get away with eating a small amount of a previously offending food occasionally, and this can be useful when you are invited out to eat with friends or business colleagues. However, some people can be lulled into a false sense of security, and when they see that they no longer appear to react to a specific food, go back to eating it daily or almost daily. Unfortunately, after a few days, weeks or months, they usually start to develop symptoms again, which may or may not be similar or identical to the symptoms they experienced prior to excluding the food from their diet.

INCREASING YOUR ABILITY TO RESIST FOOD ALLERGIES

There are a number of ways in which you can increase your adaptive capacity and so be less likely to be allergic to food. Here are a few tips that we have found to work well.

Avoid "junk" and processed foods

A diet that is rich in refined and processed foods is very often calorie-dense, nutrient-poor and loaded with various substances that do not occur naturally (colorings, flavorings, etc.) and with which the body does not necessarily have any genetic ability to cope. So it is good, sound, common sense on general health grounds, as well as in specific allergy situations, to eat wholesome, natural, unprocessed foods, fresh fruit and vegetables and to limit the amount of meat and dairy products you eat.

Ensure that you eat a good, nutritious diet in adequate quantities

(see Appendix 1)

By avoiding or eliminating certain foods from your diet, it is possible to compromise your nutrient intake to the degree that you can become truly deficient. Not only is the right type of food important, but it has to be taken in adequate quantities so that there is no excessive weight loss. Ideally, you should eat a wide range of different food items and not limit yourself to the same few foods repeatedly day after day.

Stop smoking

Smoking is a major environmental stressor. It taxes the body's ability to adapt to environmental challenges and impairs the ability of the pancreas to digest food. The simple act of stopping smoking can result in a resurgence of level of health, and an increased ability to adapt to the foods we eat.

Come off the contraceptive pill

Similarly, the Pill, for many women, is a major environmental stressor, which has profound effects on their metabolism (see page 308). Some women develop food allergies soon after going onto the Pill. By stopping smoking and coming off the Pill, a woman may substantially increase her ability to tolerate foods. Often pregnancy results in a considerable lessening of food allergy symptoms.

Avoid medical drugs, if possible

Certain types of medical drugs are associated with toxic side-effects, and this should be borne in mind if you are taking such a drug in the long term. **Be sure that you come off your drugs under close medical supervision, as reading this book is absolutely no substitute for the personal medical care of your own doctor.** Coming off drugs is discussed in more detail elsewhere (see page 133).

Keep alcohol to a minimum

Excessive, or even moderate, drinking can increase the tendency to develop food allergies.

Sort out any underlying physical condition

Certain types of infection, including chronic candidiasis (see page 346), can be associated with an apparent increased susceptibility to food allergic problems. Hormone imbalances can create the impression that there are a number of food intolerances. Correction of hormone imbalances can result in a reduction of food intolerance symptoms in genuinely food intolerant individuals, and a resurgence of health.

Bowel overgrowth (see page 210) can result in the absorption of a number of "alien" toxins into the system, and an impairment in bowel function. Correcting this condition can produce a resurgence of health, and over subsequent months food intolerance symptoms often disappear or diminish.

NUTRITIONAL SUPPLEMENTS

Nutritional supplements can be of considerable value in improving a person's level of health. We have patients who have always thought of themselves as food intolerant, yet who are in fact obviously deficient in a number of different vitamins, minerals and essential fatty acids. When treated adequately with the appropriate nutritional supplements, they experience a profound reduction in their symptoms without ever having food intolerance investigations.

Anyone who has proven food intolerances and who has a continuing low level of health, should seriously consider taking a good nutritional supplement for ninety days or so. (For details of this, see page 422.)

Deficiency of iron may aggravate cows' milk intolerance in children. In our experience, deficiencies of zinc, magnesium, and iron, together with B vitamins, are particularly common in people with food allergies.

B vitamins

Some people may be intolerant of one or more of the components of nutritional supplements themselves. For example, B vitamins that are yeast-derived can cause trouble in those who are yeast sensitive. This is one of the reasons why some people get no benefit or even get worse by going onto "natural" vitamin B complex supplements. Taking synthetic vitamin B complex preparations either in pure powder form or in a hypo-allergenic formulation can result in an improvement.

Vitamin C

Some people benefit from as much as several grams of vitamin C per day, either in tablet or powder form, despite the fact that sound evidence in the scientific literature that this is necessary is scarce. We have found this to be very useful in our clinical experience. It is sometimes worth trying different brands of vitamin C to see if there is any difference in the degree of tolerance you have to each. Vitamin C can, in theory, worsen some food allergy and inflammatory disease mechanisms, though this is probably very rare.

Vitamin A

Taking vitamin A can produce an improvement in food intolerance symptoms, possibly because it can improve the quality of the lining of the intestine.

Zinc

Zinc is so commonly deficient in chronically food intolerant people, that a supplement of between 10 and 30 mg is usually necessary and can, alone, produce a reduction in symptoms.

Magnesium

A deficiency of this element can aggravate the mechanisms of allergy and result in a wide range of symptoms (see page 54) which may be confused with food intolerance. Doses in adults should be 200–400 mg per day if proven deficient.

Calcium and vitamin D

Both of these nutrients are commonly found to be in short supply in exclusion diets, and growing children are prone to deficiency. You should consider the possibility of giving calcium and/or vitamin D supplements to a child on a milk-free diet. As we point out elsewhere (see page 46) calcium should be given with magnesium in the ratio of at least 2:1 or less. Don't overdo the calcium with respect to magnesium.

Manganese

Manganese is also essential for carbohydrate metabolism, and is often in poor supply in food intolerant people, especially those who have been on exclusion diets for prolonged periods. Low blood sugar (hypoglycemia) can be the result (see page 292).

Amino acids

We have found that 2 g of a mixed free-form amino acid can be useful in some people as it may well be that the food intolerance has been initiated or worsened by poor pancreatic secretion, which in turn causes inadequate digestion of dietary protein, so producing an amino acid deficiency.

Essential fatty acids

Some foods can inhibit certain enzymes involved in the metabolism of essential fatty acids (see page 107). Some people have reduced activity of an enzyme called delta-6-desaturase which is involved in the conversion of dietary linoleic acid to gamma-linolenic acid. Supplementation with evening primrose oil (Efamol or Naudicelle Plus) which contains gamma-linolenic acid, can reduce their food intolerance symptoms. Similarly, since animal meat is deficient in an important fatty acid called eicosapentanoic acid (EPA), supplementation with fish oil (MaxEPA) can also be helpful.

Another form of essential fatty acids that is useful to use for food intolerance is cold-pressed linseed oil. This contains substantial quantities of the two major groups of essential fatty acids. Don't forget to keep cold-pressed linseed oil in the refrigerator, with the top tightly closed. Alternatively, it can be decanted into a wide-necked jar and kept in the freezer. By doing this, oxidation and thus deterioration of the essential oils are kept to a minimum, so reducing toxicity. **Do not confuse cold-pressed linseed oil with the highly toxic linseed oil used to oil furniture.**

Digestive enzymes

On the basis that certain mechanisms underlying food intolerance can involve inadequate digestion of dietary proteins, it seems logical to use digestive enzymes in the treatment of food intolerance. In our experience, symptoms such as irritable bowel syndrome and mental symptoms respond quite well to the use of pancreatic enzymes, glutamic acid hydrochloride (or betaine hydrochloride) to replace poor gastric acid secretion, and pepsin. Smokers and the elderly may be particularly prone to poor digestive function.

DO SOMETHING ABOUT STRESS

Continuous stress in life is not conducive to recovery from any physical condition. This is particularly true of food intolerant people, who are often bombarded with a whole range of different symptoms as a result of their food intolerances. They often find it difficult to cope with diets, especially if, in addition to their food intolerance, they are also disbelieved, criticized, or put under pressure by their family, colleagues at work, or even their doctor. Sometimes professional counseling is needed to cope with these stressful situations. A considerable improvement in well-being, health and symptoms can occur simply by homing in on major areas of emotional stress. A certain percentage of chronically food intolerant individuals are reluctant even to consider the possibility that their symptoms might, at least in part, be due to stress. This is a pity because they deny themselves a very positive therapeutic way of improving their level of health.

We have found that if a particular individual is reluctant to confront this side of their illness, there are usually only two main possibilities; first, they have a definite, albeit unconscious, interest in maintaining their symptoms, and although they may consciously say they want to go through the motions of food intolerance investigations, unconsciously they want to remain ill. Maybe it suits them to be ill, in that they can get sympathy from a spouse, their family and friends, or can control them in some way. This may appear cynical, but it is common and can act as a real barrier to recovery. Second, they may actually be *unable* to confront the specific areas which are causing them the greatest stress. This can only be helped by gentle, skilled and compassionate counseling.

ADEQUATE SLEEP

Getting enough sleep, rest, relaxation, exercise and productive work are all major factors in increasing one's adaptive capacity. If we don't get enough sleep it is much more difficult to control a whole range of different aspects of our lives. Rest and relaxation are of therapeutic value in themselves. Of course, you can try specific relaxation techniques such as yoga, biofeedback or meditation, and this is to be encouraged where appropriate. Some people benefit from taking regular or occasional enjoyable exercise, perhaps because they produce certain natural chemicals called endorphins and enkephalins during exercise, which improve their sense of well-being and act as a tonic to the system. A daily walk in the fresh air is the minimum recommended.

If somebody is unemployed and sitting around the house, either because of redundancy or their illness, then they can all too easily focus on their own symptoms. Such people need productive activity of one kind or another if they are to pull themselves out of the quagmire of symptoms.

ADEQUATE SUNLIGHT AND FRESH AIR

Sunlight can have marked therapeutic effects. Fresh air itself gets one out of the house, and away from the household pollution which is discussed on page 148.

EXERCISE

This is an important part in the management of the allergic individual. Regular, enjoyable exercise will stimulate metabolism and improve morale. It may help the body cope with allergic reactions. Occasionally, strenuous exercise can precipitate a food allergy, but this is rare.

REDUCE YOUR EXPOSURE TO TOXINS

In our experience, it is well worth while screening for excess body burdens of toxic metals, and one of the best ways of doing this is by hair mineral analysis. We have noticed a small but significant percentage of chronically food and/or chemically intolerant people have excessive body burdens of lead, cadmium, aluminum and mercury. Toxic chemicals encountered in the environment should be kept to a practical minimum (see page 148).

BICARBONATE

Taking a mixture of one teaspoon of sodium bicarbonate (baking soda) dissolved in water can reduce food allergic reactions and can be repeated every few hours. It can also abort a migraine attack.

DRUGS

Occasionally, some drugs may help in food allergy. Sodium chromoglycate powder—from a capsule—can help to "block" certain food allergy reactions. The powder must be taken in water, washed round the mouth then swallowed. It should be taken before meals. Aspirin has been reported to reduce food allergy reactions but it is not very often helpful.

DESENSITIZATION AND IMMUNIZATION

In certain circumstances, when food intolerance has become "intolerable" because of a number of sensitivities, and *all* the steps above have been pursued, the sufferer can be desensitized. Certain clinical ecologists working in the field of food allergy resort to desensitization as a first line of treatment. We don't think this is an appropriate course of action in the vast majority of cases because of the expense, and the fact that the treatment dosages in certain individuals can change quite rapidly. Also, there is a danger of becoming psychologically dependent on having to be protected by the desensitizing treatment in order to be able to ingest certain foods.

The desensitizing solution is used as drops under the tongue or as an injection. Drops can be taken two or three times a day before meals, and the desensitizing injections can be taken daily at first, gradually reducing to twice weekly if possible.

If symptoms reduce within the first two or three weeks of treatment, then the treatment is considered to have been successful. There is a certain percentage of people who do not respond at all to such desensitizing treatments.

Some Problems with the Food Allergy Approach

The most obvious danger when dealing with food allergies is that a severely restricted diet can be inadequate in vitamins, minerals, amino acids or essential fatty acids.

The exclusion of grains and certain vegetables will also substantially reduce dietary fiber intake, and produce other problems such as constipation.

One of the drawbacks of going onto a diet consisting of a severely limited number of foods is that there is a tendency to develop food intolerances. If one is on only a limited number of foods, one has to consume them very frequently and this in itself can produce a sensitivity to those foods. The individual then has a return of or a worsening of his or her symptoms, and then excludes yet more foods. We have had some patients come to us who have ended up on such a ridiculous diet that they can eat nothing but rice and bananas, or even plums and sardines! This is an absurd state of affairs, and does nothing for the nutritional status of the individual!

Some food intolerant people tend to become neurotic and fixated on their condition, to the detriment of their family life and other interests. They become obsessed, talk about nothing but food intolerance, and become extremely boring to those around them. This is understandable in that they may have been suffering for many years from chronic symptoms, and have now found a way of at least controlling them, if only partially.

"LEARNED" REACTIONS

Certain individuals who have food intolerances or who, during periods of stress, develop symptoms following the ingestion of foods, may come to associate their ingestion with a precipitation of symptoms, even in the absence of genuine food intolerance. Such people are labeled "neurotic" by some doctors, but we have seen many food allergic patients who have no manifestations of neuroticism in their daily life, with the single exception of food and eating. Their problem is a *learned* response where they have "learned" to expect a particular reaction. This makes treatment very difficult and generally requires skilled counseling and/or psychological intervention. The whole process involves an "un-learning" of the individual's responses, utilizing a positive approach and optimism that their condition can and will improve.

Conclusion

Food intolerance should always be borne in mind in dealing with chronic health problems. Dealing with it can alleviate suffering. It is *not* a universal panacea but at the same time its under-recognition by the majority of the medical profession means that many people live lives of relative misery, sometimes for many years.

CHEMICAL SENSITIVITY

Dr. Theron Randolph, of Chicago, one of the "fathers" of clinical ecology, brought to the attention of the medical community the fact that individuals can actually be sensitive to inhaled chemicals, and that this can produce a wide range of clinical conditions.

Exposure to formaldehyde (commonly used in cavity wall insulation and synthetic furniture), natural gas supplied to the house, car gasoline fumes, diesel fumes, chemical additives in foods, and so on, can all cause symptoms in susceptible individuals. Many of these are difficult to avoid in twentieth-century Western civilization, which is so dependent on petro-chemical derivatives and synthetics.

Very often, people who have allergies, or are addicted to alcohol, are also sensitive to chemicals. The way the sensitivity can be diagnosed is either by skin testing or by exposing the individual to whatever chemical is being considered as a potential offending item.

Very often, people who are chemically sensitive develop "learned responses"—that is to say, they have expectations that they will feel a particular way when they smell a particular substance. However, despite this (and it is not a *true* sensitivity), there are individuals who are genuinely susceptible to chemicals in the environment.

Very often, an individual who is sensitive to chemicals in the home, for example natural gas, feels much better when they go away and stay with somebody else.

Many of these people suffer from hyperventilation (a sort of compulsive overbreathing) which can itself cause metabolic changes with the precipitation of symptoms or worsening of symptoms that are already there. This should always be borne in mind in individuals who are "exquisitely" chemically sensitive.

Doctors who are aware of the problem of chronic candidiasis (see page 346) are also aware of the fact that many sufferers are also chemically sensitive.

At least one expert in the United States considers that chemical sensitivity can be reduced by taking adequate supplements of selenium and vitamin E and other anti-oxidants (see page 83). Certainly, requirements for vitamin E are increased by exposure to ozone, present in the photochemical smog of big industrial cities.

But the answer for such people may not be simply to tackle the offending chemical. Food allergies, emotional stress, nutrient deficiencies, inadequate exercise, infection, a lack of sunlight, and excessive exposure to electromagnetics (such as living near high tension cables, pylons, etc.), can all contribute to the degree to which an individual may be chemically sensitive. Trying to solve the chemical sensitivity alone, without sorting out these other problems, can lead to environmental paranoia and fear.

In such situations, we find it important not to direct the individual's attention to the difficulties of the environment he or she lives in, but to focus his or her attention onto the positive aspects of recovery by adhering to the sort of lifestyle outlined in this book.

RESPIRATORY ALLERGIES

Of all the well-recognized allergies that affect mankind, asthma is probably the most common.

Asthma

Asthma is a type of reversible airways obstruction characterized by the narrowing of the air passages in the lungs and caused by muscle spasm and mucus secretions. This is an end result which can be caused by a number of different stimuli including inhaled allergens, ingested allergens and inhaled irritants.

Asthma is best divided into childhood and adult types.

CHILDHOOD-ONSET ASTHMA

This is closely linked with the presence of eczema, hay fever, urticaria and migraine in the victim or in his or her close relatives. People with this kind of family history are called atopic. If both parents have a history of atopy then the chances of the child being affected is fifty percent; if one parent is affected, the chance is thirty percent; and if neither parent is affected, the chance is approximately twelve percent.

Childhood asthma may very often be preceded for several months or even years by episodic coughing which later develops into wheezy bronchitis and then eventually into asthma. Such children often have a history of slow recovery from upper respiratory tract viral infections as well as a personal and/or family history of atopy.

It has been suggested that exclusive breast-feeding in infancy could protect against atopic disease but this has recently been questioned.

Interestingly, asthma is particularly uncommon in certain communities, including Eskimos, some North American Indians and Highlanders from Papua, New Guinea. Environmental and/or dietary factors may be important.

ADULT-ONSET ASTHMA

Adult-onset asthma is more common in women than men. There are two broad types. In the first there are no obvious reasons for the asthmatic attacks. In the second, there are fairly obvious trigger factors that precipitate attacks. The sufferer should avoid such triggers but, even so, new allergens will continue to be detected, to be added to the list of external or environmental causes of the condition.

SOME COMMON CAUSES OR TRIGGERS OF ASTHMA

- Inhaled allergens. Commonly inhaled allergens include the house-dust mite; animal danders; pollens, particularly grass; mold spores.
- Irritant gases—including cigarette smoke.
- Ingested allergens: foods; drugs, e.g. aspirin, colored medicines (pills, capsules and syrups); food additives; yeast and molds on food.

- Infecting organisms, either due to the infection itself or an allergy to the organism.
- Temperature changes—especially cold air.
- Changes in the weather.
- Exercise.
- Emotional stress, e.g. bereavement.
- Hormones.
- Certain chemicals in the workplace.

Inhaled allergens

In practice, taking a careful history usually enables us to determine which in the above list is the most likely cause of the asthma. This is particularly important when assessing inhalant allergens. Here are some pointers in identifying the particular allergen that we find useful when seeing people whose asthma is caused by inhaled allergens.

Allergen	*Clinical Feature*
House-dust mite	The person is worse in dusty atmospheres with soft furnishings. Often worse in the autumn, and in the morning after a night's sleep.
Feathers	Worse on contact with feather bedding or pillows.
Molds	May be worse from late summer through the autumn, but can also last all year; particularly bad in damp, warm weather, e.g. after a thunderstorm.
Occupational	Symptoms worse at work and improve at the weekend or on vacation.
Meteorological	May follow sudden changes in the weather. This could be due to pollutants, dust or molds.
Pets	Asthma after contact with cats, dogs, horses, etc.
Pollens	These usually cause asthma during the summer and are often associated with hay fever. Symptoms are worse on warm dry days.

We think it is important to assess whether the person is likely to have an inhalant allergy or not. The presence of a definitive inhalant allergen does not, of course, exclude the possibility that other *ingested* allergens may be present too. Allergies to inhalants can usually be confirmed by skin prick tests performed by a doctor.

Ingested allergens

Food. Almost any food is a potential allergen. Little good research has been done on this, but studies at St. Thomas's Hospital, London, have indicated that the most common allergens are cows' milk, eggs, wheat, artificial colorings, cheese, yeast and fish. Multiple food sensitivities are more often the rule than the exception.

Reactions to a specific food can occur within seconds or minutes, especially if they are severe. However, more often they are delayed by several hours. The use of a modified exclusion diet and the careful assessment of such patients is vital. (See Appendix 3.)

Many researchers have commented that children who have other food allergy symptoms such as eczema, urticaria, tissue swelling, abdominal pain, constipation, vomiting or behavior problems often suffer from asthma or wheezing as well.

Drugs. The occurrence of asthma following the administration of penicillin and other antibiotics is well described, but is, fortunately, relatively rare. Common drugs which may induce asthma are aspirin and other non-steroidal anti-inflammatory drugs. Aspirin-induced asthma has been reported to occur at frequencies of 0.2% to 20% of asthmatic patients. Some people are sensitive to only 30 mg and others require 300 mg. A sensitivity to aspirin is more common in those with nasal polyps. If someone is found to be aspirin sensitive and still has asthmatic symptoms even when he is not taking aspirin he may, in theory, respond to a diet which excludes foods containing natural salicylates. Such foods include many fruits and vegetables (see Appendix 3, Low Salicylate Diet, page 432).

Beta-blocker drugs (such as propranolol) used in the treatment of angina and hypertension, may also induce asthmatic attacks in those who have a tendency to asthma. Because of this they should be used with extreme caution, if at all, by such people.

Food additives. Adverse reactions (including asthma) to food additives have been well described by a number of researchers. Reactions are known to occur to the dye tartrazine, preservatives, benzoates and the preservative metabisulphite. Those who are sensitive to aspirin may also be sensitive to benzoates and/or tartrazine. (See Appendix 3, page 439.)

Metabisulphite is often used as a preservative in wine, home-made or commercially prepared. Unfortunately, the labels on wine bottles do not say so. An individual whose asthma is triggered by wine could be sensitive to metabisulphite or to the yeast content of the wine. Tartrazine sensitivity is particularly common in children. It is a food coloring widely used in sweets, puddings, jellies and squash. Metabisulphite and sulphur dioxide are used in many commercial squashes as well.

Fortunately, the majority of packaged foods now contain, by law, details of their constituents and additives. It is useful to have a source of information on these (see Appendix, page 439). These sources enable people to find out which foods contain agents to which they are sensitive.

On the positive side, certain food substances can have a *beneficial* effect on asthma. There have been reports of caffeine being an effective "cure" in young patients with asthma. The pharmacological agents biochemically similar to caffeine, such as theophylline, are of proven therapeutic value for asthmatics. Caffeine itself is metabolized to theophylline and related compounds. So an asthmatic who suddenly gives up coffee, perhaps because of insomnia or anxiety, may have a sudden or unexpected worsening of his asthma.

HAY FEVER

Descriptions of hay fever in the medical literature were very rare until some 150 years ago, and later nineteenth-century descriptions refer to hay fever being more common among the educated classes. This poses interesting questions on the causes and occurrences of allergy.

The consumption of sucrose in the United Kingdom rose dramatically in the middle of the nineteenth century. Prior to this, consumption was only a few pounds per year and this was mainly by the more affluent classes. The association between increasing sugar consumption and the corresponding increase in hay fever is an interesting one. Furthermore, grass pollen (the most common inhalant allergen in hay fever), sugar and wheat (which is the most common food allergen in adults) are all in the same botanical family of grasses. This may just be coincidence.

In our experience, few nutritional programs are of benefit, in the short term, to hay fever sufferers. We have, however, repeatedly observed that those of our patients who have symptoms of food allergy, when they have excluded those culprit foods and corrected any nutritional imbalances and deficiencies, often notice a significant reduction or even disappearance of their hay fever symptoms in the subsequent summer. This may happen because, by avoiding allergens, they reduce the oversensitivity of the airways in the lungs. In addition, if they increase their intake of certain minerals such as magnesium, and vitamin C, allergy reactions may be reduced, while eating few refined carbohydrates may have beneficial effects on essential fatty acid metabolism as well as on allergic mechanisms in general.

ASTHMA—WHAT YOU CAN DO

The following guidelines show what steps you can take to ensure that your lifestyle and environment are not contributing to your asthma.

Stop smoking

Stop smoking completely and avoid smoke-filled rooms and public places.

Avoid inhaled allergens

(a) **Dust**

House dust contains a variety of potential allergens, the major one being house-dust mite, a tiny insect that is impossible to eliminate entirely. It is concentrated mainly in bedding and it can be a frequent aggravating factor in asthma. The following advice may be useful:

- Vacuum the mattress one or two times a week. It may be useful to cover the mattress with a closely fitted polyethylene sheet. If the mattress is old and dusty, replace it with a new one.
- Vacuum the bedroom, if there is a carpet, once a week. Make sure the bedroom and other rooms are not dusty. Keeping the rooms tidy will make cleaning much easier.
- Damp dust once a week on all surfaces.
- Use a synthetic pillow and synthetic comforter. These tend to attract less dust.
- If a young child is affected by house dust allergy, do not include lots of soft, cuddly toys in the cot, bed or bedroom. These only gather dust.

- The tannin in tea chemically combines with the house-dust mite rendering it inert to the allergic patient. Strong tea (without milk) can be sprayed or brushed onto mattresses and other objects that collect dust.

(b) **Animal fur and feathers**
The hair and skin scales of animals, cat fur in particular, can sometimes be responsible for severe allergies. Firstly, if the child or adult is seriously allergic, do not buy a cat or dog. If a cat or dog is present in the house, it is important that the allergic person should avoid physical contact with the animal. The cat or dog should not enter the bedroom or living rooms, if at all possible. Make sure that bedrooms and living rooms are vacuumed regularly. Horses and other animals can also be a source of allergy.

(c) **Grasses and other pollens**
Pollens from grasses, trees, shrubs and flowers appear in the spring and summer. Tree pollen usually occurs in the early spring, and grass pollen particularly in late spring and early summer. Grass pollen sensitivity is by far the most common, producing hay fever, and exacerbations of asthma. Pollen counts are highest on warm, dry days. On such days, it may be advisable to stay indoors. Going to the seaside, away from fields, may be helpful.

(d) **Molds**
If mold sensitivity is present, it is important to check that there is not a source of mold in the house. All damp patches and mildew should be treated appropriately.

(e) **Rare and occupational asthma, e.g. to chemicals, work materials, dusts, contaminated humidifiers and farm molds.**
This requires specialist advice and treatment.

(f) **Ionizers**
Ionizers may occasionally be useful for individuals who are sensitive to inhalant allergens. An ionizer, by producing negatively charged ions, causes dust and other potential allergens to settle, rather than to remain in the air. Many large drugstores and health food shops can supply a variety of ionizers.

(g) **Desensitization**
If inhalant allergies are carefully identified, one can be desensitized to them by a series of injections given under medical supervision.

Avoid ingested allergens

(a) **Food additives**
Particularly coloring agents, azo-dyes, tartrazine and possibly related compounds found in processed foods and many medications prescribed by doctors. Also sulphites, which are used as a preservative in many drinks and foods, including squashes, wines and lettuce, can precipitate asthma. All asthmatics should avoid these.

(b) **Food allergens**
Common culprits include cows' milk in children, as well as wheat and yeast-based foods in adults. The part played by food allergens in any adult's asthma is best assessed by the use of an exclusion diet (see Appendix 3, page 429).

(c) **Aspirin**
Taking the medication can produce wheezing within a few hours. This may be accompanied by facial flushing, nettle rash, abdominal pain or watering of the nose. The individual may also be sensitive to other painkillers, such as ibuprofen, and salicylate-rich foods. These should be avoided (see Appendix 3, Low Salicylate Diet, page 432).

(d) **Sucrose and refined carbohydrates**
A diet high in sucrose and other refined carbohydrates may aggravate pre-existing allergies, and so should be avoided.

Get exercise

Exercise precipitates asthma in some individuals, but regular physical exercise may actually reduce asthmatic tendencies. Swimming classes for children seem to be particularly worthwhile, especially in a warm, indoor pool.

Supplements

The use of nutritional supplements in the treatment of asthma is not well recognized. However, some recommendations can be made:

(a) **Vitamin B6, 50–100 mg per day**
This is of proven value in reducing the level of even severe asthma, even in those asthmatics who take steroids

(b) **Multivitamins**
Some of the mechanisms involved in asthma could respond to a number of nutritional supplements, including vitamin B6; linseed oil (1–2 tablespoons per day); B-complex vita-

mins (10–20 mg per day); vitamin C (500–1000 mg at least per day); zinc (10–20 mg per day); vitamin E (600 IUs); and perhaps some trace minerals, including selenium. These may have effects upon some of the body chemicals involved in the production of asthma and, like many anti-asthmatic drugs, block or interfere with the metabolism of these agents. This is best combined with a diet avoiding sugar (sucrose), additives and low in animal fats.

(c) **Digestive supplements**
As long ago as 1931, it was shown that children with asthma can produce too little acid in their stomachs. Supplements of hydrochloric acid may be useful. Also, individuals with poor pancreatic function, (such as insulin-dependent diabetics), may respond to pancreatic supplements. You must consult your doctor about this.

(d) **Premenstrual asthma**
Many women experience a worsening of their asthma premenstrually, and treatment of this condition with a nutritional program can be valuable. Vitamin B6 (100–200 mg per day) and magnesium (200–300 mg per day), may be worthwhile. Magnesium appears to stabilize some of the allergy cells that are involved in the triggering of asthma.

Avoid stress

Stress situations are known to trigger asthma, particularly if the attacks have been associated with them in the past. Avoiding stressful situations can be helpful.

Drugs

Drugs are often necessary in the treatment of asthma (either in the form of an inhaler or as tablets) and some drugs may help particularly in those with food allergy-induced asthma. Sodium cromoglycate by mouth can be useful in some individuals with food allergic asthma.

If you appear to have asthma for no obvious cause, the first step is to ensure that you are not coming into contact with inhalants, such as house-dust mites or molds, to which you are sensitive. The next step is to make sure that you have no nutritional deficiencies. It makes sense to try a multivitamin supplement high in vitamin B6. If this doesn't work try using a type of exclusion diet. In mild cases, avoiding food additives, aspirin and other painkillers, and reducing your intake of refined carbohydrates, can produce a considerable improvement. In more severe cases, a formal exclusion diet, with the careful reintroduction of foods (see Appendix 3) will be necessary **under the supervision of your doctor.**

PART THREE

The Nutritional Management of Some Diseases and Common Ailments

INTRODUCTION

When considering the importance of nutrition to man's health, it is useful to think of the body as a biochemical machine. The quality of the fuel supply will determine not only the immediate performance of the machine, but also the way in which the machine will wear out. If you put paraffin instead of gasoline into your car you would hardly be surprised if it didn't start or work as well as it should. Similarly, the quality and quantity of our food supply profoundly affect health. An intelligent use of the vast amount of information that there already is about the importance of nutrition will allow us both to prevent and manage many current-day ills better than we do at present.

Disease Prevention

History has taught a lot about the prevention of disease, and prevention is often more economical than treatment. In the last hundred years for example, the number of deaths from tuberculosis in the UK fell from over one thousand a year to one hundred a year in the 1950s and now to only a handful of cases a year. While most people imagine that this fall was due to the introduction of mass X-rays, vaccination and the use of powerful anti-tuberculosis drugs, in fact, most of the decline preceded their introduction and was due mainly to improved housing, hygiene and nutrition.

There are many ways in which nutritional treatment can be used to manage, treat and prevent disease. These include:

- The use of individual nutrients to correct specific deficiencies.
- The use of individual nutrients in the treatment of illness either by the correction of a deficiency or, in some highly specialized situations, by its use as a drug.
- The use of multiple supplements, particularly in complex disease states or in the elderly.

- The use of specialized diets for diagnostic purposes; for example, exclusion diets for food allergy.
- The use of specialized diets in the treatment of illness; for example, the reduction or elimination of tea, coffee and cola-based drinks from the diet for women with benign breast disease.
- The use of diets or additional supplements to prevent chronic degenerative illness; for example, dietary changes to reduce cancer risk and cardiovascular disease.
- The use of dietary education in the community to prevent the occurrence of nutritional deficiencies or imbalances.

It's fairly obvious, then, that the role of diet is not simply limited to those who have diabetes or those with other "medical" diseases; we are all at risk to some extent and will benefit from using nutritional treatments in one way or another.

This part of the book looks at how these treatments can be used in many common diseases and ailments. We give many recommendations for ways in which you can help yourself. **Where treatment should not be undertaken except under medical supervision, we have said so.**

GASTROINTESTINAL CONDITIONS

The gastrointestinal tract, especially the absorptive surface of the bowel, is the interface between the individual's metabolism and one of the major aspects of his or her environment, the diet. Normal gastrointestinal function is thus of fundamental importance in the maintenance of health. Anyone with a significant malfunction of the gastrointestinal tract would find it extremely difficult, if not impossible, to maintain optimum health, however good their diet.

The Digestive Process

Food contains proteins, fats and carbohydrates, all of which must be broken down prior to being absorbed in the intestine.

The smell and the anticipation of food enhance the secretion of digestive juices in the mouth and stomach. Saliva contains an enzyme which breaks down starch, and it is produced both in anticipation of food and during chewing. It is important to chew food thoroughly because it both breaks the food up and stimulates the digestive secretions further on.

The stomach produces hydrochloric acid and pepsin which are necessary for the breakdown of proteins. A complete failure or even a reduced secretion of hydrochloric acid (which is relatively common), will reduce the activity of pepsin, and so impair protein digestion. The mechanical action of the stomach further mulches the food into a more digestible form. In the duodenum (the first part of the small intestine), pancreatic secretions are required to break the food down further. Bile salts and bile acids from the liver are added, and these are needed for the correct digestion of fats. If any of these processes is interfered with, ingested foods will be propelled down the intestinal tract inadequately prepared for this stage of digestion. This can cause symptoms that would not occur if digestive enzyme secretion and food breakdown were functioning normally.

Appetite is an important part of nutrition and normal gastrointestinal function. It influences the anticipation of food, the rate at which food is consumed and the secretion of digestive juices. There are a number of different factors that influence appetite, including anticipation, smell and taste, (impairment of either of these can result in a reduced appetite), general well-being, nutritional state, hormonal factors, drugs, and the degree to which an individual has been educated to the idea that a particular food is desirable or undesirable.

Almost any part of this complex process can go wrong and produce problems with digestion or nutrition generally.

Let us look at the most important gastrointestinal conditions starting at the top of the system in the mouth.

Nutrition and the Mouth

The lips and the mouth are the beginning of the gastrointestinal tract and any gastrointestinal, as well as general, diseases can produce symptoms and signs here.

Redness and scaling of the junction of the lining of the mouth and the lips (cheilosis) is a feature of riboflavin (vitamin B2) deficiency.

Angular cheilosis is a redness, soreness and cracking at the corners of the mouth. In the elderly, ill-fitting dentures are a common cause but nutritional factors should *always* be thought of, including riboflavin deficiency, pyridoxine deficiency, and iron deficiency with or without anemia. Folic acid deficiency can also cause it as can an infection with candida albicans (see page 404.) If you think you have angular cheilosis, it is important to see your doctor so that he can examine you for other evidence of any of the above vitamin or mineral deficiencies. He will also look for evidence of thrush in your mouth or elsewhere.

You can try taking 50 mg per day of vitamin B complex for a few weeks, as well as having ill-fitting dentures attended to, as a useful first step, but measuring serum iron, vitamins B12 and red cell folate is essential if the mouth soreness does not resolve quickly—your doctor can arrange this.

Nutritional deficiencies can also affect the tongue. A smooth, painful tongue can be caused by vitamin B12, folate, or iron deficiencies, and their appearances are indistinguishable. Vitamin B12 deficiency, however, does not produce angular cheilosis.

Severe mouth ulceration and sensitivity to gluten

Gluten is the protein found in wheat, rye, oats and barley. When somebody is intolerant of this protein and has specific changes in the intestinal tract, it is called celiac disease. However, gluten sensitivity can exist without the diagnosis of celiac disease being made (see page 208). Charles is a good example of somebody who had had severe, recurrent mouth ulceration intermittently over the previous ten years, and for which no obvious cause could be found. During the episodes of ulceration, where his throat became red and raw and he was unable to eat, he would lose anything up to fourteen to twenty-one pounds over a six week period, simply because it was too painful to eat. Blood tests showed that he was sensitive to gluten, and exclusion of gluten from his diet resulted in a complete absence of these episodes of severe ulceration for eighteen months. He became somewhat complacent about the situation and went away on vacation, where he consumed bread over a two week period and, at the end of it, experienced another bout of nasty mouth ulceration, which lasted for four weeks. Two years later he has not had any recurrence of his mouth ulceration and he sticks strictly to his gluten-free diet. It was also interesting to note that, initially, he had a drastic zinc deficiency, which often goes along with gluten sensitivity. This was corrected using a supplement of 30 mg of zinc taken last thing at night.

Tongue changes also occur in deficiencies of riboflavin, niacin and pyridoxine, but not of thiamin. Descriptions of these are given on page 404.

The presence of tiny bleeding areas under the tongue can be a sign of vitamin C deficiency (see page 404).

Oral ulceration has many causes. Aphthous ulceration (common mouth ulcers) is undoubtedly a very frequent complaint and, if recurrent, can be due to food allergy or deficiencies of iron, folic acid, vitamin B12 and vitamin B6. Try taking a multivitamin supplement and going on a modified exclusion diet (see Appendix 3, page 429).

DRY MOUTH

Failure or dysfunction of the salivary and other related glands is a feature, in animals, of essential fatty acid deficiency. Trying a course of evening primrose oil (three or four 500 mg capsules twice a day) together with high-dose vitamin C (500 mg twice a day) and B6 (25–50 mg twice a day) has been found to produce both subjective and objective improvement in some people. Supplementation with zinc (10–15 mg a day) may also be appropriate. Food allergy is another possibility too.

CANCER

Some types of early cancerous change in the mouth have responded to high doses of vitamin A and beta-carotene. **This needs to be supervised medically.**

TASTE

One important function of the mouth is to taste. A lack of taste can reduce appetite and certainly impairs one's enjoyment of food. Taste can be impaired as a result of the loss of a sense of smell, with a common cold or hay fever, or directly as a result of a disturbance of taste perception itself.

Impairment of taste perception is a well-recognized feature of zinc deficiency and is used diagnostically to assess zinc deficiency states. Poor appetite is a feature of zinc deficiency.

HALITOSIS (bad breath)

Bad breath is a very common problem and can be a social embarrassment. It is a sign of poor health and should always be followed up and treated.

This list outlines some of the most common causes of bad breath:

- food allergy/intolerance (see page 154)
- dental and gum disease
- hypochlorhydria or achlorhydria causing bacterial fermentation in the stomach (see pages 206 and 207)
- throat/nose/sinus/mouth/chest infection
- underlying illness, such as diabetes (see page 286)
- ketosis and various metabolic disorders associated with distinctive breath smell
- smoking and certain drugs and foods.

Someone who has fasted for some time will have the sweet (pear-drops) smell of ketones on their breath. This simply means that they are metabolizing fats, and are in need of a meal.

The Stomach

INDIGESTION/DYSPEPSIA

Indigestion is a vague term used to describe abdominal discomfort following eating. More specifically, dyspepsia refers to discomfort in the upper abdomen, just below the breastbone, which occurs after eating.

Many people go to their doctors complaining of indigestion. When asked if there are any dietary steps that can be taken to alleviate symptoms, the general practitioner may not always be able to give specific advice. This section is designed to advise readers as to how they can best set about minimizing their symptoms of indigestion, while at the same time pointing out those situations in which they should go to their doctor.

Gastritis is inflammation of the stomach lining without peptic ulceration (an ulcer caused by digestive-juice activity, see page 202). This form of dyspepsia should be investigated, as there can be quite severe problems if it is left untreated. If the pain radiates through to the back, or if there is associated vomiting or severe abdominal pain, then these are all good reasons for consulting your doctor.

Quite often, a barium meal X-ray will not reveal an ulcer, and looking at the stomach or duodenum with a flexible telescope (gastroscopy or duodenoscopy) will reveal either a mild inflammation of the stomach or duodenal lining, or none at all, yet the person has very real symptoms.

There are a number of contributing factors which can promote gastritis. These include smoking, alcohol and the frequent or excessive use of tea and coffee.

Some people recognize that certain foods, such as spicy or fatty foods, can make their symptoms worse. Obviously these should be avoided if this is the case.

Professor John Yudkin demonstrated, at St. Stephen's Hospital, London, that thirteen out of twenty-two patients with dyspepsia, whose X-rays showed no signs of peptic ulceration, improved substantially when they went on a low-carbohydrate diet. The results strongly suggested that sucrose (table sugar) is involved in the production of chronic gastritis, and perhaps also of gastric and duodenal ulcers. Furthermore, eight out of nine patients with hiatus hernia did better when they too excluded refined carbohydrates.

Stress has been known to affect the digestive process for many years, and this should be borne in mind in the event of persistent indigestion.

Although gastritis is commonly thought to be caused by too much gastric acid, many people with dyspepsia do not get better when they take antacids such as magnesium or aluminum hydroxide. In fact, gastritis can be associated with too little as well as too much gastric acid. In such circumstances, we have found that in a number of cases symptoms have responded to hydrochloric and pepsin supplements.

Food intolerance is becoming increasingly recognized as a cause of dyspepsia and has been associated with both under-secretion and over-secretion of gastric acid. In both events, a "gastritis"-type set of symptoms can occur.

The chronic presence in the stomach of a yeast organism called candida (see page 346) can cause gastric burning following eating, and can clear up as a result of treatment with an anti-candida medication such as nystatin. Reflux esophagitis and hiatus hernia (see page 205) can also cause dyspepsia.

Gall-bladder disease, be it stones in the gall-bladder or chronic inflammation or infection of the gall-bladder, can cause abdominal pain and discomfort just under the ribs on the right side, and even into the upper central part of the abdomen. Food intolerance has been shown to be a factor (see page 154) in symptomatic gall-bladder problems, but people with a large number of gallstones may find it preferable to have the gall-bladder removed by an operation.

Three rather more sinister, but much rarer, situations that can cause "indigestion" include cancer of the stomach, coronary heart disease (angina), and acute or chronic pancreatitis. These three should be investigated fully and thoroughly by your family doctor or specialist. **Anyone with severe or persistent pain,**

weight loss, vomiting or who develops resistant diarrhea or constipation should consult their doctor immediately.

What to do about indigestion, persistent diarrhea or constipation

1. Discuss the symptoms with your doctor; he may very well suggest that you go on a bland diet, including lots of sloppy foods such as milk and milk puddings. This isn't always a good idea, as milk has been shown to *increase* hydrochloric acid secretion in a percentage of individuals and this in turn can make the symptoms worse. We have had several patients with both X-ray-positive dyspepsia (a real peptic ulcer) and X-ray-negative dyspepsia, who have improved on the exclusion of milk products from their diet. However, there may be other foods as well as milk which could be making things worse, and a failure to improve following the exclusion of milk does not exclude the possibility of a food intolerance. Your doctor may decide to send you for a barium meal which shows up the lining of the stomach and duodenum and can demonstrate the presence of either esophageal reflux, hiatus hernia, gastric ulcer or duodenal ulcer. Another useful investigation is endoscopy in which a small telescope is passed down into the esophagus, stomach and duodenum, to enable the linings of these organs to be viewed by a specialist. The diagnosis of gastritis and ulcer can be made in this way and it has the added advantage of allowing the specialist to take a sample of any abnormal-looking tissue, so that it can be looked at more closely under the microscope and a definite diagnosis made.

Alternatively, your doctor may give you medication such as an antacid (aluminum hydroxide is commonly used). This can be useful to make a diagnosis but should not be used for long as it can interfere with the absorption of essential nutrients such as calcium, magnesium, iron and phosphorus. Dyspepsia caused by *excessive* gastric acid secretion can improve as a result of taking antacids. Antacids are readily available over the counter from the pharmacist and you can buy them without prescription. If the symptoms do not improve with antacids, then it is either because they are not in fact caused by excessive acid secretion, or because there is an ulcer so severe that such treatment is inadequate.

If your doctor suspects something more serious he may very well refer you to a specialist.

2. It makes sense to stay off those foods that you know make your symptoms worse. These may be spicy or fatty foods,

or other foods which you will be able to recognize yourself. When excluding one or more foods, it is important to ensure that you have a nutritionally adequate diet. If symptoms persist, then see your doctor.

3. Do not necessarily take milk and milk products as a treatment for symptoms. Milk, sugar, sweet foods, wheat (including wholegrain bread) and bran often produce symptoms of abdominal discomfort.

4. Cut out smoking, alcohol, tea and coffee drinking. All these are known to be causes of dyspepsia or to make it worse in susceptible individuals.

5. If antacids have not worked, try taking pepsin and betaine hydrochloride (200 mg), one to three tablets at the start of each meal (see Appendix 2). If there is an acute worsening of symptoms it may be that they are due to excessive gastric acid secretion. You should not continue to use such supplements.

6. Stay off refined foods, especially those foods containing sugar.

7. Follow the anti-hypoglycemic diet (see page 295).

8. On the understanding that there is no serious underlying condition, and if cutting out smoking, alcohol, tea, coffee, refined carbohydrates including sugar, and any foods known to exacerbate symptoms, has not resulted in the symptoms clearing up, then it may be worth while trying a modified exclusion diet, as outlined in the Appendix (page 429).

9. Eat in unhurried, relaxed surroundings. Indigestion is

A case of gastritis

Jim was a sixty-eight-year-old retired bank manager, living in retirement with his wife by the seaside. He came for advice on how to stay healthy. On questioning him he admitted to being very fit apart from a recurrent pain in the upper abdomen, just below the breast bone, for the last fifteen years. A barium meal X-ray revealed no ulcer. He turned out to be particularly fond of biscuits, sugar in his tea, ice cream and sweet, fizzy drinks. Removal of sugar from his diet resulted in a complete disappearance of this ulcer-type pain.

Non-ulcer dyspepsia has been shown by Professor John Yudkin of London University to be associated, in many instances, with sugar ingestion. Jim's condition was an example of this.

often helped by eating slowly and chewing your food well.

10. Indigestion and dyspepsia are often associated with stress, and various lifestyle factors. This makes it sensible to consider learning relaxation techniques and making adjustments in your lifestyle which will bring about a reduction or disappearance of your symptoms.

11. Indigestion and dyspepsia can sometimes resolve on the anti-candida program (see page 348).

12. Vitamin C and zinc supplements can help heal gastritis and peptic ulceration. Vitamin C should be in a buffered form (e.g. calcium ascorbate 200–500 mg per day) so as not to irritate the stomach.

PEPTIC ULCER

Peptic ulcers are breaks in the lining of the stomach or duodenum which become irritated by the acidic contents of the stomach. Exactly what causes them in the first place isn't known. Whatever the cause, they are very common. Ulcer dyspepsia is a convenient term which covers any condition with the clinical features of an ulcer, but in which the diagnosis has not been confirmed using X-rays or other diagnostic techniques. In most cases the condition starts before the age of thirty-five and it is four times more common in men than women.

Gastric ulcer

Patients with gastric (stomach) ulcers tend to have a reduced gastric acid output and the ulcers tend to occur in an area affected by chronic gastritis. The majority of these ulcers occur in the part of the stomach that leads into the duodenum. No one knows how gastric ulceration develops, but factors that have been proposed include delayed gastric emptying, over-secretion of gastric acid, damage to the stomach lining, reduced resistance followed by gastric ulceration with a parallel reduction in hydrochloric acid secretion. There is also a lot of evidence that bile flushes back from the duodenum into the stomach of those with gastric ulcers.

Certain factors appear to increase the risk of getting a gastric ulcer. They include:

- chronic gastritis
- blood group A
- increase in age
- lower socio-economic class
- cigarette smoking and alcohol

- use of drugs—aspirin, other non-steroidal anti-inflammatory drugs (such as Indocid, etc.), steroids (such as hydrocortisone, prednisone)

Duodenal ulcer

Duodenal ulcers are almost always associated with gastric over-acidity. Stress seems to play a greater part than in the development of gastric ulcers and the initial age of onset of symptoms is usually very much younger (before thirty-five years).

Factors which increase the risk of duodenal ulceration:

- gastric over-acidity
- blood group O
- psychological factors
- pulmonary emphysema
- alcoholic cirrhosis

TREATMENT OF PEPTIC ULCERATION

Emergency hospitalization is essential if the ulcer perforates or hemorrhages.

Diet

There is now some controversy about recommending a sloppy milk diet or a high-fiber diet for duodenal ulcer. This is not surprising, since milk and wheat fiber are two of the most common food items to which individuals can be sensitive. Several studies have now found that acid secretion is actually *raised* after drinks of milk and milky foods, so perhaps duodenal ulcer sufferers should avoid milk, since they are already producing too much acid.

Smoking

Smoking increases gastric acid secretion which is not conducive to the healing of a peptic ulcer. Continuing to smoke has also been shown to be a reason for failure of treatment with the drug cimetidine. Stopping smoking is probably the single most effective treatment available.

Nutritional status

Vitamin C, vitamin A and zinc, amongst other things, are important in the healing process of any ulcer, and peptic ulcers are no exception. It is important that the nutritional status of an individual be assessed if there is any suggestion that his or her heal-

Gastric ulcer and milk allergy

It has been known since the 1940s that gastric ulceration can be caused by intolerance of particular foods, but this has not found its way into routine medical practice. The case of Esme from Canterbury illustrates this well. This forty-six-year-old lady had migraines, X-ray proven gastric ulceration, and persistence of symptoms despite being put on a "sloppy diet," which consists of a great deal of milky food products which were considered to be less irritating to the stomach. She was put on a five-day lamb and pears and bottled spring-water diet, and experienced the worst migraine of her life, requiring injections of painkillers. Reintroduction of foods revealed that she was intolerant of cows' milk products and, by avoiding these, she experienced a rapid clearing of the symptoms of peptic ulceration and has remained trouble-free since. This is a good example of how treatment itself can provoke symptoms and prevent recovery. There are many factors involved in the development of gastric ulcer (see text) and it is only a very small number that are due to cows' milk intolerance.

ing rate is not as it should be. Patients with gastric ulcers, for example, are known to be at risk from vitamin B6 deficiency.

Drug treatment

Antacids are commonly used in the initial treatment of peptic ulceration. Many of these contain aluminum, the long-term safety of which is currently being questioned (see page 94).

Tripotassium dicitrato-bismuthate (TDB) seems to be comparable in success rate with the H2-antagonists.

The H2-antagonists *cimetidine* and *ranitidine*—which block the secretion of hydrochloric acid—have proved to be of great value in promoting the healing of peptic ulcers *but* they are extremely expensive and, in our opinion, they should not be prescribed unless the above recommendations have failed, or if, for some reason, they cannot be carried out. In any event they should not be prescribed for more than a few weeks since they cause profound inhibition of some essential trace elements with detrimental health effects.

Carbenoxolone is a licorice-derived substance which has been in use for many years, and has been shown to be of benefit. It has the disadvantage of causing salt retention in the body so should not be prescribed to people with hypertension, and those with congestive heart failure.

Food allergy investigations

In many instances, food intolerance is a substantial contributing factor to the development of the condition.

Vitamin E

The use of vitamin E in the treatment of peptic ulcers warrants further investigation, as recent studies have reported links between vitamin E deficiency and ulcers.

Nutritional consequences of the treatment of peptic ulceration

- Excessive use of antacids can lead to the impaired absorption of certain micronutrients (especially of iron and calcium).
- The excessive consumption of milk and antacids can produce very raised levels of calcium in the tissues and in the urine, leading to kidney stones.
- The over-consumption of milky and sloppy foods can produce obesity.
- A poor appetite in gastric ulcer can lead to reduced food consumption and even malnutrition.
- Sloppy diets in milk intolerant patients can worsen symptoms or prevent recovery.
- Some people, on stopping smoking, eat much more and become fat.

Summary of advice for patients with peptic ulceration

- do not smoke or drink alcohol
- eat regularly and basic healthy food
- eat slowly, chew well
- avoid foods that aggravate your symptoms

REFLUX ESOPHAGITIS AND HIATUS HERNIA

Reflux esophagitis is a condition in which the normally tight valve (the sphincter) between the stomach and the esophagus relaxes and lets gastric juice flow back up into the lower end of the esophagus. This causes heartburn (pain behind the breastbone). In a hiatus hernia the valve area is too high up in the chest and acid refluxes up into the esophagus. This condition is usually seen in the overweight or in pregnant women, but not exclusively so.

Smoking leads to a fall in sphincter pressure which then allows reflux to occur and thereby cause heartburn and indigestion. Alcohol increases the production of gastric acid and therefore contributes to the symptomatic problems.

What to do if you have reflux or a hiatus hernia

- raise the head of your bed or sleep with several pillows
- avoid stooping, and constricting pressure on the abdomen (from corsets etc.)
- take no food in the three hours before going to bed
- stop smoking
- avoid alcohol, or drink in moderation, always with food
- lose weight
- avoid sugar
- chew well and eat slowly

DISORDERS OF HYDROCHLORIC ACID SECRETION

Hydrochloric acid secretion in the stomach is an important part of the digestive process, and interference with this process can be a potential source of malnutrition. Hydrochloric acid is essential for the absorption of several trace minerals (most notably calcium and iron, and possibly also other minerals); furthermore, pepsin, the main gastric enzyme, must have an acid environment for its activity, and hypochlorhydria (a low level of hydrochloric acid) or achlorhydria (absence of this acid) results in a reduced activity of the enzyme.

Excessive secretion of hydrochloric acid is associated with over-acidity, gastritis and duodenal ulceration.

Many conditions can produce a gastritis with symptoms very much akin to those of peptic ulceration. Obviously it is important for your doctor to exclude major diagnoses, but once these have been excluded and you still aren't getting relief from antacids and/or a special diet (as outlined above in the section on peptic ulcers) you should bear in mind that the symptoms may in fact be due to an *underproduction* of hydrochloric acid and that the correct treatment involves the exact opposite of antacids—taking hydrochloric acid supplements.

There are a number of preparations containing medicinal hydrochloric acid, such as betaine hydrochloride (Acidol Pepsin) and glutamic acid hydrochloric (Muripsin). It is sensible to try one or other of these, but it is important to start with a small dose at the beginning of a meal and if there is a worsening of symptoms, to discontinue the therapy immediately. However, if there are no adverse side effects the dosage can be increased (according to the manufacturer's recommendations) and progress observed. A significant percentage of patients we treat in this way report an improvement in their symptoms.

People who have hypochlorhydria and achlorhydria are more susceptible to the salmonella infections which cause food poisoning, presumably because the bacteria are less easily destroyed in the stomach acid, which is what normally happens.

Gastric fermentation

In someone with achlorhydria, micro-organisms can exist in the stomach, as they are not subjected to the hostile effects of hydrochloric acid, and this can result in fermentation with the production of foul-smelling gas. This can be recognized quite readily and can be resolved by taking hydrochloric acid or (less preferably) antibiotics. It is worth trying hydrochloric acid supplements first, before resorting to antibiotics, as antibiotics can disrupt bowel microflora (see page 210).

Making a diagnosis of hypochlorhydria or achlorhydria

There are several ways in which your doctor can tell if you have one of these conditions. He'll usually be able to make a diagnosis from your clinical story, but he may do certain other tests to confirm his suspicions. A simple place to start is to do a therapeutic trial of hydrochloric acid supplements. If you get better, the diagnosis is obvious. Next, there are various ways of stimulating the acid-producing cells of the stomach to see if they are working properly. Lastly, a specialist in gastroenterology might be asked to perform radiotelemetry on you; this latter procedure involves the use of a miniature radio transmitter the size of a medicinal capsule which, when swallowed, emits radio waves at a wavelength proportional to the level of acidity in the stomach. This can be used to demonstrate whether or not gastric secretion is adequate, inadequate or excessive.

The following conditions are found to be associated with absent gastric acid secretion (achlorhydria) or reduced gastric acid secretion (hypochlorhydria).

- pernicious anemia (B12 deficiency)
- asthma
- food allergy
- iron deficiency
- osteoporosis
- bacterial bowel overgrowth
- aging
- diabetes mellitus
- rheumatoid arthritis
- underactive and overactive thyroid gland
- marijuana smoking
- fever
- pollutants (DDT)
- coffee consumption
- celiac disease
- eczema

The Intestines

CELIAC DISEASE (gluten sensitivity)

This is an intolerance to a protein called gluten which is present in wheat, oats, rye and barley.

It can show itself in young children as bowel upset, diarrhea, bloating, colic and poor growth. In adults it can appear as the irritable bowel syndrome, stomach upsets, depression, infertility, or a loss of well-being. It can occur at any age. The diagnosis is generally made by taking a sample of the small bowel. The patient swallows a capsule on the end of a piece of string and this takes a "nip" of the lining of the small bowel. The specialist can then study the sample under a microscope. Generally speaking, unless the diagnosis has been made using this procedure the condition cannot be called celiac disease. Real celiac disease causes the malabsorption of a wide range of nutrients. Recovery occurs on avoiding gluten-containing foods completely and, where appropriate, with the addition of nutritional supplements. Many doctors fail to realize that quite apart from celiac disease (where the lining of the small bowel is abnormal), people can suffer gluten intolerance although their small bowel lining is normal and this can, nevertheless, provoke quite severe intestinal symptoms. Furthermore, someone can be allergic to wheat *without* being intolerant of gluten.

COWS' MILK INTOLERANCE

This can cause a whole range of intestinal problems, especially, but not exclusively, in childhood. Symptoms resolve on cutting out cows' milk products completely.

THE IRRITABLE BOWEL SYNDROME (IBS)

The irritable bowel syndrome is a disorder in which there is pain in the colon and a disorder of bowel habit. It is also known as the irritable colon syndrome, spastic colon and mucous colitis. It is one of the leading causes of industrial absenteeism and the most common disease encountered by gastroenterologists, ranking as common as dyspepsia and peptic ulceration put together.

How you know you have it

- abdominal aching or pain
- diarrhea and/or constipation
- flatulence
- abdominal distension and rumbling

What causes it?

IBS can be provoked by a number of factors such as food intolerance, tea, coffee, alcohol, bowel overgrowth with bacteria, candida and bran (though some people improve when they take bran). Stress and other psychological factors are also thought to play a major role.

Let's look at the triggers in turn:

Food intolerance. In a study from Cambridge, food intolerance was shown to be a significant causative factor in IBS. The offending foods which provoked symptoms in the study were, in the following order of frequency:

- wheat
- corn
- dairy products
- coffee
- tea
- citrus fruits

In our experience, food intolerance is a definite factor in many cases of IBS and, if there is no other obvious cause, we think it worthwhile putting our patients on a modified exclusion diet (see Appendix 3).

Lactose intolerance is common and there are usually several pointers in the history that give the doctor a clue. It is common in children and adults from Eastern countries and often occurs after an episode of gastroenteritis. It may be caused by a deficiency of the naturally occurring enzyme lactase, which breaks down the sugar lactose in the intestines. Treatment involves the exclusion of milk and milk products from the diet.

Tea, coffee and alcohol. These drinks are known to affect gastrointestinal motility and function (see page 131 and page 133) and can give rise to the same symptoms as IBS.

Infective and parasitic organisms such as giardia, threadworms, ascaria and amoeba can produce pain and diarrhea similar to the symptoms of IBS. Giardiasis is now endemic in the UK and can be quite difficult to diagnose. Professor Gilbert at Edinburgh claims that one in five British schoolchildren is infected with parasitic threadworms, so this is particularly important in childhood.

Bowel overgrowth. The human colon contains large numbers of bacteria which live there and perform all kinds of vital functions. The number of organisms in colonic and fecal material has been estimated at ten billion per gram which means that we have more microbial cells in our bodies than we have human cells. It has been estimated that the microbial mass makes up approximately half of all the stools we pass. It is therefore understandable that any disruption in colonic bacteria can give rise to altered bowel function. Abnormal bowel bacterial overgrowth is best treated by cleaning up the diet (see Appendix 1), ensuring adequate fresh fruit and vegetable fiber, adequate fluids, ensuring regular bowel habits, avoiding antibiotics if possible, and by consuming fresh *live* yogurt and taking supplements of lactobacillus. Abnormal bacteria can flourish in the upper part of the bowel and produce abdominal pain, bloating and flatulence. Lack of acid production and a tendency to constipation are the most common predisposing factors. This can be a common cause of poor digestion in the elderly.

Candida overgrowth. The yeast, *candida albicans,* has been isolated in the stools of up to forty to fifty percent of the population. The taking of antibiotics, the disruption of digestive processes, the consumption of refined carbohydrates and the use of the Pill, estrogens and steroids all predispose to candida overgrowth in the large bowel. Though it is not generally recognized that this can give rise to large bowel symptoms similar to those of irritable bowel syndrome, we have seen a number of people in the last few years who have responded to prolonged high-dose courses of the anti-fungal agent, nystatin, and dietary manipulation geared towards suppressing the colonization of the large bowel by the excessive overgrowth of candida albicans. This is covered more fully in the section on candida (see page 346).

Bloating, flatulence and diarrhea

Susan was a forty-six-year-old journalist with two grown-up daughters. She had been suffering from bloating, diarrhea and flatulence for several years and had done the rounds of gastroenterologists (intestinal specialists). She had been told that she had irritable bowel syndrome and had been given a number of different prescriptions, none of which she liked taking and none of which seemed to do her that much good. On closer questioning it was found that she had a history of recurrent vaginal thrush, an itchy anus, hefty use of antibiotics for chest infections and a high-refined-carbohydrate diet. Her symptoms completely cleared up in five days with a low-carbohydrate, low-yeast diet and the oral, anti-yeast medication, nystatin. She continued the regime until her follow-up consultation three weeks later, at which point she stated that she was feeling better than she had done in years and her intestinal symptoms had disappeared for the first time in four years. This is a good example of irritable bowel syndrome being cleared up by treating chronic yeast infection. There are many causes of irritable bowel (stress, food intolerance, digestive enzyme insufficiency etc.) and it is only by treating one or more of the major contributing factors that relief can be obtained.

Candida allergy. Apart from the simple matter of overgrowth with candida, some people are hypersensitive to candida at various places in their body. The main places that candida takes hold are the gastrointestinal tract, the mouth, and the vagina. It has been reported that some people with the symptoms of IBS are allergic to the yeast.

It is our experience that a low-yeast and low-carbohydrate diet and, where necessary, nystatin taken orally for several weeks, can result in a considerable improvement in IBS. Candida allergy and overgrowth is discussed more fully on page 346.

Acute infective diarrhea. It has been noted that acute infective diarrhea, such as occurs in food poisoning, can trigger the symptoms of IBS, which persist long after the infective episode has disappeared.

Bran. There has been recently a substantial move towards the addition of wheat-bran fiber to the Western diet, often without a reduction in the amount of refined carbohydrate being eaten. While this is discussed in more detail in the section on Fiber (see page 123), it is worth mentioning here that certain individuals who appear to be wheat sensitive have a worsening or a precipitation of their IBS symptoms when they move over to a whole-food diet or add wheat bran to their normal diet. In these situations it is worth trying soya bran or rice bran, which is generally available from most health food stores, or on order through a local pharmacist. There are also a certain number of individuals who may have intestinal problems with a degree of malabsorption because the food rushes through the intestines so fast it cannot be absorbed. The mineral status of such people might be adversely affected.

Digestive enzyme deficiency. There is considerable evidence to show that supplements of pancreatic enzymes and bile acids can be of benefit in alleviating the symptoms of IBS in people who, because of age, smoking, diabetes or other factors, have diminished digestive enzyme functions.

Hypochlorhydria and achlorhydria (see above). Treating this, when present, may improve or alleviate IBS.

Premenstrual exacerbations. A certain percentage of women with IBS have a premenstrual worsening of their symptoms. The symptoms are often attributable to food intolerance and a failure to maintain adequate magnesium and pyridoxine intakes. These are all discussed in more detail on page 301.

Drugs, especially antibiotics. Treatment with antibiotics can give rise to symptoms similar to those of IBS. Sometimes these symptoms are due to an alteration in bowel micro-organisms, be they bacterial or yeast. These symptoms may not start until several days or even weeks after stopping antibiotic therapy, so that the relationship is not obvious. Individuals who are particularly at risk are those who have been on long-term antibiotics as a preventive in rheumatic heart disease, or on long-term tetracycline therapy for acne (see also page 275).

Stress. The intestines are very sensitive to stress, so when someone is particularly stressed they might at any time develop an irritable bowel which settles when they deal with the stress. This may be done externally, by dealing with the situation, or internally through relaxation or meditation and other mental and spiritual techniques.

Treatment of the irritable bowel syndrome

As can be seen from the section above, there are a number of different therapeutic avenues that can be taken, depending on the doctor's assessment of any given individual. Most people with IBS can be satisfactorily treated by attacking the root cause of their symptoms, without having to resort to tranquilizers or other drugs that affect the nervous system.

INFLAMMATORY BOWEL DISEASE

Inflammatory bowel disease includes two major gastrointestinal diseases, Crohn's disease and ulcerative colitis. Both can give rise to inflammation and involvement in tissues outside the colon as well as the more obvious bowel problems. The features are different though there is some degree of overlap. The cause of these two conditions is not understood and no infective agent has been isolated with sufficient reliability to be credited as the cause.

Crohn's disease

Crohn's disease is mainly a disease of white adults between the ages of twenty and forty, though it can occur for the first time in both children and the elderly.

It is characterized by abdominal pain, diarrhea, weight loss, fever, lower gastrointestinal bleeding, anal fissures and abscesses, as well as arthritis and liver, skin and eye problems in a minority of cases. It involves the small bowel only in thirty percent of patients; the colon only in fifteen percent and both the colon and small bowel in fifty-five percent.

We are now increasingly aware of the nutritional needs of people with Crohn's disease. The imbalances and deficiencies arise because the absorptive capacity of the last part of the small bowel is usually compromised to a greater or lesser degree. While the cause hasn't been fully worked out, the group of researchers from Cambridge who demonstrated the importance of food intolerance in irritable bowel syndrome have found that it can be an important factor in Crohn's disease too.

However, we advise people to be very wary of exclusion diets in such cases, as they so often have a poor nutritional status already. Avoiding sugar, sucrose and refined carbohydrates is a safe simple test to take that may produce some improvement.

It is now recognized that people with Crohn's disease are susceptible to the development of zinc deficiency. As a result, we assess the zinc status of *all* our patients with Crohn's disease. This is very important to bear in mind in children who have Crohn's disease. Their growth impairment should not be attributed solely to the steroids used to treat the condition, but to their zinc deficiency. Deficiencies of many other nutrients, including the B vitamins and vitamins A and D, occur.

Ulcerative colitis

The cause of ulcerative colitis is not understood. It has been suggested that it is the result of an allergic or hypersensitivity reaction by the colon, but there is no supporting evidence for this theory. Circulating antigens to cows' milk can be found in some people with the disease, but their significance is not fully understood. Some cases of colitis may be caused by drugs, especially aspirin, and respond to a low-salicylate diet (see page 432). There is a tendency for the disease to recur in families and there is a high incidence of eczema, hay fever, polyarthritis and ankylosing spondylitis in people with ulcerative colitis and their relatives. It shows up primarily in the twenty to forty age group and there is a female preponderance.

Characteristically, there is diarrhea with blood and mucus in the stool, and the frequent passage of stools. One fifth of sufferers have abdominal discomfort, often before opening their bowels, but the abdomen is usually not tender, except in severe cases. The degree of general bodily upset varies and is not necessarily related to the extent of inflammation of the colon. Tiredness, weakness and a lack of energy are common complaints. The diagnosis is made by colonoscopy, barium enema, or biopsy.

Inflammatory bowel disease as a group of conditions can be confused with the rather more benign irritable bowel syndrome. **It can respond to the food intolerance/chronic candida approach, but should only be so treated under medical supervision.** Nutrient deficiencies can occur and should be looked for by any doctor treating any of the conditions that come under this category.

Ulcerative colitis and salicylate allergy

Bernard, a forty-nine-year-old traveling salesman, had been troubled by ulcerative colitis for ten years. He had seen many specialists, who had tried to control his diarrhea with drugs, but, surprisingly, these had only made matters worse. Sometimes he would go to the toilet ten times a day, which would be very disruptive for his work. There were some mild deficiencies of iron and zinc, but treating him with supplements of these, and an exclusion diet, made only a minimal difference to his diarrhea. As his diarrhea had been made worse by aspirin-containing drugs, I suggested he try, as a last resort, a low-salicylate diet (see page 432). Within three days his diarrhea was less, and within seven it had ceased completely. He gained over fourteen pounds in weight and returned to full health. This was a remarkable improvement, which was confirmed by his bowel specialist. Salicylate sensitivity is a rare cause of colitis, and a specialized diet avoiding certain fruits and vegetables needs to be followed. Salicylate sensitivity more commonly causes asthma, rhinitis, and hyperactive behavior in children. Symptoms worsening after taking aspirin is an important clue, as there are no blood tests that will confirm the diagnosis.

APPENDICITIS

The appendix is a small worm-shaped portion of the bowel which is situated at the beginning of the large bowel, the cecum. In vegetarian animals, for example the rabbit, it is quite large, but in man, it is very small (the size of a small pencil).

Appendicitis is a condition almost exclusive to Western, "civilized" countries. The small, tube-like structure of the appendix may become obstructed by hard feces, and once blocked, infection and inflammation set in to produce appendicitis. Early symptoms include colicky, central abdominal pain followed by nausea and vomiting, and then the pain often shifts to the right lower quarter of the abdomen, as the inflammation spreads out from the bowel to affect surrounding structures.

Appendicitis is one of the most common causes of an acutely painful abdomen, and treatment involves removal of the appendix by operation, and attention to any infection that may have resulted from it.

Many people have a mild irritation of the appendix—grumbling appendicitis—which can occur several times over a period of months or years, before developing into acute appendicitis. Most of these grumbling appendix sufferers never get true appendicitis. While there is no dietary treatment for an acutely inflamed appendix, if you have repeated attacks of abdominal pain and nausea and have ever had suspected appendicitis, it is sensible to eat a high-fiber diet and to avoid refined carbohydrates. It appears that a high-fiber diet, especially one containing green vegetables, reduces the risk of appendicitis.

FLATULENCE

Flatulence is the medical term for the excessive production of gas, which is then passed anally (farting) or orally (belching).

Passage of gas anally (farting)

The type of food that we eat has a bearing on the amount of gas we produce. Many individuals have a lot of gas, which makes them uncomfortable, and it can be socially embarrassing. Gas is usually the result of fermentation by bacteria in the gastrointestinal tract. It can cause abdominal distention, pain, and disturbed bowel function. Increased fermentation can occur as a result of bacterial overgrowth of the gastrointestinal tract, constipation (which allows the products of digestion to sit in the colon for a time), irritable bowel syndrome, inflammatory bowel disease, food intolerance, chronic gastrointestinal candidiasis, and chronic intestinal infections with parasites. Certain foods, especially beans, can produce a lot of gas. All these conditions are made worse by inadequate digestive juice secretion by the stomach, pancreas and gall-bladder.

Those who have gas after eating beans may be helped if they soak the beans for twenty-four hours, remove the husks and cook them thoroughly.

So flatulence can either be "normal" or a manifestation of almost any gastrointestinal disease.

Belching (burping)

Belching can be a sign of a digestive malfunction, but it can also be a sign of excessive air-swallowing from eating too fast and talking at the same time. Too little gastric hydrochloric acid and pepsin can result in bacterial overgrowth in the stomach, which causes food to ferment almost immediately and produces gas which then results in distention of the stomach and a tendency to belch. If this really is a problem, it can be treated medically. Trial of a modified exclusion diet (see Appendix 3) may be helpful.

MINOR ANAL AND RECTAL CONDITIONS

Certain minor anal conditions are common and are a real nuisance. They include such conditions as hemorrhoids, anal fissures, solitary ulcers of the rectum and itching of the anus. Most of these, but particularly hemorrhoids and anal fissures, are helped in the long term by treating any constipation. The passage of hard, dry stools is likely to aggravate local bleeding from hemorrhoids and pain from an anal fissure.

Itching of the anus can be a recurrent and troublesome problem. Common causes include poor hygiene, hemorrhoids, anal fissures, threadworm infections, fungal infections in men and women (including candida), other vaginal infections in women, diabetes mellitus, anxiety and psychiatric states.

Anal itching caused by a fungal infection should be treated thoroughly with both local and oral anti-fungal agents, particularly nystatin (see page 349). If the infection returns despite such treatment, then predisposing factors such as diabetes, iron deficiency, immune deficiency states, or recurrent transmission from one partner to another should be considered.

CONSTIPATION

Constipation is usually used to mean difficulty in passing a stool; diminished frequency of opening one's bowels; or the passage of hard, dry stools.

By far the most common cause of constipation in Western societies is a lack of fiber in the diet. But there are other much less common causes including:

- drugs that affect bowel motility (such as opiates, iron tablets, certain antidepressants, lead poisoning, antacids and laxative abuse)
- irritable bowel syndrome
- food sensitivity
- diverticular disease
- any serious infection in the abdomen (such as appendicitis)
- dehydration
- obstruction to the bowel
- long periods of immobility, especially in the elderly

- stress
- depression
- painful anal conditions that make the person afraid to open his bowels

Including fiber in the diet will often help constipation and is now widely accepted practice. Here's how to do it:

- Increase your consumption of fiber-rich foods, such as wholegrains, vegetables, fruits, nuts and seeds and foods made with wholemeal flour. At the same time, reduce your intake of refined carbohydrate foods such as sweets, chocolates, cakes, white bread and white rice.
- Use fiber supplements: wheat bran, oat flakes and other high-fiber cereals are cheap and effective, or use high-fiber medicaments—these are often based on wheat bran, ispaghula husk or methylcellulose.

It is better to increase your consumption of fiber-rich foods and decrease refined foods rather than take a supplement, because you will then eat more vitamins, bulk and trace minerals. Also, wheat bran can have adverse effects in some people and worsen their constipation (see page 128).

The irritable bowel syndrome not infrequently starts off with constipation. Important features include abdominal bloating, flatulence and excessive stomach distress. Intermittent diarrhea may also be a feature. However, in some sufferers the constipation is an overwhelming feature.

Milk is also known to produce constipation and this has been well studied in children in particular. Often, the avoidance of cereal products, a reduction in dairy products and the use of high-fiber foods (especially vegetables, salads, beans and fruit) is very effective in such a situation.

Constipation may also be a feature of magnesium deficiency. Both calcium and magnesium are essential for normal nerve and muscle function, and disturbances in magnesium metabolism have been found to produce constipation. We always suspect this in women who have premenstrual symptoms (in which magnesium deficiency may also play a part), and in those on diuretics which may produce magnesium, as well as potassium, deficiencies.

Investigation and management of constipation

Constipation should never be dismissed as a trivial symptom. It makes sense, if you are otherwise well, to go onto a high-fiber diet, to increase your fluid intake and to increase your level of physical activity. Tea is not the best way to rehydrate yourself as it can cause *de*hydration and so constipation. Taking several grams of vitamin C can totally resolve constipation.

Failure of such a simple program, or the presence of complications or more sinister symptoms, makes a more formal assessment essential.

A self-help plan for constipation

- Increase fiber intake. Eat plenty of vegetables, fruit, wholegrains, nuts and seeds—reduce intake of sugar, fatty and refined food.
- Do not drink a lot of tea, which can actually cause constipation. Increase your intake of water and dilute fruit juices. Reducing salt may reduce your fluid needs.
- Take regular exercise. This is particularly important in the elderly, and those who have a sedentary lifestyle.
- Avoid the long-term use of laxatives. They do not get to the cause of the problem—and may themselves have side-effects.
- Take 1–5 g or more of vitamin C per day, and amino-chelated magnesium, 200 mg once a day.

DIARRHEA

Diarrhea is a condition in which there are loose and/or frequent, unformed stools. It is quite normal to have a bowel movement one to three times a day provided the stool is formed and does not generally contain undigested food particles. A normal stool should float in the lavatory bowl and be well formed. This is an indication of adequate fiber and bulk. If the stool sinks, it suggests an inadequate amount of bulk.

Chronic or recurrent diarrhea may be due to long-term aftereffects of antibiotics, irritable bowel syndrome (page 209), inflammatory bowel disease (page 213), worms, intestinal parasites, food intolerance, digestive enzyme insufficiency, bowel bacterial overgrowth (page 210) or any number of medical conditions which may need swift attention.

Any persistent change of bowel habit, diarrhea or constipation should be discussed with your doctor.

CARDIOVASCULAR DISEASE

This is a group of conditions affecting the heart, blood vessels and blood. They include coronary heart disease (heart attack and angina), hypertension (high blood pressure), blood clotting (excess stickiness of the blood), peripheral vascular disease (narrowing of the blood vessels, especially in the legs), strokes (obstruction of, or bleeding from a blood vessel in the brain) and high blood fat levels (which are associated with a tendency to develop the above problems). Poor circulation, varicose veins, chilblains and edema (fluid retention) are also covered.

Coronary Heart Disease

Coronary heart disease is a major cause of death in Western society. In the UK it accounts for twenty-seven percent of all deaths and is the cause of a substantial amount of illness in the general population. Associated strokes (cerebrovascular disease) account for a further twelve percent of deaths. A considerable amount of research has revealed that smoking and a high animal-fat consumption are associated with an increase in coronary heart disease. Consumption of cholesterol is not so strongly associated.

Coronary heart disease usually manifests itself as angina (chest pain on exertion) or a heart attack.

For an acutely ill person with a heart attack, the use of medications to correct heartbeat disturbances, heart failure and shock, and general intensive care are the mainstays of treatment. Nutrition has a substantial part to play not only in minimizing, and hopefully preventing, further heart damage, but also in the semi-acute situation.

There are three major areas in which nutrition is relevant to heart attacks and coronary artery disease generally:

- High blood fats (cholesterol and triglycerides) can be controlled by diet and possibly with the help of nutritional supplements.
- High blood pressure can be controlled by dietary means as well as using standard medications.
- Platelet stickiness and clotting can be reduced by dietary means.

Let us take a look at how the individual who has angina, or who has had a heart attack, can be helped by nutritional means.

First, it must be pointed out that the major factor associated with heart disease is not a dietary one, but smoking. Second, although an elevated cholesterol level is associated with an increased risk of heart disease, most people do not need to consume a very low-cholesterol diet, but simply to moderate their intake of dietary fats.

Here are some useful tips:

- Stop smoking.
- If you are overweight, lose weight to end up within ten percent of your ideal weight.
- Reduce your consumption of animal fats, such as cheese, butter, lard, suet, fatty meats and foods made with these, including many cakes, pastries, pies, processed and prepared meals. It may be helpful to use low-fat alternatives.
- Use margarine and cooking oils high in polyunsaturates, such as sunflower and safflower seed oil, but do not consume excessively.
- Ensure a good intake of green vegetables and fruit in your diet every day.
- Reduce your consumption of refined carbohydrates and sugar to a minimum.
- Moderate your consumption of alcohol to a total of two or fewer drinks per day (1 drink = 8 oz. of beer/lager = 1 glass of wine = 1 shot of spirits = 1 serving of sherry/vermouth).
- Eat at least two portions of fish per week—oily fish, particularly mackerel, herring and salmon are recommended.
- Get regular physical exercise—three or four times per week may be of help. **It is essential that you consult your doctor about this before starting.** Activities such as walking, certain sports or specialized exercise may be suitable.

Considerable evidence is mounting to support this advice. The type of dietary changes outlined above, stopping smoking and regular physical exercise can all help lower blood cholesterol levels. Furthermore, the level of your blood pressure may be reduced by changing your diet and losing weight. Researchers from the Netherlands have discovered that the risk of heart disease is substantially less in those who are consuming moderate amounts of fish on a regular basis.

SEVERE ANGINA

For those with severe angina, or people who are at high risk of a heart attack, a very strict diet composed entirely of vegetarian foods and oily fish may be beneficial (see piscine-vegan diet, page 434). A similar program, with monitored graded exercise, relaxation and counseling therapy, reduced angina by ninety-one percent in less than four weeks. **This should always be under medical supervision.**

SUPPLEMENTS FOR THOSE WITH HEART DISEASE

If you have angina or have suffered a heart attack you must check with your doctor first before taking any nutritional supplements. A recent study has shown that magnesium given intravenously to patients admitted to the hospital with a heart attack reduced their risk of dying. Many individual nutrients may help either lower blood cholesterol levels, or reduce the stickiness of the blood. These are perhaps the two most important factors that lead to a heart attack. Smoking and diet can have adverse influences on both of these. The role of individual nutrients in the treatment of raised blood cholesterol and extra stickiness of the blood are considered on pages 228 and 230.

High Blood Pressure (Hypertension)

High blood pressure is a common condition, but it is important because it is linked with an increased incidence of strokes, kidney disease and, to a lesser extent, heart attacks. Blood pressure rises gradually with age and a normal level is in the region of 140/90 mmHg. Mildly raised blood pressure is very common and is by no means serious.

Most people with a high blood pressure have no obvious medical cause. High blood pressure associated with kidney or hormonal disease, however, is well documented.

There does seem to be a genetic element in the production of high blood pressure: the relatives of patients with hypertension often have a higher than normal blood pressure. However, it may be that this evidence comes from Western societies which are socially or nutritionally predisposed to hypertension.

DIETARY SALT

Many researchers think that dietary salt (sodium chloride) intake in the West is perhaps ten to twenty times that necessary to maintain sodium balance in the body. The effects of restricting salt in the diets of patients with hypertension have been the subject of a number of trials, the results of which are not entirely in agreement. Overall, however, the evidence appears to be in favor rather than against the restriction of salt if you have high blood pressure. For those with salt sensitive high blood pressure, salt must be strictly excluded. No salt should be added at the table, or used in cooking. *All* salty foods are to be avoided. An excellent book on this is *The Salt-Free Diet* by Dr. Graham MacGregor (Thorsons, 1984). Dr. MacGregor is an acknowledged expert on this subject.

POTASSIUM

Many of the more recent studies involving salt (sodium) point to the importance of potassium in relation to sodium. One of the features of modern food processing has been not only to increase sodium salts, but to reduce potassium salts. The cooking of vegetables in large quantities of water and the addition of salt increases potassium losses, whereas steaming or cooking in minimal quantities of water, without added sodium salt, reduces such potassium losses.

It is known that vegetarians tend to have significantly lower blood pressures than omnivores. This effect is thought to be due to the higher dietary intake of potassium in vegetables.

We would therefore advise those with high blood pressure to include potassium-rich foods in their diet, to use cooking methods that will not deplete potassium content (such as steaming or cooking in small quantities of water), and to reduce the amount of salt eaten. These measures can often reduce or totally cure mild high blood pressure, even without drugs.

It appears that the effect of salt (sodium) restriction alone may be more marked in those on anti-hypertensive drugs and a combination of approaches is often required.

CALCIUM AND MAGNESIUM

The role of calcium in hypertension is complex. It is thought that, like sodium, there may be an increased influx of calcium into certain cells in hypertensive individuals. As a result, there has been considerable interest in the use of calcium antagonists to control hypertension.

Epidemiological evidence suggests that there is a link between low dietary calcium intake and hypertension. Some studies have shown that the effect is even more pronounced than that of sodium. The value of giving calcium supplements is, however, uncertain.

Calcium's coexistent and to some degree antagonistic salt, magnesium, has also been studied in hypertension. Though overt magnesium depletion may occur only rarely, people on thiazide diuretics can easily become magnesium depleted. The effect of magnesium supplementation in a group of hypertensive patients on diuretics resulted in significant further reduction of blood pressures.

OBESITY

The link between obesity and hypertension is well known. Severe obesity is linked with an increased risk of heart attack, high blood pressure and diabetes, as well as gallstones, osteoarthritis and kidney disease.

Weight reduction causes a substantial reduction in blood pressure and sometimes this is the only treatment needed. A recent study showed that in obese young men, weight reduction was more effective than the commonly used, powerful, anti-hypertensive drugs.

Whatever the controversies about other dietary proposals in hypertension, weight reduction is an important and often overlooked aspect of treatment. Stopping smoking is often followed by a substantial weight gain which may worsen high blood pressure.

SUGAR

The effects of sucrose (common table sugar) on blood pressure have been studied. Substantial increases in sucrose consumption by Western countries has, to some degree, paralleled the presence of coronary heart disease. It appears that, in some individuals at least, heavy sucrose intakes may raise blood pressure, perhaps by causing sodium retention or by a direct effect upon the stress hormones system.

ALCOHOL

There appears to be a link between alcohol and high blood pressure. People who consume small quantities of alcohol are found to have a lower blood pressure than teetotalers and those with a high intake.

Acute alcohol withdrawal causes a rise in blood pressure before there is a fall.

The reintroduction of alcohol produces a return of high blood pressure within a few days in susceptible individuals. Such people should not drink at all, or should limit their consumption to one drink a day at most.

TEA AND COFFEE

Tea and coffee both contain caffeine, as well as a number of other compounds which have profound metabolic activity. Experimental studies have shown that 200 mg of caffeine (equivalent to two or three cups of strong coffee) can produce a significant temporary rise in both systolic and diastolic blood pressures. However, evidence from an American study did *not* show an association between heavy coffee consumption and long term hypertension. Heavy coffee consumers are known to be higher consumers of cigarettes and this in turn may be associated with a lower body weight and thus a *lower* blood pressure—but smoking will increase heart disease risk.

SMOKING

Some surveys have found an association between smoking and hypertension, but others have not.

SATURATED FATS

In Finland, where the risk of coronary heart disease is amongst the highest in the world, there has been intense interest in dietary risk factors. Research into the possible association between dietary saturated fat intake in hypertension has suggested that increasing the ratio of polyunsaturated fat to saturated fat in the diet may reduce blood pressure. This is independent of its effect upon the amount of cholesterol in the blood and is apparently not related to changes in salt intake, lifestyle or other measurable effects. So cutting down on animal fats and poor quality margarines is very important.

VEGETARIAN DIETS

A number of studies have found that vegetarians tend to have lower blood pressures than do omnivores. A trial of vegetarian diets in people with normal blood pressures, carried out in Australia, showed a fall in blood pressure. Apparently such differences could not be explained on the grounds of changes in sodium and potassium intake alone.

HYPERTENSIVE FOODS AND DRUGS

Licorice is known to cause sodium and water retention and may cause elevations in blood pressure. Licorice derivatives used in the treatment of peptic ulcers may raise the blood pressure as a side effect.

Some non-steroidal anti-inflammatory drugs used for arthritis may also cause fluid retention and can raise blood pressure.

THE CONTRACEPTIVE PILL

A number of reports have suggested that oral contraceptives may cause a small but significant rise in blood pressure probably attributable to both the estrogen and the progesterone in the Pill.

TOXIC MINERALS

Lead certainly tends to produce a raised blood pressure (see page 90). The effect of cadmium is less clear, though low-level cadmium exposure may well be a factor (see page 99).

Gout, high blood pressure and hair dye

Harry arrived very fed-up with the fact that he was on pills for high blood pressure and had been told that he would be on them for the rest of his life. A mineral screening test revealed that he had a very high lead level in his system, as well as very low zinc, magnesium and chromium levels. He had a high uric acid level in his blood, indicating that he might be suffering from gout. Also, the blood tests showed his kidneys weren't working properly. It turned out that for the past fifteen years he had been using a hair dye to hide his gray hair. The dye contained significant amounts of lead which was being absorbed through his scalp into the bloodstream and was resting in his kidneys, increasing his blood pressure and his uric acid levels. Intravenous treatment with the chemical EDTA over a number of weeks, stopping using the hair dye, and taking nutritional supplements, resulted in a normalization of his blood pressure, a normalization of his kidney function tests, a normalization of his blood and hair lead levels, a return of well-being that he hadn't had for a decade or two, and he was able to stay off his drugs. One year later he was still feeling ten years younger with everything normal. This is a good example of excess lead causing kidney problems, gout and blood pressure. If he hadn't been screened for lead poisoning he would still be feeling grim and would still be taking high blood pressure tablets. There are many causes of high blood pressure and excessive lead with kidney malfunction is one of them.

EXERCISE

It appears that moderately strenuous physical exercise, enough to increase the pulse rate to 120 beats per minute, may produce a substantial decrease in blood pressure which could last from four to ten hours. So regular, possibly twice-daily, exercise could be beneficial in hypertension.

ADDITIONAL APPROACHES IN THE MANAGEMENT OF HYPERTENSION

If you have high blood pressure, you could well benefit from other non-drug treatments for hypertension. Stress can be an important cause of high blood pressure and such approaches as transcendental meditation, yoga, muscle relaxation, meditation and biofeedback have been found to be valuable. Occasionally there may be a dramatic fall in blood pressure when someone follows a modified exclusion diet for food allergy assessment (see Appendix 3).

Many doctors now agree that every person with high blood

Blood pressure, food allergy and nutritional imbalance

John was a forty-eight-year-old design engineer who, on a routine insurance check-up, had been found to have high blood pressure (170/110). Preliminary testing showed he was magnesium and potassium deficient and his chromium level was rather low. There was also evidence of mild food intolerance and it was obvious that he lived a pretty highly stressed life. By going on the modified exclusion diet, avoiding wheat, refined carbohydrates, sugar etc., and by correcting his nutritional supplements, his high blood sugar was brought under control, down to the normal range (in this case his blood pressure was around 140/85). His blood pressure occasionally went up when he was under stress, and relaxation techniques enabled him to bring his life and his blood pressure under control. This differs from the case of Alexander, who has widespread hardening of the arteries and some kidney problems, where nutritional supplementation and food allergy investigations, as well as relaxation techniques, made no difference to his blood pressure, and he had to go on drugs to treat it.

pressure should be managed by nutritional means whenever possible. Such an approach may reduce some of the other risk factors associated with heart disease, such as an elevated blood cholesterol. Furthermore, the use of diet and dietary supplements can easily be combined with drug treatments if they are necessary.

Blood Clotting in Heart Disease and Other Conditions

The formation of a clot in either a vein or an artery is a common feature of all the major diseases of the blood vessels and circulatory system, including coronary heart disease (heart attacks), cerebrovascular disease (strokes), peripheral vascular disease and clots in the leg veins.

Clots form where there is damage to the lining of the blood vessel. Then cells, called blood platelets, stick to the damaged lining and release substances which cause further clumping of platelets. Red blood cells and other materials then get caught up in the collection of platelets and a clot is formed. One of the main substances released by platelets in the initial sequence of events is thromboxane A_2. Its formation can be modified or manipulated by dietary change and the taking of certain vitamins, minerals or essential fatty acids.

So it is that nutritional intervention can have rewarding effects in people with heart disease, strokes and diseases of the small blood vessels. Because the turnover of platelets in the body is very rapid (occurring every few days), it may be possible to modify platelet function more readily and quickly than it is to modify cholesterol deposition in the arteries, which occurs over a substantially longer time.

CONDITIONS IN WHICH THE BLOOD CLOTS TOO EASILY

There are a number of conditions which increase the risk that blood platelets may become abnormally sticky and clump together.

These include:

- taking estrogens—especially the contraceptive pill—and hormone replacement therapy
- high blood pressure
- high blood fats

- diseases of the small blood vessels (related to sucrose intake and insulin levels)
- strokes
- migraine
- asthma
- rheumatoid arthritis

People with coronary heart disease don't appear to have increased platelet stickiness but rather reduced rates of "unsticking" of platelets once they do stick together. Diabetics may have increased circulating levels of various clotting factors which could explain their increased susceptibility to blood clots. The presence of increased quantities of a clotting protein—fibrin—is associated with an increased risk of heart attack.

There are several situations in which the correction of platelet stickiness is worthwhile.

These include:

- worsening angina
- minor strokes
- worsening circulation in the legs
- migraine

There are several therapeutic agents which have a beneficial effect upon blood stickiness. Those found to be of most value are:

Vitamin B6. This reduces platelet stickiness and also prevents the formation of a particular stickiness component called thrombin.

Vitamin C. Not only does vitamin C have a beneficial effect upon blood fats, particularly cholesterol, but it appears to reduce platelet stickiness in people with coronary artery disease. The dose needs to be in the region of 200–500 mg a day.

Vitamin E. Administration is known to correct a number of platelet abnormalities including increased stickiness in those who are deficient in vitamin E (such as those with cystic fibrosis). Dosage: 200–800 IUs daily. Selenium, which works with vitamin E, may also be of help.

Fish oils (MaxEPA). Taking MaxEPA in substantial quantities seems to reduce platelets sticking to blood vessel walls. This effect may be confined only to those with arterial disease. Dosage: 2–8 capsules daily.

Evening primrose oil. This has profound effects on prostaglandin metabolism, which favors the formation of substances that reduce platelet stickiness. Taking evening primrose oil or substantial quantities of polyunsaturated fatty acids with the necessary helping factors (vitamin C, B6 and zinc) could well be beneficial. Dosage: 2–8 capsules per day.

Garlic oil. Taking garlic oil can have beneficial effects on blood fats as well as on platelet stickiness.

Bromelain. This is a digestive enzyme derived from pineapple which appears to have beneficial effects on platelet stickiness.

Ginger. This has also been shown to reduce platelet stickiness. This may be an acceptable method of treatment for some patients whose blood clots too readily. Crystallized, root, or other forms of ginger (e.g. marmalade) can be taken.

The following is a safe and sensible plan if you have a condition in which too easy blood clotting is a problem:

- Vitamin B6—40 mg per day.
- Vitamin C—200–1000 mg per day.
- Vitamin E—approximately 800 IUs per day.
- Other supplements including primrose oil, fish oil—MaxEPA—or linseed oil, **under medical supervision.**

***Note:* People on anticoagulants can only take vitamin E under medical supervision.**

Other foods

Almost all fruits and some spices contain salicylates, a form of natural aspirin. Aspirin is known to reduce the clotting effect of platelets, particularly in people with strokes. Including salicylate-rich foods in your diet may also be of help. (See page 433.)

Cholesterol and Other Blood Fats

In the prevention of coronary heart disease (heart attacks), a number of risk factors have been identified. Smoking is undoubtedly the greatest, but abnormalities in blood fat levels also appear to be important. A considerable amount of the attention, both of research workers and practicing physicians, has been centered on abnormalities of blood fats and most of the public are only too aware of cholesterol and its supposedly harmful effects in heart disease.

The two main fats in the blood are cholesterol and the triglycerides. They are eaten in the diet, but what is not widely appreciated is that cholesterol is also made naturally in practically every tissue of the body, except perhaps the brain. A person's dietary intake of cholesterol may vary from 200–800 mg a day while his or her body naturally produces 2,000 mg a day.

Cholesterol is important in cell membrane structure, bile formation, steroid hormone production, and vitamin D synthesis. There is considerable misunderstanding that dietary cholesterol is bad for you.

Fats that are eaten have to pass from the intestine to the liver where they are metabolized. It takes several hours before they are cleared from the blood and if the level of cholesterol remains elevated, for one reason or another, the excess may become deposited on the lining of the arteries to produce atheroma. This narrows the artery and is one of the primary steps in the production of atherosclerosis (furring up and hardening of the arteries) and subsequent heart disease.

BASIC RECOMMENDATIONS FOR THOSE WITH HIGH BLOOD FATS

- Stop smoking
- Get some moderate physical exercise, if appropriate, including walking, swimming or some other sporting activity
- Change your diet:
  (a) cut down on sugar or cut it out altogether
  (b) reduce your alcohol intake
  (c) increase your dietary fiber intake, especially that of legumes and oats
  (d) ensure that you have a daily intake of one helping of green, leafy vegetables and one of fruit, especially apples and oranges. Garlic and onion may be helpful too
  (e) reduce the amount of animal fats you eat
  (f) reduce the amount of cholesterol you eat
- Drugs
  (a) talk to your doctor about coming off the Pill or hormone replacement therapy if you are on either
  (b) ask your doctor to consider alternatives if you are taking beta blockers or thiazide diuretics

Patients with elevated triglycerides need to avoid alcohol, sugar and refined carbohydrates in particular, as well as losing weight if they are obese.

NUTRITIONAL SUPPLEMENTS

If your cholesterol is still high after two or three months on this regime, the following supplements are of proven value. Side effects are extremely unlikely.

- Vitamin C, 300 mg–1 g per day (particularly for those with a poor dietary intake).
- Vitamin E, 400–800 IUs per day (particularly for younger people).
- Chromium—as trivalent chromic chloride solution—200 mcg of elemental chromium daily (particularly for older people). (See Appendix 2 for details.)
- Diet—further restriction of animal fats and cholesterol.
- Further measures. This could involve the use of a severely restricted vegan diet with the addition of some fish because of the content of beneficial fatty acids in certain fish (see Piscine-Vegan Diet on page 434).

OTHER SUPPLEMENTS

Specialized supplements may sometimes be used, including nicotinic acid, 3–6 g daily, and MaxEPA (fish oil), up to eight capsules a day if the triglycerides remain elevated. Evening primrose oil and MaxEPA (fish oil) can help lower elevated cholesterol levels, but medical supervision is necessary. All these measures can be combined with drugs to help lower fat levels to normal.

Strokes

A stroke is caused by bleeding from, or obstruction to, a blood vessel, usually an artery, in the brain. The disruption of the blood supply affects the nervous tissue that was previously dependent upon it. This results in damage and, usually, death of the nervous tissue though sometimes recovery can be remarkable. The major factors that lead to strokes include high blood pressure, smoking and increased stickiness of the blood. Occasionally, blood clots form either in the heart or in the major blood vessels in the neck, and, after breaking off, lodge in and obstruct the blood vessels' supply to the brain tissue. Sometimes very small, repeated strokes can occur. These are called transient ischemic attacks (TIAs).

A stroke is characterized by a sudden onset of weakness or

High blood cholesterol

Mrs. Mary H., a fifty-eight-year-old social worker, had been experiencing chest pain on exertion for the preceding two years. This had been diagnosed by a specialist as angina pectoris, for which she was given GTN tablets to take whenever she experienced the pain. She was surprised to learn that her angina was due to coronary artery disease, as she had never been a smoker, did not have high blood pressure, and there was no family history of heart disease. She was, however, slightly overweight at 140 pounds for her height of 5 ft. 5 in. Investigations showed that she had an elevated blood cholesterol of 8.5 mmol/l, the normal range being 3.9–6.7. All other routine investigations were completely normal, except that there was evidence of a mild deficiency of the trace mineral, chromium. She started on a diet avoiding animal fats, especially fatty meats, dairy produce and fried foods. Her intake of cholesterol, in the form of liver and eggs, was also kept to a minimum. Supplements of vitamin C, 1 g a day, chromium, 200 mcg per day, and multivitamins were given. After eight months, her blood cholesterol fell to 6.05 mmol/l, within the normal range. The severity of her angina has not deteriorated. An elevated blood cholesterol is an important risk factor for coronary artery disease. Ideally, all patients who have had a heart attack, or have angina pectoris, should have a fasting blood cholesterol level measured, and if it is found to be elevated, appropriate dietary and supplementary treatment should be given. Close relatives of patients who have coronary artery disease at a young age, e.g. fifty-five years or less, should also have their blood cholesterol level checked.

numbness in an arm, leg or one side of the face. Higher skills, such as speech, memory and intellectual function may also be affected. In a severe stroke, the individual can become unconscious for several hours or weeks. There is almost always some degree of recovery which, at times, can be remarkably complete. No drugs are of any real value after a stroke has occurred, and hence attention has centered on trying to prevent them.

A lack of vitamin C leads to easy bruising and bleeding, and in the elderly, particularly if they have a high blood pressure, this may easily increase their stroke risk. Some drugs are of value in helping to prevent strokes. Simple aspirin has been shown to reduce blood stickiness and stroke risk, particularly in those having repeated, small strokes (TIAs). Because many foods, particularly fruits, contain natural aspirin (salicylates) it may be that by increasing fruit consumption we have also been increasing our intake of "natural aspirin," and in this way have reduced our stroke risk.

The following advice can be usefully followed by anyone who is either at risk from a stroke or who has had one already:

- Stop smoking.
- Reduce weight if obese.
- Ensure a good intake of fresh fruit and/or vegetables *every day.*
- Follow the steps to reduce blood pressure if elevated, e.g. avoid salt, animal fats, alcohol etc. (See page 221.)
- Take supplements: vitamin C, 500–1000 mg per day. A multivitamin supplement may also be of some benefit.

Individual nutrients such as vitamin C, vitamin B6, and vitamin E may help certain risk factors in individual patients. **These should be checked by your own doctor.**

Peripheral Vascular Disease

Peripheral vascular disease is caused by narrowing of the arteries in the legs, which restricts the flow of blood to muscles in the calves, thighs and buttocks. Those affected usually have few symptoms in the early stages but later, as blood supply falls, the skin becomes pale, and cool to the touch, and hairs on the toes and legs may be lost. The most striking symptom, however, occurs when walking. The increased oxygen required during exercise cannot be provided by the limited blood supply and this results in a build-up of certain acids which precipitate pain and cramp, characteristically in the calf muscles. The sufferer can walk for a limited distance, sometimes no more than 100 yards, before the pain and discomfort stops him in his tracks. On resting, the pain eases, and he can walk again. The term "intermittent claudication" is sometimes used to describe this phenomenon. In severe cases, the blood supply becomes so impaired that gangrene develops, for which the only treatment is amputation.

The condition is almost always associated with smoking. Stopping smoking and getting regular exercise can often improve the situation, as may a change in diet. A study compared two types of diet: a high polyunsaturated, low-animal-fat diet, as is often recommended by the American Heart Association, and the Pritikin diet, which is a high-complex-carbohydrate diet and which is also low in fats.

Both were successful in increasing the distance walked by sufferers before the pain developed. The Pritikin program appeared to be the slightly more effective.

Another treatment of proven value is vitamin E. In fact, there have been nearly a dozen studies of vitamin E in peripheral vascular disease, almost all showing beneficial effects. The minimum effective dose is 300 IUs, and this must be taken daily for at least six months. Also, it might be worth trying a diet high in fish oils. **Remember, the most important thing is to stop smoking.**

Poor Circulation and Chilblains

Many patients complain of poor circulation. This can be due to an impaired blood supply, because of narrowing of the arteries, but this usually occurs in the legs, and only in those who smoke. However, poor circulation can occur in both the hands and the feet, irrespective of whether or not the sufferer is a smoker. In severe cases the fingers or toes become white on exposure to cold, and later turn red and purple as the circulation returns. This situation is known as Raynaud's Disease.

DIETARY ADVICE FOR POOR CIRCULATION

- Stop smoking.
- Follow the basic recommendations for a healthy diet (see Appendix 2), and especially include two or three portions of oily fish, such as mackerel, herring or salmon per week in your diet. Interestingly, Eskimos who eat a diet high in oily fish are renowned for their relatively good circulation.

NUTRITIONAL SUPPLEMENTS

A variety of these may be useful, including:

- nicotinic acid (not nicotinamide) vitamin B3: 50 mg three times a day, taken after meals

- vitamin C, 1 g a day
- vitamin E, 600 IUs per day
- evening primrose oil, 500 mg (4 capsules) per day and Max-EPA 4 capsules per day.
- magnesium, 200–400 mg per day

Varicose Veins

Varicose veins are a long-standing source of trouble to many people. They are much more common in Western, developed countries than in more primitive ones. A number of factors, particularly a low intake of dietary fiber, and constipation, are thought to be the causes. Obesity is another, and those who have suffered a thrombosis in the veins (blood clot) are particularly prone to them. If they have been present for a long time, and if they are severe, varicose veins may ache, and occasionally eczema and irritation develop in the skin around the veins, especially in the region of the ankle, and ulceration can occur, usually after a minor accident. Leg ulcers associated with varicose veins can be notoriously difficult to heal. Anyone with varicose veins should:

- Lose weight if they are obese.
- Wear support stockings/tights or bandage if they ache, or if there is eczema or an ulcer.

Occasionally, the restlessness and aching of the legs associated with varicose veins can be improved by Paroven, a plant extract, which is available on prescription. Other similar substances, bioflavonoids, are available in many health shops. A dosage of 500–1000 mg per day is recommended.

For those with varicose eczema or a varicose ulcer which is slow to heal, supplements of vitamin C, 2–3 g per day, and zinc 50–100 mg per day are often helpful. A multivitamin preparation may also be of benefit.

Edema

Fluid retention in the body usually causes swelling of the feet and ankles. It is particularly likely to occur in women, and is made worse by standing, and by hot weather. Being stationary for a long time, such as on a prolonged bus or plane journey, may also produce ankle swelling. More generalized fluid retention may result in swelling of the fingers, with tightness of the rings on the fingers and puffiness of the upper and lower eyelids and face. These tend to be worse after a night's rest.

Treatment of the underlying problem is necessary if fluid retention is to be resolved. In those in whom there is no obvious cause, the following things are worth trying and are often very successful:

- Stop adding salt to food at the table and during cooking. Salt helps retain water in the body.
- Cut right down on refined carbohydrates, such as sucrose (table sugar), sucrose-containing foods, honey and glucose. All these foods require a considerable amount of water to be metabolized. Often just cutting these foods out alone increases urine output as fluid is lost. This explains the rapid loss of weight that often occurs when a calorie-restricted diet is started. Most of the weight lost during these early days is actually fluid, and not fat.
- Many women suffering from fluid retention tend to be overweight, though this is not always the case. Try losing weight —it often helps.
- Avoid diuretics (water tablets). This may sound paradoxical, but though their use may reduce fluid retention initially, in the long-term it often results in *increased* fluid retention as the body compensates for the biochemical changes they cause. On stopping the diuretic, the fluid retention will get worse, but will then settle down, particularly if you follow the other measures.
- Correct any food allergies. Some food allergies produce significant fluid retention. Wheat, other grains and milk are particularly common culprits.
- Take vitamin B6. Doses of vitamin B6 (up to 100 mg per day) can be tried. This dose should not be continued for more than three months, because of potential adverse effects. It is best used along with other B complex vitamins, and a supplement of magnesium providing some 200–300 mg per day of the element.

Persistent fluid retention can be caused by heart problems which will require medical treatment.

CANCER

Cancer and heart disease are the major causes of death and ill-health in the western world.

Over the last few years, a picture of the influence of diet, and other factors, upon cancer has begun to appear. There are, as yet, no firm and proven dietary recommendations for the prevention or treatment of cancer. However, some broad guidelines are given at the end of this section.

What Is Cancer?

Cancer is a word used to describe an abnormal growth of cells which has certain characteristics. It has a tendency to spread from its original site into local or neighboring tissues and to spread to distant sites mainly by "seedlings" which travel via the bloodstream.

The term neoplasm or tumor simply describes any new growth and includes cancers, which are malignant, as well as benign or harmless tumors. Benign tumors do not spread and are almost always successfully treated by removal of the growth.

What Causes Cancer?

The causes of cancer can be divided roughly into the following headings:

- Genetic
- Environmental
  - (a) occupational
  - (b) non-occupational, non-dietary (environmental)
  - (c) dietary
  - (d) ? psychological/stress

There are certain rare genetic conditions that predispose to cancer. For example, certain types of cancer of the skin and the colon may well run in families and the early recognition and detection of such individuals is very important. But this is only an extreme minority of cancer patients. It may be that some other families also have a mild predisposition to cancer but that dietary or other factors are far more important. For example, cancer of the breast occurs more commonly in relatives of women who already have breast cancer. However, the role of diet in breast cancer is almost certain and may prove to be an overriding factor.

Exposure to certain agents is known to predispose to cancer. In particular, exposure to ionizing radiation such as was produced by the atomic explosions in Japan in the Second World War, is followed by increased risk of certain types of cancer.

Environmental factors are important causes of cancer. The major problems arise on occupational exposure to chemicals, usually petrochemical derivatives. However, arsenic, asbestos, and certain trace minerals may also cause an increased risk of cancer.

Other environmental factors may well be relevant. In the past, pollution of the atmosphere may have been a significant factor in the incidence of lung cancer, but now that pollution levels of some substances are considerably less than they were twenty to thirty years ago, this is unlikely to be so relevant.

The question has arisen as to whether certain drugs might predispose to cancer. Many drugs used in the treatment of cancer can, paradoxically, *increase* the risk of a subsequent cancer developing. The most common and relevant example is estrogens which, when given alone, without being balanced by progesterone, will increase the risk of development of cancer of the womb.

Many doctors have wondered whether social or personal factors might predispose an individual to cancer. Is there a "cancer personality"? We believe that any type of individual can get cancer, and it seems that there is no such thing as a personality that predisposes to cancer. However, it may be that stress can lead to the precipitation of a cancer in someone already predisposed (by genetic or environmental reasons) to it.

But genetic, environmental and possible psychological factors apply only to a small percentage of the population, and do not even begin to explain why cancer is one of the most common causes of death.

The majority of attention as to the cause of cancer now centers on diet.

Diet can play either a positive or a negative role. On the one hand there are certain dietary factors that predispose to cancer. On the other, there are certain nutrients, particularly vitamin A, which help reduce the incidence of certain types of cancer.

Diet as a Cause of Cancer

There are many substances in foods which are potentially cancer-producing. These are known as carcinogens and are widely found, mainly in vegetable produce. However, there are also anti-carcinogens found in foods which have the opposite effect.

There are potential carcinogens in such foods as celery, potato, certain fruits, poisonous mushrooms, coffee, certain dietary oils, alfalfa sprouts, and agents derived from moldy foods. Usually, potentially harmful agents that are found in foods such as potato and celery only occur in substantial amounts if the food is damaged, diseased or, in the case of potatoes, exposed to light. And they would probably only be a hazard if an individual ate very substantial quantities of these individual foods.

A more important source of carcinogens is the presence of the agents nitrites, nitrates and nitrosamines. These chemicals are found naturally in low concentrations in certain foods such as beets, celery, lettuce, spinach, radishes and rhubarb, but more importantly, nitrates and nitrites are used as food additives in meat products, to act as preservatives. They are converted in the stomach into nitrosamines—agents which are known to be linked to the production of stomach cancer. High levels of nitrites and nitrates are also to be found in the water supply in some areas. Increasing your intake of vitamin C and vitamin E, in the diet or with supplements, may help prevent the possible cancer-inducing properties of these agents.

Many researchers have looked at the role of calories as a cause of cancer. A high calorie intake is definitely associated with an increased risk of cancer. Whether this is due to the calories themselves or to dietary fats is uncertain. Cancers of the womb, gall-bladder and breast are more common in the obese.

Dietary fats, particularly animal fats, can play an important part in certain types of cancer. Cancer of the colon is usually more common in populations which have a high intake of fat, particularly of animal fats. High intakes of fiber may, conversely, have a beneficial effect. High intakes of animal fats result in increased quantities of bile being produced by the liver. This is then changed by bacteria in the intestines and small quantities of potential cancer-causing agents can be produced. This is particularly likely to occur in meat eaters, compared to vegetarians.

Breast cancer may also be linked with a high-fat diet. It is thought that certain types of female sex hormones, the estrogens, may be produced in the intestines, particularly in women who consume a higher animal-fat diet, or bacteria in the intestines may increase the reabsorption of estrogens that are normally excreted in the bile. The higher level of estrogens in the colon may be associated with an increased risk of breast cancer. Women who have a history of constipation have been shown to have an increased risk of early cancer-type changes in breast tissue.

The message is beginning to come across that you should not eat much fat, particularly animal fat, and that you should maintain a good intake of fiber from fruits, vegetables and grains, thereby reducing the undesirable changes in intestinal function and constipation that play a part in promoting cancer of the breast and possibly that of other organs. It has been shown that vegetarians not only produce fewer estrogens in the colon, but also have higher concentrations of substances that block the potentially harmful effects of estrogens on breast tissue.

As for protein and carbohydrates, the evidence is much less clear. A diet rich in animal protein almost always goes with a high animal-fat consumption. There has been no direct link between high intakes of refined carbohydrates and cancer, but the low level of certain essential trace nutrients in refined carbohydrates cannot be beneficial to general health, and might increase cancer risk.

Ways of cooking food may also be cancer-producing. Some studies have suggested that burning or browning food in cooking produces substances that are potentially carcinogenic. Roasting and barbecuing of meats may produce such substances in considerable quantity. Coffee contains a significant amount of burnt material, and some researchers have linked high coffee consumption with cancer of the pancreas, but this has not been confirmed by others. The cooking of fats may chemically alter them by increasing the degree of rancidity. Rancid or oxidized fats not only taste unpleasant, but may be important chemicals in the induction of cancer. Oils (linseed, sunflower, safflower) should be cold-pressed. You should keep them in the fridge and not use them in cooking. If any oil is used for cooking, olive oil is probably least harmful.

Diet and the Prevention of Cancer

So much for the bad news.

Many foods that we eat, however, contain useful amounts of certain vitamins, minerals and other agents which may well protect against cancer. Low intakes of these could increase the risk of cancer. It is important to remember that there is probably a cumulative effect: a diet that is low in nutrients may well be low in fiber and high in animal fats too. Someone eating such a diet, who is also a smoker, may be exposing themselves to a much greater risk of cancer.

VITAMIN A

Low dietary intakes of vitamin A or low to normal levels of vitamin A or beta-carotene (vegetable derived vitamin A) in the blood, have been associated with increased risks of cancers of the larynx, lung, esophagus, stomach, large bowel, bladder and prostate. It is not known whether a lack of vitamin A is the "cause" or not. Green vegetables, carrots, red and yellow fruits are all high in vitamin A and beta-carotene, from which vitamin A is produced in the body.

VITAMIN C

There is some evidence to suggest that the risk of cancer of the esophagus may be higher in those with low intakes of vitamin C. However, diets low in vitamin C will usually also be low in vitamin A and fiber and may well be high in animal fat, so a high dietary vitamin C intake may be only one factor of a diet that protects against cancer, rather than a protective factor itself. Women with abnormal cervical smears may have a low intake of vitamin C in their diet. Smoking lowers levels of vitamin C in the blood and is associated with cervical cancer.

VITAMIN E

Vitamin E works mainly as an anti-oxidant and may protect dietary fats from the chemical changes that make them rancid. Rancid fats are thought to be potentially cancer-producing.

VITAMIN B6

Those who are deficient in vitamin B6 may have changes in metabolism that produce potential carcinogens in the urine, which might predispose to cancer of the bladder. Women with cancer of the cervix have lower levels of vitamin B6 than their healthy counterparts.

SELENIUM

This essential trace element has activities similar to that of vitamin E in that it protects tissues from damage by oxygen. Low intakes of dietary selenium seem to be related to an increased incidence of breast and colon cancers. There is also evidence to suggest that people who live in areas where there is little selenium in the soil may have an increased risk of other types of cancer.

FIBER

Low intakes of fiber are usually associated with higher intakes of animal fat, so it is not easy to determine whether a low intake on its own increases the risk of cancer. However, populations who eat a high-fiber diet have a lower incidence of cancer of the colon.

OTHERS

It is quite possible that there are other dietary agents which have a protective effect against cancer. Some research suggests that these may be found particularly in vegetables. It may be that a diet high in raw or lightly cooked fruits and vegetables could reduce cancer risk not only because of its content of vitamins C, A and E, but because of other dietary constituents.

ALCOHOL

A high alcohol consumption is linked to an increased risk of cancer of the mouth, esophagus, pharynx, larynx and to some degree, of the liver. Usually, high alcohol consumers smoke more cigarettes and often have poor diets. How much is due to the alcohol itself and how much to other factors is as yet unknown.

SMOKING

There is no doubt that smoking is the major, most easily avoidable cause of cancer in the West, particularly amongst men. Since the turn of the century, the death rate for men from all types of cancer has risen by some twenty percent; but that for lung cancer has increased more than tenfold over the same time. In fact there has been an overall drop in the death rates from other cancers. In women over the same time the overall cancer risk has actually fallen a little, while that of lung cancer has increased.

It is not widely known that cigarette consumption is also related to other types of cancer, including that of the mouth, throat, esophagus, pancreas, bladder, and cervix in women.

By stopping smoking you can reduce your cancer risk in future years. Recent evidence suggests that smokers who consume a diet high in vitamin A and vitamin C have a lower risk of cancer than smokers who don't.

Diet in the Treatment of Cancer

There are few more contentious subjects in medicine than the role of diet in the treatment of cancer, though its role in the prevention of cancer is fast becoming established. But does this mean that cancer sufferers should follow a particular type of diet in the hope of controlling or minimizing their illness?

It is perhaps useful to divide use of diet in the treatment of cancer patients into four groups:

- Diet as a support for those receiving conventional anti-cancer therapy.
- Dietary advice to those with an early cancer.
- Dietary advice for those with cancer that is not responsive to standard medical treatments.
- The use of certain nutrients (e.g. vitamin C) in the treatment of cancer.

DIET AS A SUPPORT FOR PATIENTS RECEIVING CONVENTIONAL ANTI-CANCER THERAPY

Many anti-cancer drugs work by interfering with the metabolism of certain vitamins, particularly folic acid, to produce a severe cellular deficiency of this vitamin. This affects rapidly growing tissues such as the cancer cell far more than healthy tissues, and thus it is hoped kills off many of the cancer cells. Because these drugs are therapeutic poisons, it is probably unwise to take substantial quantities of vitamins and minerals at the same time. **Growth-promoting nutrients such as the B vitamins, folic acid and zinc, should certainly not be used without medical advice.**

Some people who are severely ill with cancer experience a profound loss of appetite and loss of weight and their general health may well deteriorate as a result. The use of nutritional supplements can greatly influence their well-being and also improve their ability to withstand the use of anti-cancer drugs. Such people are usually treated in a specialized hospital setting.

Patients undergoing radiation treatment who suffer side-effects such as nausea may be improved by taking vitamin B6, 40–100 mg per day, though this has not been definitely proved.

DIETARY ADVICE TO THE PATIENT WITH AN EARLY CANCER

Dietary advice for the individual who has a cancer that is either growing very slowly, or in remission, should probably be much the same as that given to healthy individuals who want to reduce their cancer risk (see page 246).

DIETARY ADVICE FOR THOSE WITH CANCER THAT DOES NOT RESPOND TO STANDARD MEDICAL TREATMENTS

Some medical practitioners have experimented with certain types of diet for such patients. Dr. Max Gerson, an American doctor, used diets with a very high intake of raw vegetables and little else. Such a dietary program can be extremely low in protein and other essential nutrients. This semi-starvation diet might have desirable effects upon the cancer, but might also have seriously detrimental effects on the individual's general health.

We are not in a position to recommend any of the severe diets used in the treatment of different types of cancer. Most of those recommended are usually fairly drastic forms of the widely accepted dietary recommendations for the avoidance of cancer. A high intake of raw fruits, vegetables, and the avoidance of animal fats and proteins form the basis of most such recommendations.

THE USE OF CERTAIN NUTRIENTS, SUCH AS VITAMIN C, IN THE TREATMENT OF CANCER

Some nutrients may have specific anti-tumor activities. The metabolism of a cancer cell is probably significantly different from that of healthy tissue and the use of massive doses of these nutrients might have a more powerful effect against the tumor cell than against its healthy counterpart. Also, high doses of certain nutrients might stimulate the body's own defenses against the cancer. This has to be balanced against the fact that others might stimulate the growth of the tumor.

Dr. Linus Pauling has been at the forefront of researching and recommending high-dose vitamin C as a treatment for certain types of cancer. It has been shown that many cancer patients have low levels of vitamin C in their plasma or in their white blood cells. The demand for vitamin C may be increased in patients with cancer, and the administration of substantial doses of

1–10 g of vitamin C may enhance some of the ways in which the body's own cells and tissues inhibit or fight the growth of the cancer. Vitamin C may also have beneficial effects by destroying various cancer-producing chemicals.

High-dose vitamin A has been used in the treatment of certain rare types of cancer, and chemical derivatives of vitamin A may be useful as anti-cancer agents though they can have toxic side-effects.

What You Can Do

In 1982, the Committee on Diet, Nutrition and Cancer, from the Assembly of Life Sciences National Research Council in America, published a report which thoroughly and extensively reviewed the literature in relation to nutrition and cancer, and came up with a list of dietary recommendations with which we heartily agree.

This is a summary of them:

- Consumption of both saturated and unsaturated fats should be reduced to approximately three quarters of current consumption, to provide a maximum of thirty percent of total calories in the diet.
- Eat more fruit, vegetables and wholegrain cereal products. Citrus fruits and carotene-rich vegetables, including cabbage, cauliflower, brussels sprouts, mustard, watercress and broccoli are to be encouraged.
- Foods containing potential cancer-causing agents, including salt-cured, salt-pickled and smoked foods, should be consumed in only minimum quantities.
- Alcohol should be consumed in moderation only.
- Also, don't forget to stop smoking!
- Follow the Rules for Healthy Living (page 398).

ARTHRITIS, OSTEOPOROSIS AND OTHER PROBLEMS WITH BONES AND JOINTS

Arthritis

The term "arthritis" means inflammation of a joint. There are many different types of arthritis, some due to infection and others due to wear and tear, but for many the cause is obscure. The two most common types, osteoarthritis and rheumatoid arthritis, cause considerable discomfort and disability. Conventional treatment with anti-inflammatory drugs often produces a good reduction in pain level, but little improvement in the arthritic process itself. As medicine's understanding of the mechanisms of arthritis improves, it has become clear that there are several important nutritional factors that influence the process of inflammation found in arthritis. It is clear that changes in diet and the use of specific supplements enable us to reduce inflammation and even to control the progression of the arthritis.

OSTEOARTHRITIS

This is the most common type of arthritis, and is particularly prevalent in old age. It is generally more common in women. A normal healthy joint such as the hip or knee is covered by a smooth layer of shiny cartilage. This can degenerate with age and result in uneven wear and tear on the bone underlying it. It is this which causes pain and stiffness of the joints to the sufferer.

Treatment

There is no single, recommended treatment for osteoarthritis, partly because there are a number of causes and predisposing factors.

In the majority of patients with osteoarthritis, it is a matter of trial and error which treatment will be of benefit to them. The following treatments may be of value:

- *Lose weight*. This is important, particularly for those who have osteoarthritis of the hips, knees and ankles. Eating less of both refined carbohydrates and animal fats forms the mainstay of any weight-reduction program.

- *Dietary manipulation of inflammation.* It may be possible, by dietary means, to suppress the inflammatory mechanisms that lie behind some of the pain and stiffness of osteoarthritis. Standard anti-inflammatory drugs affect the same area of metabolism that can also be influenced by dietary and nutritional means. Such a diet might involve substantial reductions in animal fats; the consumption of high-quality polyunsaturated fats (for example, 1–2 teaspoons of cold-pressed linseed oil per day); the avoidance of foods known to impede mineral absorption such as tea, coffee, bran and wholemeal bread; the correction of trace mineral deficiencies, particularly of iron, zinc, copper, selenium and manganese; and the use of such supplements as vitamins A, B and C, beta-carotene and vitamin E which, because of their anti-oxidant properties, may help suppress certain aspects of inflammation. **Such a program should be administered by a physician.** Results in individual cases can be quite encouraging.
- *Exclusion diets.* Anecdotal reports suggest that the avoidance of some foods can benefit individuals with arthritis. Plants of the solanacea group (the nightshades—such as tomatoes, aubergines, peppers, paprika, tobacco and potatoes) adversely affect some people and should be avoided for a trial period of one or two months.
- *Supplements*
  (a) A copper bracelet, popular with many arthritis sufferers is, surprisingly, of proven value in the treatment of both osteo- and rheumatoid arthritis. Small quantities of copper may be absorbed into the skin from wearing such a bracelet and have anti-inflammatory effects.
  (b) Nicotinamide. This has been given to patients with osteoarthritis at doses of 1–4 g per day and, again, anecdotal reports suggest that it may be of value in some cases.
  (c) An extract of the New Zealand green-lipped mussel has been tried in both osteo- and rheumatoid arthritis with encouraging results.
  (d) Vitamin E. At doses of 600 mg per day, this vitamin has been shown to be more effective than a placebo in the treatment of osteoarthritis and may be worth a trial.

Osteoarthritis is primarily a degenerative disease that occurs as we age, but mild, often undetected, nutritional deficiencies occur, too, as we get older, and these can certainly influence the process of many diseases, including arthritis. It is not easy to make broad recommendations as to which type of supplements and which dosages will be appropriate for the majority of people with osteoarthritis. However, a fairly strong multivitamin supplement, with good quantities of trace minerals may help, taken together with appropriate dietary measures and the other treatments listed above.

Osteoarthritis and infertility

Judith, a thirty-six-year-old housewife and mother of two, had noticed increasing pain and stiffness in her back and knees. X-rays had shown this to be due to osteoarthritis, which was quite unusual for a woman so young. She also complained of tiredness, mild eczema and premenstrual symptoms. Though she had had two children over ten years ago, she had not been using any contraception since then and had failed to conceive again. Investigations showed her to have deficiencies of zinc, chromium, selenium, magnesium and iron, as well as evidence of a mild diabetic tendency. Multiple nutritional deficiencies in someone so young, who was not obviously ill, was an unusual and surprising finding. Treatment with a number of nutritional supplements corrected these deficiencies and improved her arthritic symptoms considerably. However, her level of iron failed to improve and it was suspected that she might have some degree of malabsorption. It was suggested that she try avoiding dairy produce and all grains, wheat, oats, barley and rye in her diet. There was a considerable improvement in her energy level and further reduction in her arthritic pains. She was told that she could well become fertile again with her improved nutritional state and it indeed happened. On reintroducing wheat into her diet there was a marked return of her symptoms. Because of this, and the severity of her nutritional deficiencies, further investigations to assess the possibility of celiac disease were necessary. It is interesting that her arthritic symptoms improved considerably when nutritional deficiencies were corrected and her diet improved. Food allergy is known to play an important part in rheumatoid arthritis and also seems to affect some patients with osteoarthritis.

RHEUMATOID ARTHRITIS

Rheumatoid arthritis is often more severe and more generalized than osteoarthritis. It, too, occurs more commonly in women but is much more common in younger people.

It characteristically affects the hands and the large knuckle joints as well as the wrists, elbows, knees and feet. It affects the hip joints less often than does osteoarthritis. In severe cases, there is considerable destruction of joints, and other tissues, including skin, lymph nodes, lungs, the heart, and even the liver and kidneys can be affected by the rheumatoid process. Most sufferers have mild or moderate pain and swelling which usually affects the knuckles and small joints of the hands and one or two larger joints. The joints may feel hot.

Despite many theories as to its cause, nutritional factors appear to play a major part. In particular there have been a number of recent reports relating to the role of food allergy in rheumatoid arthritis. In 1981, a report appeared in the *British Medical Journal* of a woman whose rheumatoid arthritis appeared to be significantly worsened by eating dairy produce (milk and cheese). Many other foods may aggravate rheumatoid arthritis. Particularly suspect ones are wheat, oats, eggs, chicken, coffee, tea, yeast-containing foods, beef and pork. Only excluding foods in a formal way will reveal which ones are the culprits. It is possible that people with rheumatoid arthritis who are sensitive to foods have changes in blood platelets rather similar to those in people who have food allergies and migraine. We may therefore be able to influence the course of their arthritis by giving nutrients that influence platelet function (such as vitamin B6, vitamin E, vitamin C and perhaps linseed oil). This makes the following treatments worth trying if you have rheumatoid arthritis:

- *An exclusion diet* (see page 429). A standard exclusion diet can be followed for a period of up to three weeks, and, if you respond, foods can then be introduced one at a time to determine which are the culprits.
- *Zinc*. Supplements of zinc have been given with some success to patients with rheumatoid arthritis, though other studies have questioned their value. Zinc, together with certain other nutrients such as vitamins B and C, may have potentially anti-inflammatory effects and some older people with milder forms of rheumatoid arthritis appear to benefit from zinc supplements at dosages of 30–40 mg per day. Obviously, it is those who are zinc deficient who are most likely to respond.
- *Copper supplements*. Copper, together with zinc and manganese, is involved in the function of an enzyme called superoxide dismutase. This enzyme inhibits some of the inflammatory reactions that occur in rheumatoid arthritis. Ideally, levels of

copper in people with rheumatoid arthritis should be measured before copper supplements are given. A copper bracelet is of proven value.

- *Green-lipped mussel*. As reported in the section on osteoarthritis, this has been found to be effective in rheumatoid arthritis as well.
- *Nicotinamide*. Doses of 1–4 g a day may be of value. We have had little experience of this.
- *Evening primrose oil*. Beneficial effects of doses of 1–2 500 mg capsules four times daily, together with a supplement providing vitamins C, B6, B3, and zinc have been reported. Combination with a fish oil supplement, MaxEPA, may be useful.
- *Pantothenic acid*. Some reports have found low levels of pantothenic acid in the blood taken from patients with rheumatoid arthritis, and an apparent response to injections of pantothenic acid at doses of 50 mg was found to be beneficial in some cases. Oral supplementation with several hundred milligrams per day might be worth a try.
- *Tryptophan and histidine*. These two amino acids have also been shown to be of help in some rheumatoid patients. (See tryptophan warning page 106.)
- *Infecting agents*. Rheumatoid arthritis has been thought by some researchers to be due to an infection with either a virus or a bacterium. It is worth pointing out that zinc may stimulate resistance to viral and other infections.

In the management of rheumatoid arthritis, a number of different therapies can be used with varying effect. It is important to remember that different people will respond to different treatments. In young people with warm, swollen joints, the most effective single approach is, in our experience, a trial of an exclusion diet. For those who are underweight, have a poor appetite, or have had a previously poorly balanced diet, supplements should probably be tried before going on an exclusion diet. Older people often respond less well to an exclusion diet, particularly as it has to be rigorously carried out. For these people we often prefer to make use of supplements such as zinc, evening primrose oil, MaxEPA, and other nutrients such as vitamins C and B that are involved in essential fatty acid metabolism. Such supplements may have a general anti-inflammatory action, but this may take several weeks or even months for its full effect to be felt.

There is no reason why such nutritional approaches should not be combined with the use of painkillers and anti-inflammatory, anti-arthritic drugs. The more powerful drugs used in the treatment of rheumatoid arthritis may themselves call for an increased intake of nutrients.

Aches and Pains without Arthritis

A lot of us have aches and pains without there being clear evidence of arthritis. Such aches and pains have a number of causes, and if they are mild and persistent, the individual is often dismissed as "neurotic," particularly if there is no response to simple painkillers.

A fifty-year-old woman with rheumatoid arthritis

Jane was a grandmother who lived with her retired husband in the south of England. She had had some stiffness in her hands for a considerable period of time, but this became worse and she was put on an anti-inflammatory drug by her family doctor. The pain and stiffness continued to get worse, and no simple anti-inflammatory drug seemed to be effective. When she came, she was unable to rest her hands naturally in her lap because they were so hot, tender, swollen and painful, despite the fact that she was on anti-inflammatory drugs. It was evidently time to try a different tack. At that time I had never actually treated a case of rheumatoid arthritis with diet, but I had studied the medical literature on the subject, and it seemed that it was worth a go. Jane agreed to go on a five-day lamb, pears and bottled spring-water diet (see Appendix, page 429). By the end of five days (off her drugs) she was totally symptom-free, apart from a slight stiffness in a joint in one of her big toes for the first ten minutes after getting up in the morning. She then reintroduced the foods in a controlled fashion, and found that the offending food was wheat. Since that time, staying off wheat has resulted in freedom of symptoms. It is interesting to note that this was the first person I had ever put on a lamb and pears diet, and it was extremely effective. The next four people I saw with rheumatoid arthritis either received no benefit, or actually got worse from going on the lamb and pears diet—which only goes to show that each person is different!

Possible causes include:

- polymyalgia rheumatica (a painful muscular condition which mainly affects the elderly)
- an underactive thyroid
- early, generalized osteoarthritis
- osteomalacia (vitamin D deficiency)
- occasionally an early symptom of cancer
- nutritional deficiencies—particularly of magnesium, calcium, vitamin C and vitamin B6
- multiple food allergies

Anyone who has persistent muscular aches and pains should take them seriously and have appropriate laboratory investigations performed to eliminate the above possibilities.

Osteoporosis

Osteoporosis is a condition in which the bones become thin due to a loss of mineral content. Women are at particular risk after the menopause. It appears that estrogens prevent this bone loss, as women who have their ovaries removed before the menopause also have an accelerated rate of bone mineral loss. Men also lose mineral from their bones but at a slower rate than do women. Thinning of the bones leads to increased risk of fractures, particularly of the wrist, the shoulder, and the neck of the femur.

PREVENTION OF OSTEOPOROSIS

A number of studies now suggest that osteoporosis can be prevented by relatively simple nutritional and other means. Particularly useful preventive measures include:

- *Estrogen replacement*. This is only necessary for women who have had both ovaries removed or who have severe osteoporosis at an early age. Estrogens increase the metabolic need for vitamin B6 and other nutrients; supplementation may thus be necessary. We do not advocate routine hormone replacement therapy for the majority of patients with osteoporosis.
- *Calcium supplementation*. Calcium supplements to increase bone strength and reduce the risk of osteoporosis have been tried in a number of studies and form the mainstay of the nonhormonal treatment of osteoporosis. A number of studies have

shown that older women have calcium intakes below the recommended daily allowance and thus may be at risk of losing calcium from their bones.

- *Ensuring calcium absorption*. A number of things inhibit calcium absorption from the digestive tract. These include poor acid production by the stomach; the removal of the stomach at an operation; the ingestion of bran and wholemeal bread; gastrointestinal diseases that result in fat and calcium malabsorption; and a deficiency of vitamin D. Such conditions need to be sought out and treated. A supplement of 1–1.5 g of calcium as gluconate or lactate is recommended, with 0.5–0.75 g of magnesium as the oxide or aminochelate.
- *Other supplements*. With advancing years, deficiencies of vitamins and minerals become increasingly common. Though calcium has been extensively studied in osteoporosis, it is almost certain that other minerals, especially magnesium and zinc, will prove to be important. A magnesium supplement giving 0.5–0.75 g per day in conjunction with a calcium supplement is also recommended.
- *Stop smoking*. It appears that smokers have thinner bones than non-smokers.
- *Get regular exercise*. Perhaps the only advantage of being overweight is that carrying the excess load may increase bone strength and so help prevent the development of osteoporosis. Weight-bearing exercise such as walking, running, simple gymnastics or jogging, can help reduce calcium losses from the skeleton.
- *Do not take excess vitamin D*. Many people erroneously think that supplementation with large doses of vitamin D will improve the strength of the skeleton. This is definitely not true, and some studies have suggested that vitamin D in high doses, 10,000 to 50,000 IUs daily, may even be harmful. Women and old people who are at risk from osteoporosis should ensure that they have the recommended daily allowance of vitamin D either in their diet or from sunlight exposure but excess vitamin D should not be taken. A supplement of 400 IUs per day is adequate for housebound elderly people.
- *Avoid salt, sugar and coffee*. All these may have an adverse effect upon mineral balance.

Carpal Tunnel Syndrome

This condition starts as pain and tingling in the hands and fingers which may extend up into the arms. It is particularly common in women, often evident after carrying heavy shopping, and may wake them at night, or be bad on waking in the morning. Classically, there is tingling and discomfort in the thumb, index and middle finger, and the thumb side of the ring finger. This is caused by compression of a large nerve at the wrist. The nerve passes from the forearm into the hand through a "tunnel" of tissue between the wrist or carpal bones and a strap of tough fibrous tissue at the front of the wrist. Because of the compactness of the bones and connective tissue, swelling in this area compresses the nerve tissue at the wrist, producing pain and numbness in the fingers. There are many causes of the carpal tunnel syndrome, including an underactive thyroid, rheumatoid arthritis, weight gain, pregnancy and injuries to the wrist. Simple treatment involves the use of supportive splints to be worn at night. Some people benefit from injections of cortisone into the wrist and the most severe cases require an operation.

In a number of studies, researchers have shown that the carpal tunnel syndrome can occur as a result of vitamin B6 deficiency and may respond to supplementation with high doses. Doses in the region of 200 mg a day have to be used for some three months before the deficiency is corrected and the symptoms improve. This is certainly worth a try and should be combined with vitamin B complex supplements in a multivitamin.

Not all studies have shown a beneficial response to vitamin B6 and it may be better to combine this with other vitamins and magnesium.

Obviously, obese people should lose weight, and women in whom fluid retention is a problem should consider following a low-salt diet by avoiding salt in their cooking, not adding salt to their food and avoiding salty foods and snacks. Too many refined carbohydrates, too, can increase fluid retention and some people with food allergies also have fluid retention. The identification and avoidance of food allergies may also, in our opinion, be a useful approach (see page 154).

Bursitis, Fibrositis and Tenosynovitis

These conditions are characterized by inflammation and pain in soft tissues.

Rest and sometimes local application of heat or cold may be helpful. One study suggested that injections of vitamin B12, 1 mg intramuscularly daily for seven to ten days, then less frequently thereafter, may be of value in acute bursitis. Such patients had pain in the shoulder, hip, elbow, and some even had calcium deposits which were shown, on repeat X-rays, to resorb. Certainly we think this is worthy of a trial in our patients whose symptoms fail to clear by simple measures.

Gout

Gout is a cause of arthritis that particularly affects middle-aged and older men. Women are not infrequently affected, usually after menopause, and the risk of gout is increased by the use of certain drugs, especially diuretics. Characteristically, gout is thought to be a disease of the rich and the heavy drinkers, and indeed, this can be true, but by no means always. Gout is caused by the precipitation of insoluble crystals of uric acid into the joints which then become red, swollen and painful.

Gout may be helped by a number of dietary changes:

- lose weight if you are obese
- avoid alcohol completely
- avoid rich foods including red meat, game and fish roes
- take supplements—high doses of vitamin C (up to 4 g per day) increase the loss of uric acid via the kidneys; zinc, at doses of 50 mg per day, together with magnesium, 300 mg per day, can also be of benefit, in our experience. **These are best taken under medical supervision.**

Finally, some individuals with mild lead poisoning, such as plumbers, can develop gout and may benefit from treatment designed to reduce their lead accumulation. High-dose vitamin C and zinc is useful, as is a diet high in fiber.

Too much fruit consumption or the use of fruit sugar (fructose) might also aggravate gout.

Gout and renal failure

Dorothy, a delightful seventy-four-year-old lady, had been most unwell over the last four years. She had suffered from severe gout in her hands and knees, and had also been diagnosed as having an irregular heart rhythm, for which she required a pacemaker. Unfortunately, she needed a lot of drugs to control her heart problems and her gout, and these had caused considerable side-effects, to the point where she could no longer tolerate the drugs that she needed to remain healthy. More recent investigations had shown her to have a significant degree of kidney failure. She required a specialized diet, low in protein and avoiding all refined carbohydrates. Rich foods, such as game and rich meats, as well as alcohol, were avoided scrupulously, as these can all aggravate gout. She was also given high-dose vitamin C, 4 g per day, and large supplements of multivitamins and zinc. High-dose vitamin C can help lower the elevated blood level of uric acid, which is the cause of gout. With this diet, and supplements, her gout improved dramatically and her kidney function also improved. She was then better able to tolerate the drugs that she also required to maintain good health. Interestingly, she later developed eczema, which only cleared when her vitamin and mineral supplements were stopped. Fortunately, it did not return when they were reintroduced.

Back Problems

Back pain can be caused by a wide range of different conditions, including kidney and abdominal problems, as well as spinal problems. If you have severe or chronic back pain, you should always consult your doctor.

Back pain is not generally amenable to nutritional intervention. However, some of our patients benefit from the food intolerance approach (see page 154), and in certain back sufferers extremely low manganese levels have been found, which may affect their cartilage structure. Vitamin C supplementation can also be of benefit in a few people—taken in a dose of 2–5 g per day.

It seems sensible to us that those in whom there is some spinal misalignment receive osteopathic or chiropractic treatment. Exercise to strengthen the back, and swimming, are particularly helpful.

Muscle Cramps

Muscle cramps can be quite debilitating and can respond to vitamin E, 400–600 IUs per day, vitamin B6 50–100 mg twice daily, magnesium 400–800 mg daily and calcium, 800–1600 mg daily. These can be tried for one to two months. We have also found that the food intolerance approach can benefit some people.

Muscle Aches

Aching muscles are very common in people with low level health for whatever reason. The main thing is to find the underlying cause, treat it and the muscle aches go away. This may be done by "cleaning up" the diet, sorting out food intolerances and nutrient deficiencies especially of calcium and magnesium and the B vitamins. Muscle aches can be transient as in an acute viral infection but if they are more prolonged (weeks, months or years) then they are often due to one of the above or chronic candida (see page 346).

Muscle Weakness

Again this can be caused by the same things which cause muscle aches. Sometimes a potassium deficiency is a major contributing factor.

Restless Legs

Restless legs at night can be due to iron deficiency or excessive tea consumption. It can respond to correction of the deficiency; avoidance of tea and coffee. Vitamin E, 800 IUs daily, can also be of help. In some, the condition responds to specific supplements of folic acid, 5 mg one to three times daily, and this seems to be particularly helpful if the restless legs syndrome runs in the family.

DISORDERS OF THE RESPIRATORY SYSTEM

Disorders of the respiratory system occur at all ages. Common disorders of the respiratory system include acute or chronic infections and allergies.

Bronchitis

The most common acute lung infection is acute bronchitis. It can be caused by viruses or bacteria. The affected person complains of a cough, with yellowish or green phlegm. There may be a fever but this is usually mild. There is usually chest pain and there may be some soreness in the throat and chest. Smokers are particularly prone to develop acute bronchitis, as are the elderly, and such infections are more common in the winter. Antibiotics are frequently given for acute infections. From a nutritional point of view it may be worth considering high doses of vitamin C as well as supplements of zinc and vitamin B. The affected individual should avoid all refined carbohydrates and drink plenty of fluids. All these actions can stimulate the immune response to fight infection. Any additional deficiency should be corrected.

Emphysema

This condition destroys the lung tissue, usually as a part of the process of chronic bronchitis. Instead of there being lots of small air spaces in the lungs, the walls dividing them are destroyed and larger airsacs are thus formed. These are much less efficient in exchanging oxygen and carbon dioxide and as a result the amount of functioning lung is reduced. This usually troubles the chronic smoker who has a history of repeated attacks of bronchitis and/or pneumonia.

There is no definitive treatment that reverses the disease process, but it is important to try and make the most of the lungs one has. Activities such as singing, whistling, or breathing out against a partial obstruction such as a whistle or specifically designed mouthpiece, may help develop lung efficiency. Physical exercise may seem a strange recommendation for somebody who has a chronic cough and is short of breath to the point of physical incapacity. However, careful, graded physical exercise such as slow walking, building up to an increasing distance, is of proven value in improving lung function in those with chronic bronchitis and emphysema. It may also be important to ensure vitamin and mineral adequacy, particularly of the B vitamins and other nutrients involved in oxygen metabolism. Ensuring maximum efficiency of the body's metabolism in this way may help reduce the body's demand for oxygen.

Nutritional deficiencies without any obvious symptoms are very common, particularly in the elderly, and a trial of a multivitamin supplement (see page 422) for two or three months is certainly worthwhile. People whose chronic bronchitis and emphysema are characterized by excessive catarrh, may have an underlying food sensitivity or allergy. If the person also has nasal catarrh, this is particularly suspicious. The avoidance of dairy products alone, or the use of a modified exclusion diet may also be worth trying.

Cystic Fibrosis

This is a condition which affects 1 in 3,000 of all babies. Their lungs are primarily affected, and the pancreas is also affected, which results in poor digestive function, deficiencies of the fat-soluble vitamins, A, E, D and K, and also of the minerals zinc, iron, manganese and selenium.

Children with cystic fibrosis have chronic chest infections in early childhood and are often undernourished or small for their age. Occasionally, the diagnosis is not made until the child is several years old. The majority of such children used to die before reaching adult life. With the coming of powerful antibiotics, a reasonable life expectancy can now be anticipated. Nevertheless, they still require treatment with repeated courses of antibiotics, and the mucus has to be drained by laying them on their sides or backs, with the head downwards. Pancreatic problems are best treated with supplements of pancreatic enzymes. Many such children require supplements of vitamins A, D, E and K as well as zinc, which may be particularly important for those who have recurrent infections.

Asthma (see page 181)

Chronic and Recurrent Ear, Nose and Throat Infections

This includes otitis media (middle ear infection), sinusitis, catarrh, tonsillitis, quinsy, laryngitis and bronchitis. These conditions are usually caused by an infection with a virus or bacterium. If the latter is the case they may respond to antibiotics. However, the response to antibiotics is often unpredictable. In those with chronic infections, an underlying allergy is often the cause. Nutritional deficiencies, particularly of the B vitamins, vitamin C, zinc and iron, may also affect resistance to infection. We recommend the following:

- Assessment by skin tests for inhalant allergies, e.g. to house dust, animal fur, molds, and their avoidance (see pages 186–187).
- An exclusion diet (see Appendix 3, page 429). The avoidance of dairy products may be particularly valuable.
- Correction of nutritional deficiencies. A good multivitamin supplement is recommended, particularly if it is a child who is on a restricted diet.

Recurrent ear infections in children may lead to deafness and the need for an operation because of retained fluid in the middle ear. Trial of an exclusion diet is often worth considering.

In adults with recurrent bronchitis and laryngitis, stopping smoking and cutting down on alcohol are vital.

Rhinitis and Hay Fever

Symptoms include recurrent sneezing and watering of the nose, sometimes with watering and irritated eyes as well. Allergies to house-dust mite, cat fur, other animal furs and molds are very common. Some people can be allergic to drugs, e.g. aspirin. If chronic irritation occurs, polyps (outgrowths of the nose lining) can develop. Tests for the allergies can be performed. House dust should be avoided (see page 186). Exclusion diets can be helpful. Anyone with long-standing allergies, including hay fever, should follow the recommendation for a basic healthy diet (see page 398).

Severe Chest Infections

Tuberculosis and pneumonia are particularly likely to strike those who are run down, such as the elderly, or people on limited diets. Underlying nutritional deficiencies should always be considered. Remember that the main treatment for tuberculosis in the 1920s and 30s was a good diet and fresh air!

DISORDERS OF THE URINARY SYSTEM

The urinary system comprises the kidneys, in which urine is formed, and the collecting ducts, the ureters, which transport the urine to the bladder. Urine from both kidneys and ureters arrives at the bladder where it is stored before being passed out through the urethra or urinary passage.

The kidneys play an essential part in metabolism—they are not just a way of getting rid of excess water from the body. They excrete water-soluble waste products, are involved in the metabolism of vitamin D, and also in the production of hormones responsible for the normal functioning of bone marrow and control of blood pressure. Disorders of kidney metabolism can adversely affect the balance of salts and water in the body and so can produce high blood pressure.

Protein in the Urine

Many healthy people pass a small quantity of protein in their urine. This is often picked up at routine urine testing, but the individual may be aware of it already because his or her urine is excessively frothy. This is more often noticed by men. Though this is a harmless condition, some researchers have related it to the presence of food allergies. Sometimes an exclusion diet being undertaken for other reasons results in a reduction in the frothiness of the urine.

Kidney Failure

Failure of the kidneys to perform their normal function of excreting waste products is a serious condition and calls for expert management. Advice is required from a dietitian in balancing the quantities of calories, proteins, sodium, potassium, minerals and vitamins. Certain specific problems that can occur in those with renal failure may require the use of dietary supplements. Specialized forms of vitamin D may be needed for some of the bone problems that occur. In men, low sperm counts and the resultant infertility can sometimes be corrected by taking zinc.

It may be possible, by carefully manipulating the diet of those with kidney failure (whether they are being dialysed or not), to reduce the rate of progression of their disease. An interesting study by Professor John Yudkin showed that ordinary table sugar can produce changes in kidney function that could contribute to kidney damage. This means that such people would be well advised to avoid sugar if possible.

Cystitis (Bladder Infection) (see page 344)

Cancer of the Bladder

Cancer of the bladder is more likely to occur in workers in the rubber industry, and the incidence is also increased in smokers. It is thought that exposure to certain chemicals and their uptake by the body is followed by their excretion by the kidney. When there is a deficiency of vitamin B6, it is thought that more of the potentially cancer-producing byproducts are formed. Studies using vitamin B6 supplementation in patients with bladder cancer have suggested, but not yet proved, that it might reduce the recurrence rate of bladder tumors. Further studies are currently under way.

Prostate Problems

The prostate is a gland at the base of the bladder in men only, and is involved in providing some of the secretions that make semen. Certain malfunctions of the prostate can develop which can give rise to problems with urination and fertility.

CHRONIC PROSTATITIS

Chronic infection of the prostate gland due to candida, venereal and other infections, can produce pain, recurring cystitis and a reduced quality of sperm leading to infertility, and general debility. Treatment depends on the type of infective organism isolated in laboratory testing. If no infective organism is found, then food intolerance and/or chronic candidiasis should be considered (see pages 154 and 346).

However, there are a number of nutritional measures that can be taken: essential fatty acid deficiency and zinc deficiency may very well be associated with an increased susceptibility to prostatic problems. This makes it worthwhile considering taking cold-pressed safflower oil or cold-pressed linseed oil 10–15 mls twice a day, along with a zinc preparation (delivering approximately 40–50 mg of zinc) daily. **Higher doses of zinc and es-**

sential fatty acid supplements can be taken, but only under the supervision of your doctor. We have noted the reduction of symptoms in a number of patients on this regime.

PROSTATIC ENLARGEMENT

Another problem that can occur in older men is enlargement of the prostate resulting in a difficulty in passing urine. Initial symptoms include a desire to pass water urgently, having to wait for the stream to start, dribbling after finishing urination, an increased frequency of urination, and having to get up several times during the night. An extreme form of prostatic obstruction results in a total failure to pass urine at all.

There is a little evidence that increasing essential fatty acid intake and zinc supplementation can be of benefit in prostatic enlargement.

Bedwetting (see page 367)

Infections of the Urinary System

People with such infections respond rapidly to antibiotics, and nutritional therapy is really only suitable for those with recurrent cystitis. This is considered on page 344. High dose vitamin C, 5–10 g per day, can help clear up urine infections without using antibiotics. Some doctors give vitamin C, 1–2 g or more daily, long-term, to those who have recurrent urine infections. The increased urine acidity can cause discomfort in some people.

Kidney Stones

Kidney stones are collections of minerals and other chemicals that have formed insoluble crystals from substances normally present in the urine.

The stones form in the kidney and can sometimes reach substantial proportions, large ones being several inches across. The majority are small, but even then they can cause real trouble. The presence of a stone in the kidney increases the risk of infection and, in turn, some types of stones are themselves caused by infection. The kidney and ureter try to pass small stones—often with difficulty. A spasm of the muscle in the ureter caused by the kidney stone produces renal colic—a severe and sometimes excruciating pain in the loin which passes down to the groin.

Much research has been done into the factors that predispose people to kidney stones. Certain stones are caused by the presence of kidney disease or other conditions, particularly those that result in an increased excretion of insoluble calcium salts in the urine. In some cases there is a history of kidney stones in the family and it appears that there is a mild difference in metabolism in some people who have kidney stones and in their relatives. Finally, there are many dietary factors that increase the risk of kidney stone formation.

Because most kidney stones are high in calcium and oxalic acid, the major dietary and nutritional measures aimed at reducing the risk of stone formation affect both calcium and oxalic acid metabolism. Other stones are made of uric acid (as in people with gout), and other mixed minerals and amino acids in some rare instances.

Anyone with kidney stones, in particular those who have recurrent stones, should be carefully investigated to see whether they are excreting excessive amounts of calcium, oxalic acid, magnesium, uric acid, sodium and certain amino acids in the urine. Most local hospitals are able to perform those investigations routinely. Alternatively, if a stone is actually passed, and caught in the urine (with the help of a tea strainer), then an actual analysis of the stone can be performed to measure its mineral content.

Those who have recurrent stones that are high in calcium should have their blood calcium level measured to see whether it is elevated. This abnormality is found in about fifteen percent of recurrent stone-formers, and may suggest a disease of the parathyroid glands (which control calcium metabolism) that might require treatment by surgery. Blood and urine investigations for kidney disease, kidney infection, gout and, in some instances, gastrointestinal and other conditions, should be performed, to see whether any condition has resulted in a change in metabolism predisposing to stone formation. Very often these investigations are normal. The most common abnormality is a raised blood calcium. When all such investigations are normal, we turn our attention to dietary factors.

DIETARY FACTORS THAT MAY CAUSE KIDNEY STONES

In common with so many Western diseases, some of the more recent changes and additions to our diet have been implicated in the formation of kidney stones.

There appears to be little difference between the diets consumed by stone-formers and non-stone-formers, but a number of studies have shown that stone-formers react differently to certain dietary components, particularly calcium, refined carbohydrates and salt, compared with non-stone-formers. If the quantities of these three components in the diet are increased, more calcium is excreted in the urine and the risk of stone formation is increased.

There are a number of adverse dietary factors that need to be considered when it comes to kidney stone formation. These include:

- *Refined carbohydrates*. Sucrose (table sugar) can increase the absorption of calcium from the intestines and also increases its level in the urine in some individuals. Lactose (milk sugar) also enhances calcium absorption. This is obviously advantageous to the breast-feeding infant but may be disadvantageous in later life.
- *Animal protein*. The metabolic breakdown products of meat include uric acid and oxalic acid which are both involved in stone formation. Omnivores have a higher urinary concentration of calcium, oxalic acid and uric acid. Conversely, vegetarians, who have lower levels of these substances, have a prevalence of urinary stone formation of only forty to sixty percent of that of the average population.
- *Dietary calcium*. It appears that certain individuals are sensitive to an increase in quantities of dietary calcium which, in turn, may result in increased concentrations of calcium in the urine. So it seems wise to limit calcium intake, particularly from dairy products, in some stone-formers, though care should be taken to ensure that a low-calcium diet is not used long-term, as this might increase the risk of development of osteoporosis in the future. People who consume large quantities of calcium-containing antacids, together with milk, as a treatment for indigestion or peptic ulcers, can be at risk of developing high blood calcium levels and thus kidney stones.
- *Vitamin D*. This vitamin not only increases calcium absorption from the gastrointestinal tract, but also increases the release of calcium from bone, so raising blood calcium levels and predisposing to stone formation. High levels of vitamin D (greater than 400 IUs per day) are not needed by any section of the population, except for those with a proven vitamin D deficiency. Individuals who are exposed to adequate sunshine are well advised not to take vitamin D supplements at all.

- *Salt*. It appears that in some individuals, a high intake of salt results in an increased loss of calcium from the urine. There are many reasons for reducing salt consumption and it appears that in certain individuals stone formation is one of them.
- *Oxalic acid* is contained in many vegetables as well as being derived from vitamin C and to a lesser extent from protein-containing foods. Reductions in dietary oxalate may reduce the oxalate excreted in the urine and so lower the risk of stone formation. There are a number of foods high in oxalic acid. The main ones are tea, coffee, chocolate, peanuts, spinach, rhubarb, and beetroot. The metabolism of oxalic acid is, to some degree, dependent upon vitamin B6 and magnesium.
- *Alcohol*. Alcohol appears to contribute to kidney stone formation. It may increase the excretion of uric acid, calcium and phosphate as well as having adverse effects upon vitamin B6 and magnesium, which to some degree are protective against stone formation.
- *Vitamin C*. Vitamin C is metabolized to oxalic acid and there is some concern that taking high doses of vitamin C may increase urinary excretion of oxalic acid and thus kidney stone formation.

DIETARY FACTORS THAT ARE BENEFICIAL IN PREVENTING STONE FORMATION

- *Water*. Obviously, increasing urine output dilutes the concentration of minerals and other substances dissolved in it, and so reduces the likelihood of stone formation. Some experts suggest an intake of three liters of water per day, including a considerable quantity of water before retiring to bed. This is obviously unacceptable to many and may indeed be unnecessary if other dietary measures are followed. It seems good advice, however, to ensure an adequate intake of fluids. Tea should *not* be drunk, though, as it is high in oxalic acid. Hard water is high in calcium and not more than two liters per day should be consumed.
- *Fiber*. One of the beneficial effects of dietary fiber is its effect upon stone formation. Wheat and bran, both of which are high in phytate, reduce calcium absorption and have, in a number of studies, been shown to reduce calcium excretion in the urine. People with recurrent renal stones due to high concentrations

of calcium in the urine are well advised to take supplements of bran and to eat a high-fiber diet.

- *Magnesium*. Magnesium itself may be a constituent of renal stones, usually in small amounts. However, taking magnesium may increase the solubility of calcium oxalate and so reduce the chances of its precipitation in the urine. A number of studies have shown the benefit of magnesium supplementation in reducing the risk of stone formation. This is a simple, safe and effective measure—300–400 mg per day should be taken.
- *Vitamin B6*. Deficiencies or abnormalities of vitamin B6 metabolism, perhaps together with disturbances of magnesium metabolism, may reduce the ability of normal urine to keep oxalic acid in solution.

NUTRITIONAL RECOMMENDATIONS FOR THOSE WITH STONES

These dietary recommendations can be followed, no matter what type of stone you have:

- Ensure that you eat plenty of dietary fiber with every meal. Wholegrain cereals in particular are good. Eat plenty of fresh fruit and vegetables. Green leafy vegetables are high in magnesium, and may be particularly beneficial.
- Your intake of animal proteins, particularly meat, should not be excessive—40–60 g per day is enough for most people.
- Milk consumption should be no greater than two thirds of a pint per day.
- Avoid refined carbohydrates, particularly sucrose. This is found in sweets, cakes, chocolates, biscuits, puddings, jams, marmalade, soft drinks, tinned fruits, and many packed or processed foods. Certain fruits are high in sucrose, including dates and figs. A high consumption of honey is not recommended.
- Ensure that you drink plenty of water (tap or bottled).
- Reduce weight if you are obese.
- Limit or reduce your alcohol consumption. One or two drinks a day are probably not harmful, provided your diet is well balanced as above.
- Ensure that your salt intake is low by not adding salt to your food at the table or cooking with salt. Avoid high-salt foods

such as bacon, preserved meats, most packaged or savory foods and any salty tasting foods and snacks.

- Those with oxalate-containing stones, or high oxalate levels in the urine, should avoid certain foods including tea, coffee, chocolate, peanuts, spinach, rhubarb and beetroot, because they are rich in oxalic acid.

ECZEMA, DERMATITIS AND OTHER PROBLEMS OF SKIN, HAIR AND NAILS

The Skin

The health of the skin is dependent on the nutrients that it receives from the blood vessels in the underlying tissues. A characteristic of the skin is that it is particularly susceptible to outside influences, such as contact with irritating substances including detergents or chemicals. It is also sensitive to exposure to sunlight. In the treatment of skin disease, considerable emphasis has been placed upon the use of creams and ointments applied locally to the area of diseased skin. While this undoubtedly has a value, it also has distinct limitations. Little importance has been placed on the role of nutritional factors upon skin quality. Deficiencies of many vitamins and minerals result in skin changes, and a considerable number of skin diseases can be treated by using nutritional methods which get to the root of the problem. Although there are many skin conditions which respond to a nutritional program, **those that are listed in this chapter should best be treated by consultation with your own general practitioner.**

ECZEMA

Eczema is characterized by inflamed, red, itchy skin eruptions which often, but not always, contain small bubbles just under the skin surface. In severe cases these break on the surface producing a weeping, itchy rash.

The term "dermatitis," which simply means inflammation of the skin, is almost interchangeable with the word eczema, and is usually reserved for conditions where the cause is an external irritant.

Contact dermatitis or contact eczema

This is a very common type of dermatitis. Often the sufferer is all too aware that an external factor is the cause, but has been unable to identify it. It is usually a chemical, perfume, plant, metal, or even an item of clothing.

People with poor quality skin are particularly likely to develop such problems, and the Advice for Poor Skin may be of special benefit to them (see page 278).

We recommend that you ensure adequate supplies of vitamins B and C, and of zinc in your diet, and avoid an excessive consumption of animal fats. Supplementation with certain vegetable oils, particularly sunflower, safflower or linseed may be beneficial.

Atopic eczema

Eczema often occurs in association with asthma, hay fever, urticaria and sometimes migraine, either in the same person or in his or her close relatives. Such families are said to be atopic. There is thought to be a definite constitutional disorder which accounts for the findings of atopic eczema in some one to three percent of the population.

In the last few years, work from the Hospital for Sick Children in London has increased our understanding of the cause of eczema considerably, and has demonstrated that many children with eczema have food allergies. A child will often develop eczema when it is weaned from the breast and cows' milk or other foods are introduced. Delaying the onset of weaning and in particular the avoidance of common eczema-producing foods such as cows' milk, eggs or fish, will often reduce the risk or delay the onset of eczema.

Nutritionally, people with eczema are more likely to have a zinc deficiency and to have associated disturbances in the metabolism of essential fatty acids. Both zinc and essential fatty acids, which are derived from dietary vegetable oils, are probably important in maintaining skin quality and health.

Clearly there is no single treatment for all cases of eczema. Some people will have to avoid foods that offend them; others will have to avoid particular environmental agents; and some may need to take certain vitamins, minerals and oils to improve their skin quality. In others, treatment may be even more complex.

WHAT TO DO

The approaches to childhood and adult eczema are somewhat different. The severe exclusion diets used in adult eczema are not always suitable for children and care should be taken when using them.

Children

Diet. Young children should not be put on rigid exclusion diets without expert guidance. However, the avoidance of common allergens such as cows' milk, eggs, fish, cheese, food additives and sugar, can fairly easily be undertaken. Safe foods such as meat, vegetables, fruit and rice can be eaten instead.

If the eczema started just after the child was weaned, you should be particularly suspicious of recently introduced foods. A mother can trace back the foods that have been recently introduced, and avoid them in the future. If the eczema clears, then careful reintroduction of individual foods at approximately one new food every four or five days may help identify the offending food. However, eczema caused by foods in the mother's diet can occur in breast-fed infants. An exclusion diet under careful supervision may then be indicated for both mother and baby.

Milk allergy and eczema

James was seven years old and had had bad eczema since birth. This had required several admissions to the hospital and almost constant use of skin creams to keep the eczema under control. He was put on a milk- and egg-free diet resulting in a resolution of his eczema. Reintroduction of eggs did not produce an exacerbation or a recurrence of his skin problem, whereas milk did. The interesting point about this boy is that he is able to tolerate reasonable quantities of Carnation Milk—a form of condensed milk. This illustrates that the process of heating to the temperatures used in the preparation of Carnation Milk can change the allergic properties of a substance.

Supplements. Evening primrose oil may be safely given either by mouth or rubbed into the skin from which it is absorbed into the bloodstream. A 500 mg capsule, two or three times a day, can be beneficial for eczema in the body's creases and folds. It can be combined with a dietary approach as well.

Vitamins and minerals. The use of a children's multivitamin supplement including calcium is particularly advisable if the child is undergoing any kind of dietary restriction. The addition of zinc (5–10 mg per day), is perfectly safe and can be a very effective treatment for children under the age of two years (1–2 mg per kg of body weight). Children over this age can be given 15 mg. **Don't go on with zinc supplementation for longer than three months without medical supervision.**

Dietary oils. Reducing animal fat intake from dairy products, the fat from meat and fried foods may also be helpful. Also, remember that poor-quality margarines may be chemically no better than animal fats. Include high-quality sunflower, safflower or linseed oil in the diet.

Adults

There are certain differences in the approach to adults with eczema. First of all, it is important to exclude a possibility of con-

Eczema and zinc deficiency

Arthur, a forty-four-year-old postman, had developed severely itchy red patches on his legs and arms. He had never had asthma, eczema, or any allergies as a child, and couldn't understand why, at this age, he should now develop eczema. His wife, a keen reader of magazines and books on health and diet, wanted him to start an exclusion diet to see if he had food allergies. He was most reluctant to do this and give up some of his favorite foods! Investigations showed him to have a very low level of zinc in his sweat, 90 parts per billion, normal range 360–910. He was treated with large supplements of zinc sulphate, 220 mg twice a day, together with multivitamins and evening primrose oil, 500 mg six times a day. His intense skin-itching improved markedly over the next four weeks, and disappeared almost completely after eight weeks. He was delighted with the results, particularly because he did not have to go through an exclusion diet. Deficiencies of zinc and vitamin B may be particularly important, as they affect the metabolism of essential fatty acids, a lack of which may contribute to the development of dry skin and eczema. Correction of such deficiencies with the use of evening primrose oil and, where necessary, an exclusion diet, can be very effective, both in adult and childhood eczema.

tact dermatitis, which is very much more common in adults than in children.

In most cases of non-contact eczema, the most dramatic and usually the first approach is to try a strict exclusion diet for seven to ten days. The response can be remarkable. If you have no luck using this approach, take zinc, multivitamins and evening primrose oil, together with a low-animal-fat diet. This is worth trying for a few months. Any associated conditions such as thrush or other infections should be treated.

Magnesium and vitamin B6 deficiencies, which are found not infrequently in women with premenstrual symptoms, might cause allergic symptoms and should certainly be thought of if any allergy problem, including eczema, is worse premenstrually.

The use of local ointments, including steroid creams, will not generally strike at the root of the cause, but some people who have widespread eczema do need such treatment, particularly in the short term, until more definitive treatment can be used.

URTICARIA (NETTLE RASH)

Urticaria, nettle rash, or hives, are all names for a characteristic skin rash. It is a collection of red, raised, intensely itchy patches, some of which may have areas of white scattered among the redness. The rash lasts for several hours, but not usually longer than a day. Treatment with antihistamines usually produces dramatic relief. There are several types of urticaria. Some occur in response to physical exercise or emotion, some in response to allergies to foods, especially those containing natural salicylates (see page 432), drugs, coloring agents (e.g. tartrazine), or reactions to fungus infections or candida; and yet others occur following contact with animals or following the sting of nettles, jellyfish or insects.

It's often easy to identify the cause. Try to remember what foods you have eaten in the preceding few hours, particularly if you have had an unusual food such as shellfish or strawberries, or one containing unusual additives. If you have had similar reactions before, a good memory is a most useful approach to making the diagnosis. Skin or blood tests can be done to identify the offending agent. If you have recurrent, frequent bouts of urticaria, an exclusion diet or a low-salicylate, low-yeast, additive-free diet will be helpful (see Appendix 3).

SEBORRHEIC DERMATITIS

Seborrheic dermatitis is a red, greasy, scaly rash which is mildly irritating and usually found on the face, around the nose, chin and forehead, behind the ears, between the shoulder blades, or on the chest, over the breastbone, in the armpits, groins and under the breasts in women. Mild forms are extremely common. Vitamin B6 and vitamin B2 deficiencies frequently aggravate or sometimes can even be a cause of seborrheic dermatitis. An effective treatment program includes the following:

- the use of a strong supplement of vitamin B
- the avoidance of refined carbohydrates, particularly sugar
- a reduction in animal fat consumption
- try a supplement of cold-pressed linseed oil, 1–2 tablespoons per day
- coming off the contraceptive pill sometimes helps, too

Seborrheic dermatitis allergy and vitamin B6 deficiency

Betty was a sixty-four-year-old retired postmistress who had suffered from mild asthma all her life. Over the last year, however, she had been troubled by a red, greasy, itchy rash on her face, which was easily noticed by her friends. She had become withdrawn and shy because she found her new appearance to be socially embarrassing. Treatment with steroid ointments produced only temporary benefit and never cleared the rash completely. When I saw her, the diagnosis was classical seborrheic dermatitis, the appearance of which can be due either to vitamin B2 or vitamin B6 deficiencies. In fact, she had clear laboratory evidence of quite marked deficiencies of both of these, together with zinc deficiency. Her blood tests also showed evidence of an allergy reaction. Treatment with vitamin B resulted in a fifty percent improvement in the rash within four weeks, but there was clearly something else to be done. After trying a variety of diets, it became clear that coloring agents, particularly tartrazine (E102), aggravated her rash. Interestingly, this coloring agent may have an adverse effect upon vitamin B6 status, and can also be a factor in asthma. A trial of strong vitamin B supplements is worth considering in patients with red, greasy facial skin, and vitamin B6 alone is of proven value in the treatment of asthma.

ACNE

Acne, the scourge of teenage years, is characterized by three types of skin changes. These are blackheads, pustules (yellow spots) and papules (red spots). They are usually found on the face, though they may extend onto the shoulders, back, arms and chest. A wide variety of medical and non-medical treatments has been suggested and the response is rather variable.

Standard medical treatment with long-term antibiotics and ointments can be highly effective, but has disadvantages. For severe cases, powerful drugs derived from vitamin A or hormonal treatments can be used, but again there are significant risks.

Certain nutritional factors aggravate acne. Preparations containing iodine, such as kelp, definitely do so. Certain cough mixtures and tonics are rich in iodine and should also be avoided. Iodized table salt is not a problem in this respect.

Treatment with zinc in high doses is of proven benefit and has been found to be as effective as antibiotics. We recommend amounts no greater than 30–40 mg of zinc per day for about three to four months. Recently, supplements of selenium in the region of 200 mcg per day have been shown to help young men with acne. **This requires medical supervision.**

The avoidance of refined carbohydrates and a reduction in animal fats, combined with a multivitamin supplement and moderate doses of zinc, often proves very effective. Some individuals do not, however, respond. Many girls are acutely aware that if they eat sweets or chocolates they can rely upon a worsening of their skin the following day. The adverse effect of sucrose and glucose, within one hour of their consumption, on resistance to bacterial infection has been well described (see page 122), and the strict avoidance of such foods makes a lot of sense. Occasionally, an exclusion diet produces marked improvement and is well worth considering. Alternatively, try a fish and vegetable diet (see Piscine-Vegan diet, page 434).

PSORIASIS

Psoriasis is a common condition characterized by the presence of red, scaly plaques which are found on the arms, legs and trunk. Very rarely does it affect the face, though it can, and often does, affect the scalp. It is most often found on the points of the elbows and knees and mild forms are quite common. The cause of psoriasis is unknown and individual sufferers respond to a variety of treatments. Standard treatments make use of coal tar preparations, mild steroid creams, and specialized treatments with ultraviolet light.

Recent research on psoriasis has suggested that the metabolism of certain derivatives of dietary oils in sufferers may change subtly. It might thus be possible to produce an improvement in psoriasis by making long-term dietary changes. Psoriasis is not caused by a food allergy, and a response will not occur within a few days. The dietary changes on the following page may, however, be worth trying:

Arthritis due to psoriasis

A twenty-eight-year-old store manager had suddenly been affected by a very painful, swollen right knee. This was a severe type of arthritis which can occur in association with a skin condition called psoriasis, which had also troubled him for a few months previously. His arthritis had failed to respond to powerful drugs and injections of steroids into the knee. He was becoming particularly worried as, if he did not improve within the next two months, he would be likely to lose his job, a prospect that he and his wife did not relish. Interestingly, he also related the pain in his knee to a car accident that had occurred two years previously. A hair analysis showed a borderline level of zinc and, because some patients with psoriasis may have zinc deficiency, he was started on large doses of zinc, as zinc sulphate, 220 mg twice a day. This produced a gradual and sustained improvement in his knee, which became less painful and less swollen. He also had some stress counseling, which helped him uncover the hidden trauma of his car accident. After two months there was practically no evidence of any remaining arthritis, and the psoriasis that he had had on his body and the palms of his hands had almost completely cleared. He was delighted with the response and was able to return to work and retain his job. He found it hard to believe that his arthritis could improve just by taking zinc, but when he stopped it on two occasions the pains in his knee returned within two months. He has maintained himself on a supplement providing 30 mg of elemental zinc per day. Patients such as this, on prolonged high-dose zinc therapy, should always be under medical supervision, as copper deficiency can occur as a side-effect.

- Reduce your animal fat intake.
- Ensure that you eat plenty of fresh vegetables and fruits.
- Take high doses of zinc (30–40 mg a day), possibly together with other nutrients. One of us (A.S.) has seen two cases of widespread psoriasis clear completely after long-term, high-dose zinc administration. He has also seen two cases of psoriasis affecting the palms of the hands and the soles of the feet improve significantly though not clear completely, again following high-dose zinc administration. **This sort of treatment should be carried out under medical supervision because of the potential adverse effects of high-dose zinc.**

LEG ULCERS

Persistent ulceration of the legs is not an infrequent problem, particularly in the elderly and those who suffer from varicose veins.

The essentials in the treatment include the control of infection, elevation of the leg, and the use of pressure bandages to reduce the high pressure found in the veins adjacent to the ulcer. This high pressure prevents normal healing.

Despite these measures, many leg ulcers are slow to clear.

Studies have shown that vitamin C and zinc are both of proven value, sometimes reducing healing times by half.

Try:

- vitamin C, 1 g per day
- zinc, 30–60 mg of elemental zinc per day

Ensuring a healthy diet (see page 398) and the correction of any other nutritional deficiencies is very important. Local applications of vitamin E have been used, but these are probably less effective.

SKIN INFECTIONS

Skin may be infected by bacterial, viral or fungal organisms. Bacterial infections include abscesses, boils, and superficial skin infections such as impetigo which produces yellow, crusting, infected patches, usually on the faces of children. All such conditions usually respond either to antibiotics applied locally, in the form of ointment, or by mouth. In individuals with recurrent infections, or infections that are slow to clear, attention to the diet to ensure adequate nutrition is important.

INJURIES TO THE SKIN

Old people often bruise easily and this may be an early sign of vitamin C deficiency. Smokers are known to have lower vitamin C levels than non-smokers. Spontaneous bruising may be an indication of underlying blood disorders, and appropriate medical investigations and treatment are necessary.

BURNS

Burns and scalds of the skin require considerable response from the body's repair and wound-healing mechanisms. The demand for such nutrients as vitamin C and zinc also increases and their supplementation seems appropriate, particularly in the elderly and those with extensive burns.

FLUSHING

Facial flushing occurs in response to a number of causes. These include alcohol, drugs, and vitamins (vitamin B3 in the form of nicotinic acid), at menopause, in those with food allergies, and in some people with an overactive thyroid. Some individuals appear to be particularly sensitive to alcohol, especially those who have diabetes and take certain oral anti-diabetic drugs. Hot flushes occurring at the time of menopause may respond to vitamin E and other appropriate treatment for menopause symptoms (see page 307). People who have intermittent flushing for no obvious reason may have a hidden food allergy. It's worth trying an exclusion diet.

ADVICE FOR POOR SKIN

- Eat a good basic diet (see page 398).
- Take a good general multivitamin and mineral supplement.
- Avoid contact with caustic substances.
- Take 1 teaspoonful of cold-pressed linseed oil daily.
- Find a soap that suits you.
- Get treatment for any specific skin conditions.

Nails

Many skin diseases, particularly eczema and psoriasis, can also affect the nails, causing the smooth, regular surface to be replaced by ridging or pitting of the nail surface. A number of nutrient conditions can also affect nail quality.

BRITTLE AND SPLIT NAILS

Splitting and brittleness of the nails is a frequent complaint, particularly of people who often have their hands in water. Deficiencies of iron and zinc may also affect nail quality. Iron deficiency produces thinning of the nail, with a characteristic shape. The normal rounded, downward curve is replaced by a flattening of the nail which may be upturned (spoon-shaped nails). This may be particularly obvious on the thumbs. It is seen with chronic iron deficiency and can even occur if the person isn't anemic. Evening primrose oil may also help people with poor-quality nails.

WHITE SPOTS ON THE NAILS

The exact significance of white spots on the nails is as yet unknown. They can be a sign of zinc deficiency. White spots often clear following supplementation with zinc.

INFECTIONS OF THE NAILS AND NAIL BED

Acute and chronic infections of the nail and nail bed can occur. These go by the common term "whitlow." An acute infection is caused by a bacterium which usually enters because of a break in the skin due to a hangnail or trauma. An acute swelling, redness and pain occur at the side of the nail, which often resolves with the discharge of pus. A chronic infection of the skin and flesh around the nail is more often found in individuals who have repeated contact with water, such as housewives, bartenders, and nurses. It is often due to a chronic infection with candida albicans, and responds to the repeated application of anti-fungal ointments to the nail-bed area. In people with chronic paranychia, predisposing conditions such as diabetes, iron and perhaps zinc deficiencies should be considered, particularly if such infections are repeated.

Anyone with recurrent nail or nail-bed infections should follow the basic healthy diet (see Appendix 1) as a minimum treatment. Vitamin C and B, iron and zinc (to improve resistance to infection) are also worth trying. Vitamin E rubbed into the skin around the nails also seems to help.

Hair

HAIR LOSS

Hair loss is most noticeable from the scalp, but can occur in other areas, for example, the legs. Some hair loss is natural with age, not only on the scalp but also on the limbs, chest, armpits and pubic area. Excessive hair loss can occur if the skin itself is affected by conditions such as eczema, psoriasis, or seborrheic dermatitis. Some people with excessive hair loss from the scalp may actually have eczema or psoriasis of the scalp and may only be aware of it because it shows up as hair loss. There are many other causes of hair loss.

Deficiencies of certain nutrients are associated with poor hair growth, including deficiencies of iron and zinc. Certain drugs, particularly the Pill, anticoagulants and certain anti-cancer drugs can also produce hair loss.

Women with excessive hair loss should be checked for iron and zinc deficiencies. Supplements, if necessary, should be taken for several months. Vitamins B and C deficiencies and lack of protein can lead to hair that is easily lost.

In women, thinning of the hair might well respond to a different nutritional approach. Women normally have a small quantity of testosterone and other male sex hormones in their blood, and higher levels are found in some individuals, especially around the time of menopause. Vitamin E, at a dosage of 600 IUs per day, reduces elevated levels of one of these male sex hormones in women. Furthermore, vitamin C at a dosage of 1 g per day may, under some circumstances, enhance the effect of female estrogens. Having said this, neither vitamin C nor vitamin E has ever been tried formally for premature thinning of the hair in women or men.

There is no effective treatment for hair loss in men, but an application containing biotin, niacin and an emulsifier called polysorbate, has apparently been used with some success. We have not had any clinical experience with this regime, but in theory it might be of some value as niacin increases the blood supply to the scalp and certain drugs which act in a similar fashion can also stimulate scalp hair growth.

Sometimes hair loss from the scalp occurs in an isolated patch–alopecia areata—the cause of which is unknown. Fortunately, many cases recover spontaneously though it can take several months. Again, there is little proven treatment, but doctors in Poland have tried long-term, high-dose zinc and reported a successful response in two patients. **Long-term, high-dose zinc supplementation should always be carried out under medical supervision.**

GRAYING OF THE HAIR

Loss of hair color is an almost inevitable feature of aging. In rats, a deficiency of vitamin B5 (pantothenic acid) results in graying of the hair which is reversible by correcting the vitamin deficiency. However, in humans, no such response has ever been demonstrated. Graying of the hair in the twenties may be associated with an increased risk of celiac disease, thyroid disease, diabetes, pernicious anemia, and other autoimmune diseases. It is quite probable that there are a number of nutritional factors which have yet to be identified in those who have graying of the hair at an early age. Very often, those who gray at an early age keep a healthy head of hair well into late adult life. We have noted several people who, having received nutritional treatment for other conditions, have found the graying of their hair has lessened. Correction of vitamin B12 deficiency is particularly important.

DANDRUFF

Dandruff is an all too common complaint in which the skin of the scalp scales and flakes, resulting in the familiar mantle of white specks on clothing, headrests and pillows. The scalp is sometimes itchy and irritating, which causes the sufferer to scratch and increases the loss of dandruff scales. There has been a lot of debate as to the cause of dandruff, but a leading British dermatologist, Professor Sam Shuster from Newcastle-upon-Tyne, feels that the evidence in favor of its being due to a fungal infection is overwhelming. It could be that a general "antifungal program" could be of value in the treatment of dandruff, particularly if combined with the use of an anti-dandruff shampoo. Such a program would include the avoidance of excessive quantities of refined carbohydrates, a reduction in intake of animal fats and hydrogenated margarines, the correction of deficiencies of zinc and vitamin B, perhaps supplementation with vitamins C and E, and the use of supplements of oils high in polyunsaturates, particularly cold-pressed sunflower and linseed oils. Any such treatment would have to be prolonged for three or four months, as the fungus is likely to be located deep in the hair follicle and it would take this time for it to grow out from hair completely. Such a dietary and supplement program would be likely to improve skin quality in general. One messy, but sometimes successful, treatment is to apply cold-pressed linseed oil at night and wash off with shampoo in the morning. (Use an old pillowcase!) Try this three times a week. Selenium-containing shampoos such as Selsun and Lenium are an effective treatment for many forms of dandruff. Here selenium is being used as an antifungal agent and not as a nutrient. Toxicity can occur if you don't follow the manufacturer's instructions.

DISEASES OF THE EYES

Disease of the eyes runs from minor problems such as conjunctivitis to serious conditions that threaten sight. Throughout the world, undoubtedly the most common cause of blindness is a deficiency of vitamin A. It has been suggested that half a million children each year lose their sight because of a deficiency of this single nutrient. Such children are often malnourished and living in underdeveloped countries.

In the Western world, blindness is more likely to occur as a result of such conditions as cataracts and glaucoma, which are both thought to be degenerative changes. Medical treatment for such conditions is useful but only of limited value, and definitive treatment often involves surgery. Their prevention may well involve nutritional changes, though we do not currently know how useful nutritional methods could be.

A number of eye conditions, however, *are* known to respond to a nutritional program.

Night Blindness

Poor vision at night is usually caused by a deficiency of vitamin A or of zinc. In vitamin A deficiency, night blindness is often the earliest feature, but may not be very obvious to the person who has it. They may dislike driving at night or find that they have to have a really bright light in the evening for reading. A deficiency of vitamin A at this level is only likely to occur in certain liver diseases, malnutrition, particularly in the elderly, or impaired digestion leading to malabsorption which may also cause a zinc deficiency. If there is no satisfactory and quick response to vitamin A supplementation then a zinc deficiency could be the problem. Zinc is probably involved in the metabolism of vitamin A in the retina at the back of the eye.

Tobacco Amblyopia

In smokers, a rare form of blindness can occur in association with a vitamin B12 deficiency. Urgent treatment with specialized vitamin B12 injections (as hydroxycobalamine) is effective.

Central Retinal Vein Thrombosis

The eye receives its blood supply from a group of blood vessels that enter and leave at the back of the eye through a hole in the retina. Sometimes a blood clot forms in the vein through which the blood normally leaves the eye. This results in the disruption of blood flow and a loss of vision. This condition occurs in elderly people who also have diabetes or high blood pressure. Taking certain nutrients such as vitamins C, E and B6, selenium and fish-oil derivatives might reduce the risk of thrombosis.

Retinal Hemorrhage

A fine network of blood vessels passes over the retina supplying it with oxygen and other nutrients. If one of these blood vessels breaks, there is a loss of vision in the corresponding area of the retina. This may produce a blind spot, or, if it affects the central point of the eye, there may be a loss of fine vision in one eye. Such hemorrhages are more likely in the elderly, and sometimes occur with hypertension. Nutritional management of the hypertension (see page 222) is certainly beneficial.

Retinal Detachment

Sometimes the retina becomes detached from its blood supply, and thus perishes, causing blindness. The loss of vision is usually partial, affecting, for example, the upper or lower field of vision of one eye. In dogs, retinal detachment can be caused by an acute zinc deficiency, but no similar research has, to our knowledge, been performed in humans. The retina has a very high zinc content as well as a lot of vitamin A. It is hoped that this will interest future researchers enough to look at the zinc status of those with degenerative eye conditions, including retinal detachment.

Diabetic Retinopathy

In diabetes, there are many changes in the blood vessels at the back of the eye and it is quite possible that a number of nutrients could be of value in this condition. Supplements of vitamin C, for example, have been shown to reduce the fragility of blood vessels in diabetics. They may also benefit from supplements of vitamin E, selenium, vitamin B6, zinc, essential fatty acids and bioflavonoids.

Cataracts

These cause a clouding of the lens of the eye, usually in old people. Diabetes certainly accelerates such changes, but occasionally cataracts develop in younger people and even in babies. When cataracts develop in relatively early adult life, the person needs careful investigation because disturbances in calcium or sugar metabolism can be a cause of the premature formation of cataracts. Those with these conditions can be treated by a specialized nutritional approach.

It is not known whether the ordinary type of cataract that develops particularly in the elderly can be affected by nutritional factors. It was once thought that deficiencies of riboflavin (vitamin B2) might be relevant, but this appears to have been recently disproved. There is a possibility that vitamin E and selenium could influence the rate of normal degeneration in the lens of the eye, but this is a subject that needs further research.

Minor Eye Conditions

The following, less serious, eye conditions sometimes respond to nutritional approaches:

A DISLIKE OF LIGHT

This is sometimes a feature of a migraine headache, which in turn may be related to food allergies (see page 154). Sometimes a deficiency of vitamin B2 can cause this problem. Such people often have red eyes.

CONJUNCTIVITIS

This is inflammation of the front of the eye which becomes red, watery, gritty and painful. It is often caused by an infection, and responds to antibiotic eye drops. Occasionally, it is caused by an allergy, for example to pollen, and shows up with the other features of hay fever in which case vitamin C (as potassium ascorbate) eye drops may help. If the redness of the eye is confined to the ring around the front of the eye, it is a feature of vitamin B2 deficiency. Food allergy can cause repeated conjunctivitis, too.

RED EYELIDS

Soreness, redness and cracking of the outer corners of the eyes can be caused by a deficiency of vitamin B2 or B6 and usually responds promptly to treatment. Inflammation along the margins of the eyelids often occurs in the elderly, particularly if there is deformity of the eyelids. (Sometimes it goes along with severe dandruff and greasy skin.) In this latter case, a nutritional approach can be helpful. Reduce your animal fat intake, take cold-pressed vegetable oil (e.g. linseed oil) and take supplements of vitamins C and B and zinc.

Eczema of the eyelids can also be caused by candida allergy (see page 346).

PUFFINESS OF THE EYELIDS, AND PROTRUSION OF THE EYES

These occur in some people who have an overactive thyroid gland. This obviously requires appropriate medical treatment. An underactive thyroid gland can also produce puffy bags under the eyes. The individual also usually has a rather puffy face and their voice may deepen. For many people with normal thyroid glands, puffy bags under the eyes are a persistent complaint and are sometimes associated with food allergies. In children the skin may be smooth, distended and shiny, giving rise to the name "allergic shiners." A full or modified exclusion diet may well help to identify the cause of the problem, particularly if other food allergic symptoms are present such as rhinitis, asthma, eczema, catarrh, mouth ulcers, malaise, muscular aches and pains, digestive complaints and headaches. It is usually the presence of three or four of these symptoms (including puffiness of the eyes) that makes us suspicious of a food allergy or intolerance.

DRY EYES

This can be a persistent and disturbing complaint.

In its most severe forms it may accompany conditions such as rheumatoid arthritis and other related, though rarer, forms of arthritis. Dryness of the eyes may go hand in hand with mouth dryness.

A Scottish trial reported on seventeen people with dry eyes receiving vitamin C, 3 g a day, and vitamin B6, 50 mg a day, for a period of at least two months. Ten of the seventeen showed a significant improvement. Such an approach certainly seems worthwhile.

Some people may also have an allergy especially to wheat and other gluten-containing grains, such as rye, oats and barley. Deficiencies of vitamins A and B2, or an essential fatty acid deficiency (see page 107), can also cause eye dryness. Allergy to house dust or pets can cause eye irritation.

DIABETES MELLITUS

There are essentially two types of diabetic: those who require insulin—Insulin-Dependent Diabetics (IDD); and those who can be managed with diet and oral agents—Non-Insulin-Dependent Diabetics (NIDD). About forty percent of all diabetics are on insulin, forty percent on drugs and twenty percent require only dietary management. All diabetics, however, do need dietary advice.

Insulin is needed for the normal metabolism of glucose. After a meal, blood glucose rises and as a result insulin is released from the pancreas. This helps the cells to take up the glucose and use it so the level of glucose in the blood falls back to normal. Young diabetics often lack insulin; older ones have insulin, but their bodies fail to respond to it normally.

Thirst, passing lots of urine and weight loss are the most common symptoms of diabetes.

Though there are a number of known glandular and other diseases which predispose to the disease, the precise cause of the majority of diabetics' faulty glucose metabolism is unknown. Research in this field has been intense and a number of studies have suggested that in children with diabetes either a virus toxin or a self-generated poison causes the destruction of the insulin-producing cells in the pancreas. In older people there is no lack of production of insulin, but it appears that the fat and muscle cells do not respond to its presence. The sugar levels remain high in the blood instead of being taken up by the cells.

Diet and Diabetes

There have been considerable changes and variations in the dietary advice given to diabetics over the years. The advice now given by the British Diabetic Association probably represents the majority of opinions in this area and sets out realistic goals for most diabetics. The recommendations are as follows.

If you are diagnosed as being diabetic you should:

- Match your energy intake to your individual requirement and lose weight if you are obese.
- Exclude, where possible, simple sugars (glucose, sucrose) from the diet.
- Obtain half or more of your calories from unrefined carbohydrate, putting special emphasis on fiber-rich foods.

- Restrict dietary fat to thirty-five percent of your calories overall, principally by reducing saturated (animal) fat.
- Continue with your dietitian's advice on the estimation and distribution of carbohydrate "exchanges" or "portions." This is especially true for insulin-dependent diabetics.
- Reduce your salt intake.
- Moderate your alcohol intake.
- Use artificial sweeteners in moderation and then only as a part of a calorie-controlled reducing diet.

There is considerable scientific research to support these recommendations and interest has centered mainly on the type of carbohydrate and the type of fiber that is best included in the diabetic diet. However, to be realistic, it can be difficult to make such changes quickly and some diabetics will probably need the help of a dietitian with such a diet until it becomes a natural way of life.

Weight reduction plays a crucial part in diabetic control. Weight reduction appears to increase a diabetic's lifespan and may be valuable for helping the other conditions such as hypertension that often go hand in hand with diabetes. Physical exercise can also help in diabetic and blood sugar control.

Foods differ in their effect on blood sugar. An aim of the diabetic's diet is to prevent excessive swings of blood sugar level. Those foods that appear to produce the least rise in blood sugar include all the legumes (particularly soybeans), most fruits (except bananas and raisins), wholegrain rye bread, buckwheat, wholewheat pasta, and the sugar fructose (fruit sugar). Diabetics are encouraged to eat these in particular.

CHROMIUM

Interest in chromium has been increasing considerably in recent years, particularly since research which documented the relationship of chromium deficiency in Western populations to atherosclerosis (hardening of the arteries) and diabetes. Chromium deficiency has been found in both children and adults with diabetes.

There is now a considerable number of studies investigating effects of chromium supplementation in diabetics. The majority show benefits, particularly for the elderly non-insulin-dependent diabetic.

Unfortunately, it is difficult to test for chromium deficiency as such investigations are not available at local laboratories. In view of the low toxicity of chromium and its cheapness, it seems to us that the best test is a therapeutic trial. The most readily available and most convenient form is chromic chloride which contains trivalent chromium (see Appendix 2). The absorption of chromium from chromic chloride is extremely poor—perhaps less than one percent. It also seems that in order for chromium to be biologically active it must be combined with nicotinic acid (vitamin B3) and a number of amino acids. This composite compound is known as the Glucose Tolerance Factor (GTF). This is thought to bind with insulin to improve the utilization of insulin by cells. Chromium GTF is found in high concentrations in ordinary brewers' yeast (brewers' rather than baker's).

It therefore seems reasonable to suggest that either chromium chloride solution or 20–30 brewers' yeast tablets per day be taken by *all* elderly diabetics. Chromium is considerably cheaper and notably free from side effects when compared with the usual anti-diabetic drugs.

VITAMIN C

Vitamin C has a very similar chemical structure to that of glucose. Vitamin C deficiency is known to occur in diabetics and its administration may improve the fragility of blood capillaries and reduce elevated cholesterol levels. Smoking can substantially depress vitamin C levels and a diabetic who smokes, has a raised blood cholesterol and perhaps a history of small strokes or easy bruising, might greatly benefit from vitamin C supplementation (as well as stopping smoking). Doses of 250–1000 mg per day are necessary.

VITAMIN B6 AND B12

Both these nutrients can be of value to the diabetic and supplements can improve blood sugar control. Pregnant diabetics may particularly benefit from 100 mg of B6 per day for three weeks.

OTHER MINERALS

Other minerals such as zinc, magnesium and potassium, are particularly important to diabetics. Increased losses of zinc in the urine are known to occur and a diabetic who has symptoms of zinc deficiency (such as eczema, acne, recurrent infections including thrush, or poor growth in a child) should have tests of zinc status done to see if there is a need for zinc supplements.

Magnesium deficiency can be a complicating feature of diabetes, particularly in those diabetics who have ketoacidosis which probably results in increased magnesium losses in the urine.

ESSENTIAL FATTY ACIDS (EFAs)

EFAs are dependent upon a particular enzyme which requires in particular vitamin C, zinc, vitamin B6 and vitamin B3 as well as other nutrients. It is suspected that in diabetics the metabolism of EFAs is reduced as a consequence of the raised blood glucose or insulin deficiency. The use of specialized supplements which bypass this chemical block may well be justified, and evening primrose oil, or MaxEPA, may benefit diabetics with specific complications of diabetes.

DRUGS

Some drugs may worsen diabetes, especially diuretics (water tablets). They may do this by producing a potassium or magnesium deficiency.

Diabetes and food allergy

Henry was a middle-aged architect who had diabetes mellitus (where the blood sugar goes too high). It had been fairly poorly controlled with diet, but he did not need to take insulin. On preliminary screening it was evident that he was deficient in zinc, magnesium and chromium—all common findings in diabetics. Putting him on supplements of these essential trace elements resulted in a considerable improvement in his blood sugar control level, although it was not ideal. Checking his vitamin B6 level revealed a marked deficiency of this vitamin, another common finding in diabetics. Giving him supplements of vitamin B6, as well as vitamin C and the B vitamins, resulted in a further improvement in his blood sugar control, but it was still not right. Then, putting him on a stricter diet excluding those foods to which he was allergic resulted in a dramatic improvement in his diabetes. Exclusion of these foods improved his blood sugar control in a way that was not dependent on the carbohydrate content of the foods that he was consuming. He started to feel better than he had done in a number of years and his blood sugar control became normal so long as he avoided the offending foods and continued to take his supplements of zinc, magnesium, chromium and vitamins C and B. Whenever he violated his diet by taking an offending food, his blood sugar level shot up. This is an interesting illustration of how blood sugar levels are controlled by a number of different factors which, if not taken into account, can result in poor diabetic control.

Nutritional Approaches to Diabetic Complications

Diabetes can produce some very serious, even life-threatening, complications. Let us look here at a few individual complications and see which of the nutrients above could be of value.

Going onto a high-fiber, high-complex-carbohydrate, low-animal-fat, low-refined-carbohydrate diet and a careful control of blood sugar by oral drugs or insulin together with appropriate nutrients is likely to minimize the risk of complications. This is the current view held by many diabetologists and good diabetic control is central to the treatment of the complications.

NEUROPATHY

Diabetes is very often complicated by a disease process in the nerves which causes tingling and numbness, particularly in the legs. It can also produce impotence, fainting on standing up, and bladder and bowel disturbances. It is thought that metabolic abnormalities may cause these problems. Supplements of vitamin B6, 100 mg per day, and injections of vitamin B12 have been beneficial according to some reports. Recently, a study of evening primrose oil suggests it, too, may be of benefit.

DIABETIC LEG ULCERS

Leg ulcers are not at all uncommon in diabetics. They appear to be caused by blood vessel problems, neuropathy and a generally reduced resistance to infection and obesity. Both vitamin C and zinc are of proven value in the healing of resistant leg ulcers. This makes it sensible to take vitamin C, 1–3 g per day, and elemental zinc, 20–80 mg per day, in conjunction with other nutrients, including chromium.

RAISED FATS IN THE BLOOD

Elevated triglycerides are a common feature of diabetes and the restriction of alcohol and refined carbohydrates may be particularly beneficial. Reduction in the blood levels of both triglycerides and cholesterol may reduce the risk of coronary heart disease for which diabetes is a serious risk factor. Diabetics who have a heart attack are known to have a considerably worse outlook.

Therapeutic agents of value include vitamin C, 300 mg–1 g per day, trivalent chromic chloride, an increased intake of polyunsaturated fatty acids and their derivatives (evening primrose oil

500 mg, six capsules per day and MaxEPA 10–20 g per day). Weight reduction is of paramount importance.

PERIPHERAL VASCULAR DISEASE

Diabetes is often characterized by disease affecting small blood vessels, whereas that associated with smoking and generalized arteriosclerosis more commonly affects large vessels. There are reports of the beneficial effects of vitamin E in this small-vessel disease, but trials have not been done specifically on diabetics. Of proven value in peripheral vascular disease has been the use of a low-animal-fat, high-fiber diet and also a low-fat, high complex-carbohydrate diet.

DIABETIC KIDNEY DISEASE

Kidney problems are not uncommon in diabetes, particularly in those with long-standing diabetes. Stopping smoking and improved diabetic control may be particularly important.

EYE PROBLEMS

Diabetes produces eye problems characterized by bleeding and the proliferation of tiny blood vessels. These can eventually lead to blindness and so are well worth treating where possible.

Diabetics with retinopathy have different fatty acid constituents in their blood platelets compared to healthy people and diabetics who do not have retinopathy. These alterations in fatty acid concentrations are likely to produce changes in level of certain body chemicals called prostaglandins, which in turn lead to increased platelet clumping in diabetics. On the basis of analysis of platelet fatty acids, it seems that consuming salmon, mackerel, herring and linseed oil may be particularly beneficial for diabetics. Trials of vitamin E on platelet clumping in diabetic retinopathy suggests that it, too, may be of benefit. Dosages should probably be in the region of 200–600 IUs per day. Use of specialized absorbable preparations of vitamin E (micellized) may, because of improved absorption, be particularly desirable. The fragility of blood vessels in patients with diabetic eye disease has been shown to be improved by vitamin C. 200–500 mg per day is suggested. It is quite possible that other nutrients such as bioflavonoids, trace minerals such as magnesium, and essential fatty acids play a very important role in diabetic retinopathy. Correction of deficiencies and use of appropriate supplements is suggested.

HYPOGLYCEMIA

Hypoglycemia, or low blood sugar, is a condition of considerable importance in nutritional medicine. Failure to recognize it, or to believe that it exists, can lead to erroneous diagnoses and inadequate or wrong treatments. Unfortunately, this is all too often exactly what happens.

It is important to bear in mind that there are basically three types of hypoglycemia:

1. Severe hypoglycemia as a result of organic disease, such as an insulin-producing tumor of the pancreas or liver. This can produce coma, and can be life-threatening. It obviously needs to be investigated fully, so that the underlying tumor can be removed surgically, if that is possible.
2. Diabetic hypoglycemia. This occurs when an insulin-dependent diabetic gives him or herself too much insulin, resulting in an excessive fall in blood glucose levels. How insulin works is described below.
3. Reactive hypoglycemia. This is the condition which we will discuss in this section, and is basically that form of low blood sugar that is brought about by less severe metabolic problems than the previous forms. It is nevertheless important in that the range of symptoms can be wide and the detrimental effects on the lives of sufferers can be devastating.

Reactive Hypoglycemia

Blood sugar, under normal circumstances, is controlled within reasonably close limits. When the blood sugar is consistently too high, the person becomes a diabetic (see page 286) and when it goes too low, the person is said to have hypoglycemia. The hormone insulin, secreted by the pancreas, reduces blood sugar levels by driving glucose into the cells. With inadequate insulin, blood sugar is high and the person has diabetes mellitus. Hypoglycemia is often associated with the production of too much insulin resulting in too much sugar being driven into the cells. The blood sugar level is then reduced to too low a level. This does not matter quite so much for the muscle cells and the other cells in the body as it does for the cells of the brain, because glucose is required by the brain if it is to work normally. It is, therefore, hardly surprising that many of the symptoms of hypoglycemia are related to mental function.

Glucagon is a hormone also secreted by the pancreas which is released into the bloodstream in response to a low blood sugar level. The action of glucagon is to bring about the release of glucose into the bloodstream from glycogen stores in the liver.

SYMPTOMS OF HYPOGLYCEMIA

The main ones are:

- weakness
- faintness
- palpitation
- fast heartbeat (tachycardia)
- anxiety, cold sweats, panic attacks
- irritability
- insomnia (especially night waking and nocturnal fridge raiding)
- hunger, nausea
- vertigo
- behavior problems and mood swings
- mental disturbance
- allergic reactions
- epilepsy in susceptible individuals
- migraine and headaches
- personality disorders (hysteria, hypochondriasis)

Symptoms are most common at mid-morning and mid- to late afternoon, usually two to five hours following food. Exercise may provoke symptoms but food or glucose may not provide definite relief. Between attacks, sufferers often report feeling run down and functioning below par.

It's easy to see how somebody suffering from symptomatic hypoglycemia can be dismissed simply as neurotic. On the other hand, those with genuine psychological problems should not be classified as hypoglycemic without good reason.

CAUSES OF HYPOGLYCEMIA

Refined carbohydrates

One of the most common contributing factors in hypoglycemia in the West is excessive refined carbohydrate consumption. Foods containing sugar and glucose rapidly increase blood sugar levels and can result in the excessive production of insulin. Some doctors are under the misconception that if a person has a low blood sugar they should simply have a cup of tea with a few teaspoonfuls of sugar. This is wrong. While this might well produce relief of the symptoms for a while, it encourages a vicious circle; a low blood sugar, refined carbohydrate ingestion, excessive insulin secretion, followed by a low blood sugar. One approach to treatment of low blood sugar is the elimination of refined carbohydrates from the diet. Additionally, you can eat complex carbohydrates which may have a very beneficial effect. This is discussed in more detail later on. The principle of this is that complex carbohydrates take longer to digest, so there is not such a rapid increase in blood sugar, with a lesser insulin response. This approach is used in the management of both diabetes and hypoglycemia.

Chronic stress

Very often, individuals who are bothered by symptoms of hypoglycemia are under chronic stress of one sort of another. This makes it very easy for the doctor to attribute all the symptoms that the patient may be complaining of to anxiety or neurosis. However, on testing, the individual may be found to be hypoglycemic and the diagnosis of hypoglycemic becomes valid. Nevertheless, controlling chronic stress can be a very useful approach to the treatment of genuine reactive hypoglycemia.

Food intolerance

There is some evidence to show that specific foods can actually produce an abnormally low or high blood sugar, irrespective of the carbohydrate content of the food.

So a very sensible part of the management of hypoglycemia can be the management of food intolerances. A high-protein, low-carbohydrate diet which excludes wheat and dairy products, two of the most commonly offending foods in adults, has been found to be of proven value in the management of hypoglycemia.

Too much or too little thyroid hormone

Both underactivity and overactivity of the thyroid gland can result in a low blood sugar. So anyone with hypoglycemic symptoms should see their doctor about the possibility of their thyroid gland being over or underactive.

Deficiencies of nutrients

Deficiencies of several nutrients—chromium, magnesium, potassium, manganese, zinc, and the B vitamins—are all associated with an increased tendency to hypoglycemia. A broad spectrum vitamin B complex supplement, chromium GTF (see Appendix 2), zinc, manganese, magnesium and potassium supplements, can improve reactive hypoglycemia and glucose tolerance.

Drug effects

Several drugs, including metronidazole, which is used in the treatment of vaginal trichomoniasis and parasitic infestation of the intestines, can cause hypoglycemia. Anyone who experiences symptoms of hypoglycemia when on any drug therapy should bear in mind the possibility that the drug is actually precipitating the symptoms by way of its toxic effects directly or by its blood-sugar-lowering effect.

Missed meals

People who miss meals, especially infants and young children, often experience hypoglycemic symptoms. This makes it important to have regular meals so that the hypoglycemic symptoms are avoided. Quite often fights within families occur at the time of day when meals should have been taken, but for some reason or other, have not. Similarly, problems at work can be worsened by one or other of the workers being hypoglycemic.

Excessive tea and coffee consumption

Both these substances cause an increase in the release of insulin from the pancreas, and thus can cause hypoglycemic symptoms. As a result, anyone who has hypoglycemic symptoms should avoid drinking tea and coffee.

Cigarette smoking

Cigarette smoking increases the release of both glucagon and insulin, and an initial response can be too much sugar followed by hypoglycemia. Very often a smoker requires "topping up" every hour or so with a blast of nicotine, and this can be a short-term remedy for hypoglycemic symptoms.

Alcohol

Alcohol is very definitely a cause of hypoglycemia. Most alcoholics are quite severely hypoglycemic, and a part of coming off alcohol should include the use of an anti-hypoglycemia diet.

THE TREATMENT OF HYPOGLYCEMIA

1. *Avoid refined carbohydrates*. This is a cornerstone of treatment and is an *extremely* important rule to follow. Anyone

who has hypoglycemic symptoms or has been given a diagnosis of reactive hypoglycemia should avoid refined carbohydrates *totally*.

2. *Eat a high-protein/low-carbohydrate diet, or a high-complex-carbohydrate diet.*
3. *Eat small, frequent meals.* Whichever diet they follow, some individuals do very much better by having small, frequent meals rather than a few large ones. This is especially true of people on the high-protein, low-carbohydrate diet. Those on a high-complex-carbohydrate diet tend to do better with fewer meals in that their blood sugar levels are maintained over a longer period of time due to the slow release of sugar into the bloodstream from the complex carbohydrates.
4. *Tryptophan supplements.* Some individuals on a high-complex-carbohydrate diet do very well with tryptophan supplements, 500–1500 mg daily.
5. *Niacinamide* (nicotinamide) (vitamin B3) (see Appendix 2). Some people do very well on niacinamide supplements, 1000–3000 mg per day. This is especially true of those who wake up at night around 2–3 a.m. with hypoglycemic symptoms. It should be emphasized that this is niacinamide, and not niacin. **Any individual who is having high-dose niacinamide should have their liver function tests reviewed every month or two by their doctor.**
6. *Nutritional supplements.* A nutritional supplement program for hypoglycemia should include:
   - B complex 20–100 mg per day
   - nicotinamide 1000–3000 mg (but see warning above)
   - tryptophan 500–1500 mg per day (with complex carbohydrate regimen)
   - chromium GTF 200 mcg per day or 200 mcg of chromium in the form of a chromic chloride ($CrCl_3$) which can be made up by your pharmacist
   - zinc 15–25 mg daily
   - manganese 5–10 mg daily
   - magnesium 200–400 mg per day
   - potassium 500–1000 mg per day or more
   - vitamin C 2000–3000 mg per day or more
7. *Glycerine.* Some individuals who get quite severe hypoglycemic symptoms, especially at night, benefit by taking

5–15 mls of glycerine before retiring. This is available from the pharmacist without a prescription. Glycerine itself is an intermediate metabolite of fat and carbohydrate metabolism, and the mechanism by which it works in hypoglycemia is probably that it facilitates the slow release of glucose from the liver into the bloodstream over a number of hours. This method should not be overused, but it can be a useful short-term measure.

8. *Cut out tea and coffee*. Tea and coffee both stimulate insulin release. If you are suffering from too much insulin or hypoglycemia, an addiction to tea and coffee can be the trigger factor. It may be that some people's high insulin levels are so sensitive that they are unable to tolerate any tea and coffee at all.
9. *Avoid alcohol*. Alcohol is a factor causing hypoglycemia, and should be avoided if you are trying to manage hypoglycemia. Hypoglycemia itself can increase a desire for alcohol and treatment of hypoglycemia can facilitate recovery from alcohol addiction, mild or severe.
10. *Cut out cigarette smoking*. Trying to manage hypoglycemia while you are still smoking can lead to considerable problems, and cutting out smoking is a useful tool in the treatment of hypoglycemia.
11. *Adequate rest*. Individuals who are hypoglycemic, especially those who wake at night, may actually be exhausted and do not have any way of getting adequate rest and sleep. This tends to create a vicious circle, with resultant difficulties in the management of hypoglycemia.
12. *Physical exercise*. Regular exercise can improve blood sugar control dramatically. Exercise should be started slowly and built up.
13. *Management of hyperventilation* (uncontrollable overbreathing). Hyperventilation can exacerbate existing symptoms, and this can make management of hypoglycemia really difficult.
14. *Stress management*. As is the case in so many different physical conditions, an element of stress can be either a cause or a result of hypoglycemia. In either event, learning to deal with stress is of paramount importance in terms of improving symptoms.

Low blood sugar, fatigue, irritability and depression

Jim was a thirty-six-year-old television company executive who commuted one and a half hours to work every morning and back again every evening. He had become extremely fatigued, even to the point of it affecting his performance at work. Nutritional supplementation, food allergy approaches and relaxation techniques had failed to produce any significant improvement in his condition. There were periods in the day when he felt worse than others: mid-morning, late morning, mid-afternoon and during his trip home in the evening. A glucose tolerance test revealed that he had a profound drop in his blood sugar between one and four hours after ingestion of glucose. His problem was too much secretion of insulin driving his blood sugar down too far, resulting in fatigue and mental symptoms. Taking a cup of tea with sugar, a sweet biscuit or a piece of chocolate, resulted in a temporary lift, but, often a worse feeling afterwards, and it certainly was no cure for the overall problem.

Eliminating refined carbohydrates (sugar, white bread and flour, etc.), eating small frequent meals and keeping higher carbohydrate foods within moderation, while also continuing his nutritional supplement program with extra magnesium and chromium (both helping to maintain his blood sugar level), resulted in a remarkable improvement in his symptoms. His condition totally resolved when he realized that he did not really like his job and changed it for one he enjoyed more. Low blood sugar affects physical and mental function. It is made worse, in the long run, by eating sugary, sweet things, drinking tea and coffee, stress, and magnesium, vitamin B6 and chromium deficiency.

OBESITY

Obesity is one of the most common health problems in the Western world. Estimates suggest that some twenty-five to thirty percent of people in Western communities are overweight or obese. Of course, there is a considerable debate as to what is a healthy weight and what is an unhealthy weight.

Generally speaking, overweight is defined as a condition in which an individual's weight is ten to twenty percent greater than the acceptable range. Obesity is the term used when the individual is twenty percent or more above the ideal weight.

There are many reasons for wanting to lose weight, not the least of which is cosmetic in a society that stresses slimness so much. The adverse effects of obesity have been well documented and include: reduced life expectancy; increased blood pressure; increased risk of coronary artery disease; elevated blood fats (cholesterol); a reduced ability to take exercise; an increased risk of gallstones, diabetes, varicose veins, hiatus hernia, constipation, post-operative inflections, poor wound healing, osteoarthritis, and, in women, an increased risk of irregular periods and period pains, hairiness and cancers of the breast and womb.

There are some positive benefits to being obese and these include a reduced risk of osteoporosis—thinning of the bones—and an increased tolerance of cold weather.

In the vast majority of cases, obesity is caused by consuming more calories than are needed to maintain normal weight. Certain diseases, such as an underactive thyroid, are an occasional cause of obesity. But some overweight people strongly believe that they consume the same amount or even less food than do their thin counterparts and recent research has shown this to be true. The idea that the obese individual is always greedy is now outdated.

The health risks of obesity are increased if either one or both parents are obese. Obesity often starts in childhood and this, in turn, increases the risk of that individual remaining overweight into later life.

Interestingly, there appear to be two different types of body fat. The ordinary subcutaneous fat (fat which is under the skin) is mainly a store of energy. When excess calories are consumed, either in the form of fat, carbohydrates or protein, they are chemically converted into fats which are then in turn stored in fatty tissue. A different type of fat, brown fat, is not simply a store of energy, but is metabolically very active. Such fat is found between the shoulder blades and around the kidneys and it appears that its function is to burn up excess energy and provide heat. Obese individuals may have relatively inactive brown fat. Some researchers suspect that this may be the cause of obesity. It is quite possible that a number of nutritional factors including the balance of vitamins, minerals and essential fatty acids may influence the activity and metabolism of brown fat.

Losing Weight

If you are overweight or obese, it may be desirable for you to lose weight either for cosmetic reasons, or because of an associated medical problem. A necessary prerequisite for losing weight is a desire to do so. Many books, magazines and local and national societies give advice and help for those who want to lose weight. A summary of our recommendations for weight loss is as follows:

1. *Eat less.* It is important that you cut your calorie consumption. However, equally important is not just how much you eat, but what you eat.
2. *Avoid fatty foods.* Fat contains as many calories as carbohydrates and protein. Avoid fatty meats and dairy products (particularly cheese), and use low-fat alternatives such as skimmed milk and low-fat yogurt. We do not recommend the use of low-fat margarines unless they are high in polyunsaturates. It may be better to use a good polyunsaturated margarine sparingly (about 50 g/2 oz per week).
3. *Avoid sugar and refined carbohydrates.* Such foods as sweets, chocolates, cakes, biscuits, puddings, jams, marmalades and alcohol are all high in refined carbohydrates and calories. Their content of essential nutrients such as vitamins and minerals is usually low.
4. *Eat nutritious foods.* These include vegetables, salad foods, fruit, peas, beans, lentils and good sources of protein—e.g. lean meat, eggs, fish, whole grains, nuts and seeds.
5. *Eat regularly.* Skipping meals is no way to lose weight. Three or more regular meals a day are essential.
6. *Avoid food cravings.* Swings in blood sugar, or eating irregularly, may result in food cravings. The correction of deficiencies, particularly of chromium, magnesium and the B vitamins may help in blood sugar control (see Hypoglycemia, page 292).
7. *Food allergy.* It has been our experience that many patients with weight problems lose weight easily when on an exclusion diet. We have been particularly suspicious of wheat, oats, barley, rye and dairy products as being important in this respect. Often, a diet which is low in fat and refined carbohydrates and avoids grains and dairy products, seems to be successful when other diets have failed.
8. *Supplements.* It is advisable that those on a restricted calorie diet ensure the adequacy of their intake of vitamins and minerals by taking an appropriate supplement (see Appendix, page 422). Also, essential fatty acid supplements may be required (see page 113).

9. *Exercise*. Physical exercise is a useful way of increasing calorie needs by the body and of reducing weight. Furthermore, it serves as a stimulant to the metabolism and is a morale booster. There is now a considerable body of evidence that shows that exercise greatly enhances the weight-losing effects of any slimming diet. Exercise should be taken at least three times a week for a half to one hour.

Adhering to the above advice, with an appropriate diet, often helps an individual lose weight. Remember that in the first week or two, you may lose several pounds in weight, but in the long term, weight loss may average out at only between two and five pounds per month.

MENSTRUAL PROBLEMS

Premenstrual Syndrome (PMS)

A lot of confusion has surrounded PMS over the years because of a failure to define the condition accurately. Dr. Katharina Dalton, from London, has defined PMS as "The appearance of symptoms in the premenstruum and their disappearance in the postmenstruum." Unlike almost all other medical conditions, the diagnosis is based on the cyclical nature of symptoms rather than on the actual symptoms themselves. More than 150 symptoms have been described in PMS and some women suffer from only one. More usually, though, half a dozen or so symptoms are the norm.

SYMPTOMS OF PMS

The most common symptoms have been categorized by Dr. Guy Abraham, who has been at the forefront of nutrition research in relation to PMS. He and his colleagues have subdivided PMS into the following four categories:

- PMS-A anxiety, irritability, nervous tension and mood swings.
- PMS-B weight gain, swelling of the extremities, breast tenderness and abdominal bloating.
- PMS-C headache, craving for sweets, increased appetite, heart pounding, fatigue and dizziness or fainting.
- PMS-D depression, forgetfulness, crying, confusion and insomnia.

Other symptoms include oily skin, acne, clumsiness and feelings of violence or even suicide in severe cases.

It is also well recognized that certain conditions, including asthma, epilepsy and alcoholism, are aggravated premenstrually. We think that any woman of child-bearing age, with a significant medical condition, should be closely questioned by her doctor as to whether her symptoms are worse premenstrually. This often provides a useful clue as to the possible cause of her symptoms.

A number of studies have been performed to determine the frequency with which premenstrual symptoms are experienced by women from different countries in different age groups.

It seems that about fifty percent of women of child-bearing age experience at least some symptoms premenstrually. Probably only about half of them feel that their symptoms are severe enough to warrant treatment or medical attention. Countries such as Greece and Japan have a lower frequency of symptoms, and this may well be related to dietary differences.

There are certain risk factors for PMS. Increasing age and increasing numbers of children increase the chances of PMS. Young women and girls in their teens and early twenties appear to suffer more from painful periods which frequently improve as they get older, often to be replaced by the appearance of premenstrual symptoms. Our experience is that the most severe and difficult cases of PMS are to be found in women in their forties. Often, severe premenstrual symptoms merge with the appearance of menopausal symptoms, with no respite for the sufferer.

DIET AND PMS

There are many theories as to the cause of PMS. Some doctors feel that it is purely a psychological reaction or that it is a hormonal disease just as thyroid disease or diabetes are. These approaches don't allow the patient to do anything about the condition themselves, nor do they explain the rapid increase in the incidence of PMS in Western societies.

Over the last 100 years there have been marked changes in dietary and social habits—increased consumption of sugar, alcohol, tea and coffee, dairy products and animal fat; a lower intake of magnesium and only borderline intakes of other essential nutrients. Many more women smoke now than did at the turn of the century. Any or all of these changes may have played a part in the production of premenstrual symptoms.

Dr. Abraham has shown that the dietary intake of nutrients in women with premenstrual symptoms is often less than in healthy women with no PMS. He has also found that women with PMS often have low levels of magnesium, which may play a crucial role in influencing hormonal metabolism as well as affecting blood sugar control.

Tea, coffee, chocolate, cola-based drinks and medications containing caffeine can all aggravate symptoms such as anxiety, insomnia, tremulousness, and breast symptoms. It appears that avoiding them significantly reduces the occurrence of breast tenderness, as does stopping smoking.

A high intake of salt often aggravates fluid retention and breast tenderness. Many authorities consider that our current salt consumption is too high and may predispose to high blood pressure. A woman with premenstrual symptoms is extremely unlikely to have significant premenstrual fluid retention if she is on a low-salt diet.

Fat consumption may well be important as a cause of PMS. Research suggests that PMS sufferers cannot efficiently metabolize the essential fatty acid, linoleic acid—which is mainly found in good quality vegetable oils—into its normal by-products, perhaps because of a subtle interaction between derivatives of linoleic acid and certain menstrual hormones. This "block" could occur because of dietary deficiencies of nutrients essential for its conversion. Such nutrients include vitamin B6, magnesium, zinc, vitamin C, vitamin B3, and chromium. A diet high in animal fats would not favor the efficient metabolism of essential fatty acids. Abraham has shown that countries that have a high intake of vegetable-produce tend to have a lower incidence of PMS.

Poor blood sugar control is often a problem in women with PMS. Many women notice an increase in appetite and/or food or sugar craving in the week or so before their period, and this may contribute to their weight gain and fluid retention.

Some women on the Pill are known to have impaired blood sugar control, which can be improved by taking vitamin B6. A diet high in sugar and sweets doesn't help the situation, neither does smoking, alcohol consumption or excessive tea and coffee drinking. Poor blood sugar control may also be made worse by the use of diuretic drugs. Women with these symptoms are well advised to cut down or avoid tea, coffee, alcohol and cigarettes; to use alternative contraception to the Pill; to eat regular, small meals, with a good protein intake, particularly from vegetable sources; and to ensure that they get enough vitamin B, magnesium and trace elements in their diet.

There are many reasons why dietary factors might contribute to, or even cause, PMS. A detailed discussion is outside the scope of this book, but all of the above dietary factors can influence brain or hormonal metabolism in such a way as to produce premenstrual symptoms.

TREATMENT OF PMS

The treatment of premenstrual syndrome includes one of the widest ranges of therapies ever proposed for any single condition. This gives some idea of the confusion that exists both in the medical profession and in the public's mind as to what PMS is, how it is caused, and how it is best treated.

The following treatments are either proven or accepted by a significant number of medical experts. The list includes vitamin B6, evening primrose oil, multivitamin and mineral supplements, progesterone therapy either by mouth or as vaginal pessaries, estrogen implants, the Pill, vitamin E, diuretics (particularly spironolactone), bromocriptine (a powerful antihormonal drug), lithium, tranquilizers, antidepressants and painkillers.

Quite an impressive list but many of them are ineffective in any one woman.

Improving your diet plays a crucial role in the treatment of PMS and often does away with the need to take drugs, hormones or even nutritional supplements.

The following dietary recommendations have been made by Abraham.

Basic dietary recommendations for all PMS sufferers

- Limit the consumption of refined sugar, salt, red meat and alcohol.
- Eat fish, poultry, whole grains and legumes as major sources of protein, and rely less on red meat and dairy products.
- Reduce or abolish tobacco consumption.
- Consume only minimal quantities of coffee, tea, chocolate, and cola-based drinks.
- Reduce the intake of fats, avoiding particularly animal fats, fried foods, and hydrogenated margarines. Consume only good-quality margarines high in polyunsaturates.
- Increase the intake of fiber in the form of complex carbohydrates such as green, leafy vegetables, legumes and fruits.
- Reduce weight, if you are obese, by avoiding refined carbohydrates, reducing animal fat intake, and increasing fiber intake.

- If you experience sugar or food craving, eat regularly, with high-quality protein snacks, e.g. nuts, seed, peas, beans and lentils, as well as animal protein such as eggs, fish and meat.

Certain other things are of proven value, including:

- Regular outdoor exercise. Daily walks, or exercise such as swimming or aerobic exercise.
- Stress reduction. Severe sufferers of PMS may put a considerable strain upon family and personal relationships and the increase in domestic tension will only serve to aggravate their symptoms further (see below).
- Work situations. Mental confusion or clouding are not uncommon premenstrual symptoms and many women find that they become indecisive in the week or so before their period. If you have severe or moderate symptoms, avoid making major decisions at this time of the month.

Nutritional supplements for PMS

While there is no perfect nutritional supplement for PMS, many women derive considerable benefit from certain nutritional supplements. Here is what we suggest:

Multivitamin supplement. Take a supplement providing approximately 100 mg of vitamin B6 per day, together with the B vitamins, vitamin C, and preferably magnesium and trace elements, every day throughout the month. One multivitamin supplement, Optivite, is of proven value in treating PMS and even corrects the hormonal abnormalities found in severe sufferers.

You could take vitamin B6, 100–200 mg alone. This helps many, but a more balanced supplement is preferable.

Evening primrose. 500 mg capsules 4–8 per day. This should be taken during the two weeks before your period, but if you have no response, you can take it throughout the month. It is best combined with a multivitamin and trace mineral supplement.

Try vitamin E. 300–500 IUs per day. This can be of particular value for women with premenstrual breast swelling and tenderness.

Take magnesium. Because so many women with PMS are found to be magnesium deficient, a magnesium supplement providing some 200–300 mg of elemental magnesium per day should be taken throughout the month. This is best combined with a multivitamin supplement.

While the purely dietary recommendations we outlined can be followed by any woman with PMS, the above supplements should be taken preferably after consultation with your general practitioner.

Appropriate treatment with nutritional supplements should continue for at least three months before deciding whether or not they're doing you any good.

IMPORTANT NOTE

If your symptoms do not improve or are very severe, you must see your doctor. Some hormonal or gynecological problems can have symptoms similar to those of PMS yet require medical or surgical treatment.

Premenstrual syndrome and fluid retention

Veronica, a forty-year-old housewife and part-time shop assistant, had experienced severe premenstrual fluid retention and irritability for the past ten years. She had noticed that her weight could increase by some 6 to 7 lbs. in the week before her period. Treatment with diuretics that produced a loss of water were only of temporary benefit. She had a very low level of magnesium, 1.6 mmol/l, normal range 2–3. This is a common finding in women with PMS, and can be worsened by some types of diuretic drugs. Her fluid retention responded to a very-low-salt diet, 25 mmol per day, and was worsened if she consumed salty foods or ate foods containing wheat. Adhering to her diet and supplements of a specialized multivitamin, Optivite, and additional magnesium, resulted in a correction of the magnesium deficiency, improvement in her fluid retention, and loss of premenstrual symptoms, without the need for her to continue with her drugs. Stopping her oral contraceptives helped clear her symptoms completely.

Painful Periods (dysmenorrhea)

Painful periods (dysmenorrhea) for which no medical cause can be found, often resolve following a pregnancy or by going on the oral contraceptive pill. We have had numbers of women as patients who have been helped with supplements of calcium, magnesium, vitamin E, zinc or essential fatty acids; even so, it may take several months to settle down. Treatment of any food intolerance or chronic candidiasis may also help; osteopathic or chiropractic treatment, especially of the lower lumbar region, can also be helpful in some cases. We do *not* recommend the use of the Pill for the treatment of dysmenorrhea.

Heavy Periods

Heavy periods can be caused by hormonal problems (including thyroid problems) or structural problems in the uterus, and vitamin A supplementation has been found to be effective. It has been shown that some women do well on supplements of iron, zinc, vitamin B6 and vitamin A. Heavy periods can cause iron deficiency, but some women have a return to normal periods following iron supplementation. Bioflavonoids may also be useful. Women who are being treated for chronic candidiasis (for other reasons) often notice that their periods get heavier for two or three months but then settle down to normal. Food intolerance may also need to be treated.

Infrequent, Scanty or Absent Periods

These are probably normal in some women, yet may reflect hormone problems in others. They can occur because of slimming diets, when taking excessive physical exercise (such as jogging or athletics training), or after being on the Pill. By going onto a good, basic diet, and correcting any nutritional deficiencies with a broad spectrum nutritional supplement program (see Appendix 2), you should find your periods return to normal within two or three months if there is no underlying medical problem.

Vaginal Bleeding between Periods

While this can sometimes occur when you start on the chronic candidiasis program (see page 346) or if you are on the Pill, **always go to your doctor and have a check up as it can be a sign of a medical problem requiring urgent attention. Any woman who has vaginal bleeding after menopause should go and see her doctor immediately.**

MENOPAUSE

Menopausal symptoms include fatigue, hot flushes and sweating as well as the emergence of food intolerance symptoms. Hormone treatment can be given, but sometimes this can be avoided by ensuring adequacy of nutritional status, supplements of vitamins B and E, zinc and essential fatty acids (e.g. evening primrose oil), and the treatment of candidiasis and underlying food intolerance may also be helpful.

Vaginal Thrush (see page 352)

SIDE-EFFECTS OF THE PILL

The oral contraceptive pill prevents pregnancy by preventing ovulation every month, as well as thickening cervical mucus which inhibits its penetration by sperms.

The hormone(s) contained in the Pill can have side effects which include increased risk of cancer of the cervix, breast and liver, blood clots in the legs, stroke and heart attacks, increased blood pressure, diabetes, gall-bladder disease, migraine, food allergies, fluid retention, weight increase, thrush and depression.

Women who smoke and are overweight run additional risks of stroke and heart attack if they take the Pill.

The Pill also affects the way in which the body uses and needs certain vitamins and minerals, as we shall see.

The Influence of the Pill

It is well known that the contraceptive pill has many medical side effects and we are unhappy about prescribing it routinely. However, what is little discussed is its effects on nutrition. It is becoming increasingly apparent that the status of many vitamins and minerals is altered by the Pill and that this can have considerable repercussions on the health of the woman who takes it.

VITAMIN A AND THE PILL

Women on the Pill have increased circulating levels of vitamin A. The increase seems to happen immediately on starting the Pill and takes approximately three months to return to normal levels after stopping the Pill. Vitamin A has been shown to be harmful to both animal and human fetuses, though there is no clear evidence in humans that raised vitamin A levels as a result of oral contraceptive use are associated with an increased risk of having a malformed baby. Nevertheless, the observation that it takes three months to recover from this effect on vitamin A is a further argument to suggest that it is wise to stop taking the Pill at least three months before conceiving.

VITAMIN B1 AND THE PILL

There is some evidence to suggest that the Pill interferes with vitamin B1 metabolism, increasing the woman's requirements for the vitamin and possibly causing vitamin B1 deficiency symptoms (see page 12).

VITAMIN B2 AND THE PILL

Numerous reports have shown vitamin B2 deficiency in women on the Pill, especially if they have been on it for more than three years.

VITAMIN B6 AND THE PILL

Many studies have been done on the effect of oral contraceptives, particularly the estrogen component, on tryptophan and vitamin B6. There are several clinical manifestations of altered vitamin B6 status which have been described in oral contraceptive users, including psychiatric symptoms (particularly depression), impaired glucose tolerance, cancer of the urinary tract, and peri-oral dermatosis.

The effect of the Pill on carbohydrate metabolism has been well studied. The age and individual predisposition of the woman are risk factors, as are also the duration, type and dose of the Pill used. The giving of vitamin B6 to women taking oral contraceptives who had demonstrable vitamin B6 deficiency and impaired glucose tolerance, results in an improvement in their glucose tolerance.

It has been shown quite clearly, and has been our own observation in clinical practice, that many women on oral contraceptives do well on a supplement of pyridoxine in the order of 40–100 mg per day.

VITAMIN B12 AND THE PILL

It appears that the Pill adversely influences vitamin B12 in women, but without producing anemia.

It is possible that some of the psychiatric effects of oral contraceptive usage, which are not responsive to vitamin B6 supplementation, could be responsive to vitamin B12.

FOLIC ACID AND THE PILL

One potentially serious problem of Pill use is the possibility that it may interfere with blood cell formation by altering folic acid and vitamin B12 metabolism.

Studies clearly demonstrate that oral contraceptives reduce

folic acid status, but the indiscriminate use of folic acid supplements has been discouraged on the grounds that vitamin B12 status may also be abnormal and that excess supplements of folic acid might possibly mask or worsen neurological symptoms caused by a faulty vitamin B12 status.

Coming off the Pill and conceiving at once is also a source of concern. There are two reasons for this. First, normal pregnancy alters folate status and this could be worsened if lowered levels of folate persist from previous Pill use. Second, a compromised folic acid status has been linked with the occurrence of congenital abnormalities (see page 26). Women who use an oral contraceptive within six months of conception have been shown to have lower than normal red blood cell and plasma folate levels in the first three months of pregnancy. This eventually corrects itself as pregnancy proceeds. There is thus a case for taking folic acid supplements prior to conception if you have been on the Pill. Perhaps the most sensible advice is not to become pregnant for three to six months after coming off the Pill. There is also a case for taking a supplement of 5–10 mg of folic acid daily both before and around the time of conception.

It is sensible, too, to increase your intake of foods which are rich in folic acid while on the Pill, and after discontinuing it, for the months prior to conception. Green vegetables and liver are high in folic acid.

It is also worth bearing in mind the fact that zinc deficiency, which can be associated with oral contraceptive usage, also compromises folic acid absorption. Increased occurrence, in Pill users, of cellular abnormalities of the cervix may be related to impaired status of folic acid.

VITAMIN C AND THE PILL

It appears that vitamin C requirements are increased by the use of the oral contraceptive. It would therefore be sensible for women taking the Pill to increase their intake of foods which are rich in vitamin C (see page 28).

There is some discussion within expert circles as to whether or not vitamin C supplements should be taken. In our opinion, 100–500 mg a day would seem entirely appropriate, not just from the point of view of oral contraception, but for other reasons as well, all of which are discussed in more detail on page 30. However, there is an effect of vitamin C on oral contraceptives which should be clearly understood. It has been shown that doses of 1 g a day of vitamin C increase the concentration of estrogen (ethinylestradiol) in the plasma by increasing the availability of the hormone. The effect of this could be to change a low-dose estrogen pill into a high-dose one, and increase the adverse effects of the Pill. There is thus a potential risk in taking high doses of vitamin C when on the Pill.

VITAMIN D AND THE PILL

There appears to be no change in the vitamin D requirement of women taking oral contraceptives.

VITAMIN E AND THE PILL

Plasma vitamin E levels seem to be lowered by about twenty percent in women taking oral contraceptives. Some workers have recommended a daily supplement of 10 IUs of alpha-tocopherol to restore plasma levels.

However, further work has to be done to be sure of the exact requirements for vitamin E supplementation (if there is any at all) in oral contraceptive users.

VITAMIN K AND THE PILL

This vitamin is hardly ever measured directly in the blood—an assessment of vitamin K status usually involves the measurement of plasma prothrombin, or the blood clotting factors VII, IX and X. Women taking the oral contraceptive show striking increases in levels of prothrombin and factors VII, IX and X. In other words, their blood is much more likely to clot.

Given that oral contraceptive users are at a significant, albeit small, increased risk of developing cardiovascular disease (especially thrombosis), vitamin K status could well be very important. While the estrogen component of the Pill has been implicated as a possible culprit, other factors such as the age of the woman and whether or not she smokes could also be important.

Some women with heavy periods are put on the Pill to control their problem. Since both vitamin A and vitamin K can reduce the bleeding it is possible that the effect of the oral contraceptive is simply to reverse increased requirements for vitamin A and vitamin K. That is to say, if a woman has heavy periods because she doesn't meet her body's needs for vitamin A or vitamin K, then the Pill may act by increasing plasma vitamin A or by increasing the production of vitamin-K-dependent plasma clotting factors. We do not advocate the use of the Pill to control heavy periods when there are other less toxic methods available. We recommend supplements of vitamins A and B6 (see page 307).

MINERALS AND THE PILL

The Pill has been shown to influence a woman's mineral status, but it is not yet fully understood just how many of the ill-effects of oral contraceptives are mediated by their effects on mineral metabolism.

Copper

It has been known for many years that serum copper increases during pregnancy and it has also been found to go up in women taking oral contraceptives.

Zinc

Low plasma zinc has been known for twenty-five years to occur in pregnancy, and it is also recognized that women on oral contraceptives have low plasma zinc, though not to as great an extent as in pregnancy. It is possible that this may be a result of increased serum copper and ceruloplasmin (the copper-carrying protein in the blood) concentrations.

Iron

Iron deficiency anemia is a common disorder in fertile women. It is usually caused by heavy periods, pregnancy, a marginal diet or excessive tea and coffee drinking (see page 131). Oral contraceptive usage can lower serum iron, but usually increases it because women on the Pill have reduced menstrual blood loss.

Magnesium

We are not aware of any conclusive studies that show the direct effect of oral contraceptives on magnesium status, but in our own clinical experience, women who are recovering from oral contraceptive usage are invariably magnesium deficient as judged by their serum, hair, sweat, or red blood cell magnesium levels.

The Pill for Teenagers?

The decision to use the Pill should not be taken lightly. In our opinion it has been prescribed far too liberally by the medical profession, partly in response to considerable public demand.

Girls who have only recently started having periods and are going through the growth spurt and maturation of sexual organs that accompany this, have considerable nutritional demands put upon their bodies. It is well recognized that pregnancies among girls in their early and mid-teens are associated with increased problems. This is partly due to the fact that they may be borderline or even overly deficient in certain essential nutrients. The same can be said of girls starting the contraceptive pill. Many girls who have just started having periods have a marked zinc deficiency and deficiencies of other nutrients. The Pill puts further metabolic stresses on an already compromised system. The long-term effects of starting the Pill in the early teens have not yet been established. However, the incidence of cancer of the cervix appears to be related to the age of onset of oral contraceptive usage and the age of first intercourse.

In our opinion, to put a young girl on the Pill, possibly for many years, may well turn out to be a crime of considerable

The birth control pill and depression

Anthea was eighteen years old and very depressed. She had no interest in life, was critical of her family and boyfriend, and held herself in low esteem. At the consultation she was accompanied by her mother, who was very concerned about her as she had been a bright, vivacious girl with a good sense of humor and a zest for life. But over the previous year her personality had changed remarkably. On closer questioning it was discovered that she had been put on the Pill eighteen months earlier to help her with her painful periods. She was fine for the first four to six months, but then gradually started to go downhill. She thought it might be the Pill, so after a year she came off for a couple of months, but with no obvious improvement, so she discounted it as the cause and went back on it. Nutritional assessment showed her to be low in magnesium, zinc and vitamin B6, and high in copper—all features common in those who take the oral contraceptive pill. Coming off the Pill, improving her diet and taking a nutritional supplement (see Recovering from the Pill, below) resulted in a return over the next two months, of the previously happy, vivacious Anthea.

The Pill does cause these symptoms in susceptible girls and women, and it often takes more than just coming off the Pill for a couple of months to recover from the marked biochemical disturbances resulting from the Pill. Also, there are nutritional actions that can be taken to help painful periods (see page 306), thus, in most instances, removing any need to go on the Pill, something which should, in our opinion, be avoided if possible.

magnitude. Far better to educate girls about alternative forms of contraception, the liability of going on the Pill, and the increased risks of cancer.

When defending the virtues of the Pill, the point is often made that the risks of pregnancy can be medically more severe than taking the Pill. This may be so in the short term; the psychological and social consequences, for an unmarried teenager, of becoming pregnant are obviously profound. However, on the basis of the evidence to hand, we believe that prescribing the Pill to a young teenager should be strongly discouraged and in fact avoided wherever possible.

Recovering from the Pill

The best course of action for any woman who has felt unwell on the Pill, or who is coming off it with a view to conceiving, is to follow the recommendations for a good, healthy diet (see page 398).

Also, it is well worth taking a nutritional supplement for several months.

A basic program we recommend includes the following daily supplements:

Vitamin B1	10–50 mg
Vitamin B2	10–50 mg
Vitamin B3	10–50 mg
Vitamin B5	50–100 mg
Vitamin B6	50–100 mg
Vitamin B12	200–400 mcg
Folic acid	400 mcg–2 mg
Inositol	50–75 mg
Choline	50–75 mg
Vitamin A	not needed usually by women on the Pill
Vitamin C	250–2000 mg (or more)
Vitamin E	50–200 IUs
Magnesium	100–200 mg (or more)
Zinc	5–15 mg (or more)
Manganese	3–5 mg
Copper	don't take any
Iron	depends on individual's iron status

Higher doses may be required by some people.

Post-Pill failure to menstruate

Pamela was thirty-six and unmarried. She had been on the Pill for twelve years until three years ago, since which time she had not menstruated. She lived with a man and wanted to become pregnant but had failed to do so. Nutritional assessment showed her to be low in a number of minerals, including zinc, as well as in a number of B vitamins and vitamin C, despite a reasonable diet. She also drank a fair amount of wine on a daily basis. On taking a broad multivitamin and mineral, extra zinc and B vitamins, and cutting out the alcohol, she menstruated within two months.

This case illustrates the fact that the Pill suppresses normal hormonal function and that there is a strong nutritional link. Appropriate diet and nutritional supplementation can help bring about normal menstruation after the Pill. Alcohol further compounds the adverse nutritional effects of the Pill and should not really be taken by anyone who wants to become pregnant.

INFERTILITY

Infertility in Women

When it comes to diseases of the reproductive organs resulting in infertility, very little can be done by way of nutritional intervention.

Infertility in women can be caused in a number of different ways. Here are just a few:

- male partner's sperm incapable of bringing about conception (see page 317)
- failure to have intercourse
- poor nutritional state
- blockage of fallopian tubes
- pituitary gland failure
- ovarian failure
- after-effects of the Pill
- other hormonal imbalances
- endometrial failure

- sperm antibodies
- hostile cervical mucus
- recurrent miscarriages
- chronic illness or infection

A very poor nutritional state (as is found in anorexia nervosa or severe malnutrition, see page 390) results in a failure of ovulation and a failure of menstruation. It might be thought that a diet sufficiently poor to cause infertility would only be found in developed countries in times of severe food shortages caused by wars and their aftermath, but this is not so. There are minorities of women, even in the most prosperous communities, who are infertile because of poor nutrition. As many as fifty percent of women attending clinics complaining of a loss of periods are there because of the effects of dieting.

Gross hormonal imbalances of the pituitary, thyroid, and ovarian glands may or may not be amenable to nutritional intervention, and should be investigated by the appropriate specialist physician; at the same time, however, it is well worth embarking upon a good, healthy diet.

If the cervical mucus is hostile, the woman produces antibodies to her partner's sperm, and nutritional intervention cannot be of use, though it is quite possible that cervical mucus may become hostile due to the accumulation of toxins in the system that are being excreted by various routes including the cervical mucus.

Recurrent miscarriages can be caused by, among other things, essential fatty acid deficiency, zinc deficiency, manganese deficiency, vitamin E deficiency, and overload with toxic elements, and it is these areas that we are looking at in this section.

Formal infertility investigations should be conducted under the supervision of a competent infertility specialist.

While undergoing these investigations, it is well worthwhile going onto a sensible diet (see page 398) avoiding refined carbohydrates and foods with artificial additives, cutting out smoking, cutting out alcohol, taking regular, mild or moderate, but not excessive, exercise, taking a broad-spectrum multivitamin and mineral supplement and being sure not to take excessive amounts of vitamin A, which has been shown to cause congenital malformations.

RECURRENT MISCARRIAGES

Recurrent miscarriages can be due to immunological causes and this should be investigated thoroughly by a gynecologist. However, certain nutrient deficiencies such as those of zinc, manganese, essential fatty acids and vitamin E have been linked to an increased tendency for spontaneous miscarriages and it is worth bearing this in mind when thinking about the likely causes of a miscarriage. Other causes of miscarriage include diabetes, thyroid problems, fibroids and particular infections such as cytomegalovirus, chlamydia, herpes and chromosomal abnormalities or anatomical problems of the womb.

POST-PILL AMENORRHEA

Some women don't have periods for some time after coming off the contraceptive Pill, especially if they have been on it for a long time. You should follow the plan described in "Recovering from the Pill" (see page 314). It is advisable not to become pregnant within three to six months of coming off the Pill.

Infertility in Men

Infertility usually relates to some failure of the sperm-producing mechanism. This is a complex business that takes several months and is very susceptible to outside influences, including dietary ones.

CAUSES OF MALE INFERTILITY

Male infertility can be caused by structural problems within the reproductive system, disruption of the pituitary secretion of the gonadotropic hormones, immunological factors (such as the production of antisperm antibodies), toxic factors and other environmental illness as well as nutritional factors.

Before trying to deal with an abnormal sperm count nutritionally, it is important to exclude the common medical conditions associated with an abnormal sperm count. This is best done by an infertility specialist.

It is well known that food deprivation in a man results in infertility. Evidence from desperately poor populations, those ravaged by war, and from victims of concentration and prisoner-of-war camps shows that a prolonged lack of food leads to a loss of sex drive as well as to structural changes in reproductive tissue. Having said this, large amounts of food are not necessary for fertility, because birth rates remain high in poor, even malnourished populations.

Severe obesity can also be associated with impotence and/or a poor sperm count. It may be that sperm production is impaired in grossly obese men if the scrotum is surrounded by folds of fat which raise the temperature of the testicles. Most importantly, obesity may be psychologically handicapping in cultures that associate virility and attractiveness with slimness, and the disease-states that frequently accompany obesity, such as hypertension and osteoarthritis of the lumbar spine and hips, may interfere with sexual performance.

Also, in the extremely obese, testosterone levels in the plasma are low, and female hormones elevated. Both of these result in poor-quality or too few sperms.

NUTRIENTS ASSOCIATED WITH SPERM PRODUCTION

Several studies have shown that giving nutritional supplements has improved the sperm count. The nutrients that appear to be essential for normal sperm formation include:

- arginine
- essential fatty acids
- zinc
- chromium
- selenium
- vitamin E
- vitamin A
- B vitamins
- vitamin C

Arginine

The head of the sperm contains an exceptional amount of this amino acid. A marked reduction in sperm count was observed in three men fed an arginine-free diet for nine days.

Essential fatty acids

It has long been known that a deficiency of essential fatty acid is associated with impaired function of the gonadal in experimental animals. Semen is rich in prostaglandins which are derived from essential fatty acids, but their precise role in male reproductive processes is unknown. Some men with low fertility of unknown cause have low levels of seminal prostaglandins. With the increasing interest in the role of essential fatty acids in human health and diseases, it is quite possible that disordered essential fatty acid metabolism will be identified as a significant cause of low sperm counts, though at the moment there is no evidence to confirm this.

Zinc

The role of zinc deficiency in sperm formation has been well studied. Zinc deficiency has been found in men with low sperm counts and zinc supplementation can improve sperm counts and sexual performance in such individuals. Furthermore, zinc therapy raises the level of testosterone in the plasma of zinc deficient men. Effective treatments have involved giving 50 mg of elemental zinc per day for weeks or months. Don't forget that sperm formation takes almost three months, so you shouldn't expect an increase in sperm count following the start of zinc therapy for at least this time.

Impotence and zinc deficiency

Alfredo had had a part-share in a beach bar on the Costa Brava in Spain. During the three years that he had been involved in this business, he had become alcoholic. What had worried him most was that he had become impotent and was unable to develop or maintain an erection. He was told that this was because he was alcoholic, and he instantly gave up drinking. However, after nine months with no alcohol he was still impotent. At this point he was assessed for zinc status and he had one of the lowest zinc levels that we have ever seen. Over a period of eight weeks he was given zinc supplementation, and came back into the consulting room for a follow-up visit jumping with joy, saying that his manhood was back! Zinc is intimately linked with sexual function, and zinc deficiency is associated with loss of libido, reduced sperm count and, in extreme cases, impotence.

Other nutrients

Studies in animals have shown that chromium, selenium and vitamins E, A and B have marked effects on the function of the reproductive organs and the formation of sperm. Though no studies have been done on humans, it seems likely that deficiencies of these nutrients are relevant to male infertility.

WHAT TO DO ABOUT INFERTILITY

Any infertile couple should be medically investigated if they want to conceive. Several sperm counts should be done, and conclusions should not be drawn on one sample alone as there is considerable variation from one sample to the next.

Several nutrients have been found to be involved in enhancement of sperm formation but there are no broadly based nutritional studies to confirm the validity of the following recommendations. These recommendations are, however, based on sound common sense, and some scientific evidence. The risk of toxicity or unwanted effects is minimal, and there is some chance that sperm quality and sperm count may be enhanced, and thus fertility increased.

- Stop smoking.
- Give up alcohol.
- Ensure that you have no excessive toxic exposure to lead, arsenic, aluminum, cadmium, herbicides, pesticides etc.
- Wear loose underpants and trousers so as to keep the testes cool.
- Get adequate rest and exercise to minimize fatigue.
- Ensure that there is no obvious medical cause for the abnormal sperm count.
- Look at any other symptoms that might be amenable to nutritional intervention or a food allergic approach.
- Handle environmental stress.
- Take nutritional supplements:

  vitamin C, 200–500 mg per day,
  arginine, 1.5–2 g per day for three to six months in divided doses,
  free-form amino acids, 500 mg of the major amino acids twice daily,
  lysine, 500 mg daily,
  zinc, 50 mg of elemental zinc per day,
  a multivitamin and mineral to include 7,500 IUs of vitamin A; 200–400 IUs of vitamin E; chromium 50–100 mcg; selenium 50–100 mcg.
- Live healthily (see page 398).

LOSS OF LIBIDO (REDUCED SEX DRIVE)

This can occur as a result of physical illness or because of psychological problems.

The following advice may be helpful:

- Lose weight if obese. Excess fat tissue in men can result in increased levels of female sex hormones.
- Get fit. Take regular physical exercise.

- Correct any nutritional deficiencies. Vitamin B and zinc are particularly important in sex hormone metabolism and your sex drive.
- Do not drink excessively. Men with alcoholic liver disease can lose their sex drive and lose the ability to achieve or maintain an erection.
- Go on vacation to reduce domestic and work tensions.
- Live healthily (see page 398).

If these measures are unhelpful, then medical investigation is necessary to assess the presence of thyroid and other hormonal conditions in the elderly.

PRECONCEPTIONAL CARE

The nutritional status of the father and the mother in the weeks and months preceding conception can influence the outcome of a pregnancy. As much of the crucial development of the fertilized egg into a baby occurs in the first eight weeks of pregnancy, many women are pregnant without realizing it. Their nutritional and toxic status during these critical weeks can determine whether or not the baby will develop normally. Similarly the quality of the father's sperm can be influenced by both nutritional and toxic factors. Excessive burdens of toxic metals such as lead, mercury and cadmium can adversely influence the quality of the sperm and subsequent conception. Smoking and alcohol can increase the number of sperm abnormalities, and can also reduce the sperm count.

Anyone reading this section who is pregnant and has not taken any of the precautions outlined in the following pages should be reassured by the fact that the vast majority of pregnancies result in a healthy, normal baby. The purpose of this section is to provide information for those who are not yet pregnant, so that they can maximize their level of health in order to make the most of being pregnant and producing the healthiest possible baby.

Things which are known to increase the risk of congenital malformation are:

- Poor nutritional status
  (a) protein/amino acid deficiency
  essential fatty acid deficiency
  inadequate carbohydrate intake

vitamin deficiency
mineral deficiency
(b) low body weight
slimming diets

- Drugs
  (a) legal—the birth control pill, anticonvulsants, etc.
  (b) illegal—marijuana, etc.
- Toxins
  (a) social—tobacco
  —alcohol
  —tea and coffee
  (c) environmental—lead, mercury, cadmium, etc.
  —organochemicals
  —mycotoxins (toxins from fungi)
  — food additives
- Infections
  rubella
  toxoplasma
  mycoplasma
  syphilis

Aside from congenital malformations, the health of the mother before pregnancy is obviously important when it comes to determining whether or not she will be well during pregnancy. This is discussed in more detail in the section on pregnancy.

Nutrient Deficiencies and Birth Defects

It has been shown in animal studies that deficiencies of vitamins B1, B2, B12, folic acid, and vitamin A, and a range of minerals are all associated with an increased tendency to produce congenital abnormalities.

Extreme deficiencies of these nutrients result in infertility and a failure to conceive. But there is a shady area between the extremes of poor nutritional status and infertility, and good nutritional status with fertility and normal reproduction where we find women who may be fertile, but are at risk of producing an abnormal child. It is this area that is the target of dietary and nutritional intervention in preconceptional care.

Vitamin A is interesting in that vitamin A toxicity can actually cause congenital malformations, so it is very important that no woman should take this vitamin in excess if she intends to become pregnant. Choline and vitamin E deficiencies enhance the toxicity of vitamin A. We advise no woman who intends to get pregnant or who is actually pregnant to take any supplement that contains more than 7,500 to 10,000 IUs of vitamin A per day.

Essential fatty acids are also necessary for correct fetal development, as they are intimately involved in the development of each cell in the body, and are specifically important in brain development.

Extreme protein or carbohydrate deficiencies are rare in the West, but women on slimming diets should be wary of getting pregnant if they are on a nutritionally inadequate regime.

NEURAL TUBE DEFECTS

This is a condition where the development of the spine and spinal cord is incomplete. Women who have had one NTD baby have a higher risk than average of producing another. Studies have shown that if these women take a multivitamin and mineral supplement including folic acid around the time of conception the risk of producing a second NTD baby is reduced.

CLEFT PALATE

Cleft palate is a congenital abnormality which is relatively common. It has been shown that women who have had a previous child with this condition can reduce their risk of having further children with cleft palates by taking vitamin and mineral supplements around the time of conception. In one study, such women were given a daily supplement for three months before conception and the first three months of their pregnancies. In eighty-five supplemented pregnancies, there was only one recurrence of cleft palate. In 212 unsupplemented pregnancies (women who did not take the vitamins) there were fifteen recurrences.

DOWN'S SYNDROME

As yet, there is no evidence that preconceptional care can prevent a child being born with Down's syndrome. However, good nutrition will always be a woman's best safeguard against congenital malformation of the fetus and increase the likelihood of its developing normally.

Environmental Toxins

Some of the toxins known to be associated with the development of birth defects are toxic metals, methyl mercury, lead, cadmium, organochemicals, DDT, dioxin, agent orange, polychlorinated biphenyls, drugs (anticonvulsants, thalidomide and many others) and calcium, vitamin A and vitamin D in excess.

Heavy metals, including mercury, lead and cadmium have been associated with the development of congenital malformations, increased rates of miscarriage and stillbirths. It is quite probable that mothers and fathers, if exposed to lead in sufficient quantities, can produce children who have not only congenital malformations, but also defective mental development. It is our opinion that anyone attending a doctor for preconceptional advice who may be at risk, (e.g. living in a city or industrial environment) should be screened for toxic metals either by a blood test or, preferably, a hair mineral analysis, as the latter shows low-level toxic accumulation of these toxic metals better.

The Birth Control Pill

Gross metabolic disturbances occur as a result of taking the Pill (see page 308). You should therefore discontinue the Pill for *at least* three months before conception and use other forms of birth control, such as a condom, instead. At the same time, it may well be worth taking a nutritional supplements program.

Alcohol

The fetal alcohol syndrome is a condition in which the baby's skull (and in extreme circumstances, the limbs) do not form properly and its immunity and mental development are defective. There is controversy as to whether women should drink *at all* around the period of conception, and while it is evident that some women are more susceptible to the effects of alcohol, in terms of producing a baby suffering from fetal alcohol syndrome, than others, we advise no alcohol at all around this time.

An adequate intake of vitamins and minerals, amino acids and essential fatty acids will give a marked degree of protection against the ill-effects of alcohol.

Maternal Smoking

Smoking during pregnancy causes an increased risk of problems in the perinatal period, and is also associated with reduced birth weight, which of itself can be a risk factor for future problems. As a result, we advocate strongly that all women planning to conceive should stop smoking.

Premenstrual Syndrome (see also page 301)

Women who experience premenstrual syndrome almost always have a problem with poor nutritional status as regards zinc, magnesium, and vitamin B6, to name but a few. Often there is a problem with food intolerances, especially of dairy products, yeast and wheat, and this should be seen as a health problem worth sorting out before becoming pregnant.

Food Intolerances

Some women have food intolerances, and it seems only sensible to avoid consuming large amounts of these particular foods when considering becoming pregnant. Infertility and congenital malformations are more common in women with celiac disease. This may very well be due to marginal absorption of zinc and other essential micronutrients, and this should be assessed before becoming pregnant. Lesser degrees of food intolerance can still result in the malabsorption of micronutrients which can compromise the development of the fetus.

Recommendations for Preconceptional Care

Start this program at least three to six months before planned conception. The basic recommendations are:

For men:
- stop smoking
- reduce or stop alcohol consumption
- improve your diet (see below)
- take nutritional supplements (see page 422)

For women:
- stop smoking
- stop alcohol consumption
- improve your diet (see below)
- take nutritional supplements (see page 423)
- stop oral contraception
- sort out food allergies
- rubella screen
- toxoplasma screen
- toxic metal screen
- handle any health problems
- stop all drugs and medicines unless essential

For men and women, to improve your diet:

- avoid refined carbohydrates, processed foods and foods with artificial additives
- eat an adequate amount of protein
- eat plenty of fresh fruit and vegetables (especially dark-green, leafy vegetables) and whole grains
- cut down on tea and coffee drinking
- get regular exercise
- try to deal with stress

PREGNANCY AND BREAST-FEEDING

The physiological and metabolic changes during pregnancy are very pronounced and nutrition plays a large part in the normal progression of pregnancy with a healthy mother and child at the end.

We saw in the preceding section on preconceptional care just how important nutrition and the toxic environment are in relation to the development of a normal baby. Those women reading this section who have already conceived without having carried out any of the recommendations in the chapter on preconceptional care should not be alarmed though. While it is naturally important for those at risk to ensure that their diet and nutritional intake is adequate and that they are not loaded with environmental toxins, it is important to bear in mind that the vast majority of pregnancies result in the birth of a healthy baby. Also, take encouragement from the fact that there is a lot that you can do between now and the time that the baby is born.

Nutritional Requirements

Ideally, conception should take place when the mother is taking an adequate quantity of all nutrients, and is free from toxins. We saw how to work towards this in the previous section. Many physicians say that there is no need for nutritional supplements prior to or during pregnancy if one has a "good, balanced diet." We believe that this is incorrect, based on our nutritional assessments of many mothers-to-be who apparently have what is generally accepted as a sensible diet. It should be remembered that food intake in pregnancy increases by fifteen to twenty percent, but the requirements for folic acid, vitamin B, vitamin C, calcium, zinc and magnesium increase by thirty to one hundred percent. Your diet therefore has to be very good to start with.

Nutritional supplementation does *not* aim to replace a healthy, sensible diet, but on the other hand, a healthy, sensible diet does *not* necessarily guarantee nutritional adequacy for each individual, as each of us has such different nutrient requirements.

There is controversy as to what constitutes a safe and sensible supplementation during pregnancy. There have been reports of isolated nutrients given in high doses causing congenital abnormalities. We feel that high-dose vitamins and minerals are not sensible during pregnancy as the appropriate trials have not been done to prove their safety. However, we do advocate taking a multivitamin and mineral supplement, which supplies a broad spectrum of nutrients in small or moderate dosage. And if someone actually has a documented nutritional deficiency, in our opinion it would be negligent not to give the appropriate supplement.

IMPORTANT NOTE

If you intend to take nutritional supplements during your pregnancy, you should consult your own doctor first.

ZINC AND IRON

The report *Nutrition in Pregnancy* by the Royal College of Obstetricians and Gynecologists does not advocate the use of zinc supplements during pregnancy. In our experience, in view of the hazards of being zinc deficient (see page 66) in pregnancy, and in view of the recognized poor zinc intake in both the UK and the United States, it seems sensible to take a *moderate* supplement of zinc as well as other nutrients—10–15 mg is adequate for a daily dose.

It has been the general vogue in medicine in recent year to give folic acid and iron routinely during pregnancy. The wisdom of this is now being questioned, as both iron and folic acid inhibit the absorption of dietary zinc and possibly also of other nutrients. Quite apart from the fact that so many women complain of constipation with iron supplements, the fact that one is doing something that can inhibit the absorption of zinc is something to be wary of, as dietary zinc seems to be barely adequate, or low, in so many women, and because zinc is so important for the development of the fetus (see page 66).

Iron and zinc absorption are inhibited by both tea and coffee, as is discussed elsewhere, and in view of the fact that iron stores are normally compromised during pregnancy, it seems sensible to keep tea and coffee consumption during pregnancy to a minimum around meal times, in order to make the most of whatever iron is present in the meal. By taking a slightly acidic drink such as orange juice, you can enhance iron absorption substantially. Alternatively, you can take a vitamin C supplement (50–100 mg) at meal times, and this will enhance the absorption of iron.

SPECIAL GROUPS

Vegetarians and vegans should receive supplements of vitamin B12 during pregnancy and breast-feeding if there is any chance of deficiency occurring. Women who have been on such diets for more than four years are particularly at risk.

Colored women may easily develop vitamin D deficiency and, if city dwellers, should receive a supplement providing 400 IUs per day while pregnant or breast-feeding. A calcium supplement providing 500–1000 mg per day is recommended, and chapatis should be avoided in the diet.

Normal Pregnancy

Pregnancy usually lasts forty weeks from the date of the first day of the last period, and during that time women put on weight. If you become overweight, we do not necessarily suggest that you lose weight, as this can put the pregnancy at risk. Instead, we suggest you cut out refined carbohydrates (if you haven't already done so) and eat plenty of fresh fruit and vegetables, together with an adequate protein intake.

Our recommendations for the management of a normal pregnancy are:

- Diet
  - avoid refined carbohydrates
  - avoid foods with artificial additives
  - eat plenty of fresh fruit
  - eat plenty of fresh vegetables (especially green, leafy ones)
  - take adequate protein—60–80 g daily
  - avoid known food allergens
  - keep tea and coffee consumption to an absolute minimum
- Stop alcohol.
- Stop smoking.
- Take nutritional supplements where necessary.
- Attend regular antenatal check ups.
- Exercise for pregnancy.

- Get adequate rest.
- Get adequate fresh air.

If a woman is drinking alcohol when she finds that she is pregnant (and it is usually better to stop drinking altogether *prior* to conception) then we advocate stopping immediately. The same applies to cigarette smoking, as problems during pregnancy, low birth weight, and also increased number of respiratory tract infections during the first year of life are more common in children born to mothers who smoked during pregnancy.

Drugs should be avoided in pregnancy wherever possible. You'll have to rely on your medical doctor as to when drugs are required. **The general rule is: Do not take any medications or drugs during pregnancy unless they are absolutely unavoidable.**

As part of a general commonsense approach, you should not expose yourself to large quantities of environmental toxins such as chemical sprays (including hair sprays) etc. as there is no guarantee that these will not cross the placental barrier, be absorbed by the fetus and have a detrimental effect on its health.

Previous Pregnancy Problems

Any woman who has had problems in previous pregnancies should seek specialist medical advice on how to deal with them. Such things as early morning sickness, pre-eclampsia, diabetes occurring in pregnancy, premature labor, recurrent miscarriages and so on, should always be dealt with by a specialist.

STILLBIRTHS

Stillbirths are usually associated with either failure of the placenta or some kind of problem occurring during the actual delivery. Professor Bryce-Smith and others have shown that there is a higher than normal content of cadmium and lead in the bones of stillborn children. In our limited experience in dealing nutritionally with women who have previously had a still-born child, without exception they have been *extremely* zinc deficient. This is of interest in that zinc is an antagonist to both lead and cadmium. This once more reflects the importance, in certain instances, of seeking advice after previous problems.

Allergy and Pregnancy

The degree to which the mother's exposure to allergens affects the baby is not yet clear but we still recommend where possible the avoidance of known allergens, whether they be food, chemical or inhalant. Sometimes allergies become less troublesome during pregnancy, but this is no reason to be complacent. In others, allergies are precipitated or worsened by pregnancy.

Early Morning Sickness

Early morning sickness and nausea during pregnancy are extremely common and for many women it is an early sign that they are in fact pregnant. Whether or not this is a normal physiological variation of pregnancy has been disputed, but we consider it to be a sign of nutritional or hormonal imbalance. Despite this, the vast majority of women progress to a normal delivery and a normal child. Nausea and vomiting in pregnancy are no indication on their own that the pregnancy is heading for problems. They respond quite well to the hypoglycemia approach (see page 292) and vitamin B6, 50 mg once or twice a day, and magnesium 200–500 mg daily. Cutting out dairy products completely may be helpful for some women. Prolonged vomiting during pregnancy can cause severe vitamin B deficiency. Some doctors have found intramuscular vitamin B6 50–100 mg daily, plus 5 mg vitamin K intramuscularly, to be very helpful.

Early morning sickness of pregnancy

Ruth was delighted that she was pregnant, but four weeks after her missed period she started to develop morning nausea and vomiting which made her feel absolutely ghastly. Supplements of 200–400 mg of magnesium and 50–100 mg of vitamin B6 brought about a marked improvement in the condition. Additionally, by having a drink of orange or apple juice by her bedside, she found that taking a few mouthfuls before getting up in the morning was quite helpful. This presumably prevented the excessive drop in blood sugar which often accompanies the nausea and vomiting of pregnancy. In the past, some doctors have found that vitamin K injections have been very useful in alleviating the nausea and vomiting of pregnancy, though we have had no experience with this.

Pregnancy Diabetes

Some pregnant women develop abnormal carbohydrate metabolism. It appears that the stress of pregnancy results in a failure to regulate blood sugar adequately.

Some women who develop pregnancy diabetes go on to get true diabetes later in life, but more often than not the woman recovers completely within six weeks of delivery and there is no further evidence of diabetes.

Pregnancy diabetes, if left untreated, is associated with a higher risk of death in the newborn.

There have been several studies showing that women with pregnancy diabetes who are put on a diet and given 100 mg of pyridoxine daily for two weeks, have a considerable improvement in their diabetes.

Thrush and Cystitis (see pages 342 and 344)

Insomnia

Some women find it difficult to sleep during pregnancy and this may very well relate to nutrient deficiencies (see page 387), but there are usually other considerations, such as physical discomfort.

Dyspepsia

Many women who are pregnant get dyspepsia, a discomfort at the bottom of the breastbone at the top of the abdomen. This may very well be caused by the baby's pressing on the abdomen and can sometimes cause discomfort and difficulty, especially at night. If this is a problem, it may be worth propping yourself up in bed, and not eating too late at night. Excessive use of antacids, especially those containing aluminum, should be avoided during pregnancy as there is some evidence to suggest that the aluminum which gets absorbed can be toxic. A small amount of sodium bicarbonate (a quarter of a teaspoonful dissolved in water) can often bring relief, but this should not be relied upon heavily, or taken around meal times, as it can neutralize gastric acid which is necessary for the digestion of food and the absorption of a number of essential nutrients.

Constipation

Many women get constipated during pregnancy. Sometimes this is caused by the iron supplements that they are routinely given by their obstetricians (see page 327). In most cases, extra vitamin C, 3–5 g per day, plenty of dietary fiber in the form of fruit and vegetables, adequate liquid, and exercise, can all cure the condition effectively.

Varicose Veins

Quite a number of women develop varicose veins during pregnancy and there is some evidence that a vitamin B6 shortage can be a predisposing factor. Other predisposing factors are constipation, and increased pressure on the veins.

Premature Labor

Some women go into labor prematurely and have to be hospitalized and treated with drugs that stop the contractions of the womb. There is some circumstantial evidence to suggest that calcium and magnesium supplements, as well as essential fatty acids, can be of benefit in this situation. We suggest 1–2 g of calcium in the form of calcium gluconate or aminochelate per day and magnesium 500–750 mg as the carbonate or aminochelate per day. Additionally, 2–3 g of evening primrose oil daily may help. The reduction of stress, adequate rest and appropriate medical treatment should be included in the above regime.

Toxemia of Pregnancy

Toxemia of pregnancy is characterized by the appearance of protein in the urine, soft tissue swelling, weight gain, and increasing blood pressure. Such a situation is very important to detect, and is one of the reasons why it is so important to attend antenatal visits routinely right through to the end of pregnancy.

There is evidence to show that women who have suffered from pre-eclampsia have markedly lower levels of vitamin B6 than those who had a normal pregnancy. Whatever the mechanism, it appears that a deficiency of B6 predisposes to the development of toxemia. Studies have shown that those women who receive a supplement of 10 mg of vitamin B6 daily during pregnancy have a significantly lower incidence of pre-eclampsia than those who do not.

Calcium, 1 g once or twice a day, along with magnesium, 400–800 mg once a day, and vitamin B6, 10–50 mg per day, in addition to paying attention to food allergies, can be very helpful in toxemia. There is also good evidence that pregnant women should take at least 500 mg of magnesium daily, in addition to whatever magnesium they may be obtaining from their diet. One expert reports that numbness, tingling, loss of sensation in the fingertips, weakness of handgrip, impaired flexion of the fingers, pain in the finger joints and nocturnal paralysis of the arm, may all respond to vitamin B6 supplementation in pregnancy. It has also been observed that *severe* muscle spasms in the legs and feet are improved or relieved with 50–450 mg of B6 daily. Oral calcium, 1000 mg twice daily for two weeks, magnesium, 400–800 mg once daily, and vitamin B6, 50 mg once or twice daily, can eliminate or reduce the frequency and severity of muscle cramps during pregnancy. Paying attention to food intolerance (especially cows' milk products) may also be helpful.

Carpal Tunnel Syndrome

Carpal tunnel syndrome can also occur as a pregnancy-related condition. It responds to vitamin B6 (see page 255).

The Delivery

The delivery of the baby is one of the most exciting things that can happen to a couple, and some women get particularly anxious about it. Education in what is actually going to happen during pregnancy, the mother and father attending antenatal classes together, and the father's presence at the delivery, can all help reduce concern about the delivery itself.

Postnatal Depression

Recent research reveals that this can be due to lack of vitamin B and calcium—perhaps influenced by a lack of magnesium, too. Any woman experiencing depression after the birth of her child should ensure that she has a good diet, adequate rest and emotional support. Any nutritional deficiency should be thoroughly corrected.

Breast-feeding

Nature has provided mammals with breasts to feed their young and it has been presumptuous of man to think that he can replace breast milk provided by nature with milks of his own formulation. Cows' milk is ideal for calves—it was not designed for human beings. So it is hardly surprising that children who are given formulas derived from cows' or other non-human milks, quite often run into trouble. Many obstetric units have also got into the pernicious habit of whisking the newborn baby away from its mother and placing him or her in the nursery to be fed a mixture of water and glucose—the latter often being derived from corn.

Certain trace elements, amino acids and essential fatty acids are present in human breast milk that are not available in the same form elsewhere. Biochemistry is not yet sufficiently advanced to be able to identify every single substance in maternal breast milk—there are more than 200 known substances in it. Modified cows' milk doesn't come anywhere near replicating human milk except in the main nutritional elements. We feel that breast milk must be the best food for a baby, and that breast-feeding should be encouraged for at least three to six months and preferably longer.

Having said this, with today's modern diet and lifestyles, it doesn't mean to say that a mother's breast milk is the perfect, sole nutritional source for her baby. She too is exposed to toxic chemicals in the air, in the water she drinks, and in the food she eats. We are all also exposed to foods that have been contaminated with sprays, insecticides, pesticides, herbicides, preservatives and so on before they reach our plates. Obviously, some of these toxins are passed into maternal breast milk and then on to the infant, where they may, in susceptible babies, cause problems. To be fair, cows' milk too contains many of these impurities—sometimes in far greater quantities—mainly because cows eat foods that are much more heavily contaminated with noxious substances.

Some women, too, run into problems with breast-feeding and have to resort to bottle-feeding. Whenever this is the case, every effort should be made on the part of the attendant midwives, health visitors, physicians, family and friends, to encourage and support the mother through whatever problem is threatening her ability to continue to breast-feed. If such a situation arises, and bottle-feeding becomes inevitable, then the decision has to be made and the appropriate actions taken. This is discussed later in the section on Bottle-Feeding.

ALLERGY AND BREAST-FEEDING

Infantile colic is very often due to cows' milk intolerance. This is more common in bottle-fed than in breast-fed babies. However, breast-fed babies are not immune. If a mother is drinking cows' milk, certain of the proteins derived from cows' milk appear in her breast milk, are absorbed into the gastrointestinal tract of the baby, and can then cause problems in susceptible infants. So if a baby has eczema, wheezing, skin problems, digestive problems or sleep disturbances, he or she might be reacting to certain of the foods that the mother is eating. (Apart from dairy foods, other suspects include wheat and citrus fruit.) Under these circumstances, it is worthwhile keeping a food diary and noting on which days the baby has problems and on which days there are none. By comparing the onset of the baby's problems with the foods taken by the mother over the previous twenty-four hours, it may be quite possible to identify the most likely offenders. It is then a question simply of eliminating the suspect foods over a period of time and seeing if there is any improvement in the baby. It is important to mention here that you shouldn't compromise your overall nutritional intake by excluding these foods. While nutritional supplementation with vitamins and minerals during breast-feeding may be entirely appropriate, it is no substitute for a nutritionally adequate diet.

If it appears that your baby reacts to a wide range of foods that you are eating, it may be worthwhile going onto a rotated diet and avoiding those major food allergens which you have isolated, identified or even suspected. **You'll need the help of a dietitian with this to ensure that your nutritional intake is adequate.**

Breast-feeding and infantile colic

Gloria was delighted to have given birth to a healthy 8 lb. boy until she found that it was no fun spending so much time in the middle of the night pacing up and down the bedroom trying to pacify Jason, who seemed to spend most of his time shrieking, with his face screwed up in a wrinkled ball. The family doctor had said that it was colic and had given a preparation to help settle him, but this was ineffective. On closer questioning it was found that Gloria had been drinking more than a pint of milk a day during pregnancy to try to ensure that she was providing the baby with enough nourishment to grow properly in the womb. Gloria had had eczema as a young girl and there was a strong history of asthma and eczema in the family. By cutting out milk from the diet, Gloria was delighted to observe that Jason slept peacefully. This is a good example of how a baby can be intolerant to a given food that the mother is eating, and which passes through the breast milk. Naturally, she was given advice as to how to make her diet nutritionally adequate even though she wasn't having cows' milk products while breast-feeding. She was given calcium and magnesium supplements too.

By following the above regimen, we have seen infantile colic, sleep disturbances, skin problems, and restlessness all settle beautifully.

NUTRITIONAL REQUIREMENTS DURING BREAST-FEEDING

Your nutritional requirements are higher during breast-feeding than at other times, including during pregnancy, particularly for calcium, magnesium, zinc, B vitamins, folic acid, and other vitamins as well as minerals such as manganese, copper etc. It is vital that you eat a sensible diet and if there are signs or symptoms of deficiencies then the appropriate supplement should be considered.

If you do have known food intolerances, it seems sensible to avoid a significant consumption of these substances while you are breast-feeding.

FOODS TO GIVE A BABY ON WEANING

Whatever foods you give to your child, it seems sensible to vary the diet as much as possible. In this way, he or she won't become dependent on one particular food and the likelihood of developing an intolerance to one or more foods is also reduced. If there is any suspicion of a family history of food intolerance, then we advocate avoiding the introduction of cows' milk or wheat until nine months and even then, only from time to time. It is also worthwhile keeping a food diary, noting which foods are introduced and when. This may be invaluable retrospectively if a baby produces some kind of reaction which could initially be attributed to infection or upset, or flatulence or whatever, though may in fact be a food reaction. If you also note when particular problems start, you can quite often identify the offending food, exclude it from the baby's diet, and have a healthy, happy baby once again. The most common deficiency in the first year of life is iron. Give baby lean meat and vegetables (especially greens) which are nutritious, safe foods, rather than over-emphasizing milk and wheat. Other good foods to introduce are rice, potatoes, fruit and avocados. Nuts, sweetcorn, wholemeal bread, bran and mushrooms are often poorly digested.

BOTTLE-FEEDING

Babies who are bottle-fed probably do better, especially if there is an allergic history in the family, if their formulas are rotated, using one every three days of cows' milk formula, goats'-milk-derived formula, soya-derived formula, and, in exceptional circumstances, grain-derived formula. In this way, the likelihood of developing an intolerance to any one of them is reduced.

Benign Breast Disease

A major clinical problem and the most common form of cancer in women is breast cancer, on which considerable research has been performed. Because of the awareness of breast cancer many women are exceptionally conscious of minor breast discomfort or breast lumps and often go to their doctor with them. The vast majority of breast conditions are not sinister—the most common by far is fibrocystic disease.

FIBROCYSTIC DISEASE

This term is in common usage yet means different things to different experts. Usually there are feelable lumps in the breast, often associated with pain and tenderness, which fluctuate with the menstrual cycle and that become progressively worse until menopause.

For some time fibrocystic disease of the breast has been considered to be a small but significant risk factor for cancer. This is probably only true in a small percentage of women. Definite risk factors for cancer of the breast include a family history of breast cancer, an early start to having periods, a late menopause, and a heavy consumption of meat.

Any woman who goes to her doctor with painful breasts should have a full and careful assessment, including a thorough history, to find out whether the symptoms are cyclical or noncyclical; the presence or absence of other premenstrual symptoms, and thorough examination to assess not only the breasts, but also the presence or absence of discharge from the nipple, and an assessment of her hormone state.

In particular, your doctor will be careful to assess whether there is any possibility of the pain or the lumps being due to a cancer of the breast. Sinister signs would be a well-defined mass; local enlarged glands, especially in the armpit; a bloodstained nipple discharge; inversion of the nipple or nipple tethering; or an abnormality of the overlying skin. Any of these need urgent further assessment.

Once your doctor has satisfied himself that you don't have a cancer he then has a number of treatments that he can use.

Drug treatments include the prolactin-antagonist bromocriptine and the drug danazol. Both drugs are expensive and not without side-effects.

Many less drastic nutritional programs have been suggested.

Dietary recommendations

- Reduce dietary animal fat.
- Increase polyunsaturated fatty acids, particularly those derived from fish such as mackerel, herring and salmon.
- Avoid tea, coffee, chocolate, cola and other caffeine-containing substances as well as drugs and medicines containing caffeine.
- If you have a long-standing constipation, abdominal symptoms, PMS and breast discomfort, we would be suspicious of a food allergy, particularly to wheat. A trial of an exclusion diet is sometimes recommended (see Appendix, page 425).

The use of supplements

Over the last few years, a number of nutritional supplements have been used in the treatment of benign breast disease and some of them look particularly promising:

- Vitamin E, 400–600 IUs per day.
- Vitamin B6, 50–200 mg per day in conjunction with vitamin B complex, 25 mg per day.
- Evening primrose oil, 500 mg capsules, 4–6 per day.
- Magnesium, 200 mg per day.
- Zinc, 10–40 mg, particularly if premenstrual symptoms are present, if the woman is on a poor diet, or evidence of deficiencies is found. Women with elevated levels of the hormone prolactin may respond to zinc treatment.
- Cold-pressed linseed oil, 1–2 tablespoons per day, or evening primrose oil, 500 mg capsules, 4 to 8 per day in conjunction with vitamin C, 600 mg, plus B vitamins and zinc if appropriate. MaxEPA could also be of help.
- Iodine supplements, e.g. kelp 4–6 tablets per day.

Remember, if your symptoms are persistent, consult your doctor.

INFECTIONS

All through history, infections have always been a major cause of death throughout the world. Now, in Western society, infections have mainly been controlled by three factors: improved nutrition, the provision of a clean water supply and effective sewerage, and mass immunization programs.

To understand the role of nutrition in helping fight infection, we need first to look at the normal mechanisms involved in resistance to infection.

Unlike organs of the body, such as the liver or kidneys, the immune system which fights infection is not concentrated in any special location—it is distributed throughout the body. It is composed of different types of white cells which are found in the lymph glands, the liver, the spleen, the blood, and bone marrow, and there are small collections of many different types of white blood cells in almost every tissue and organ.

Essentially, there are two different types of white cells. The first are called granulocytes. These contain "granules" of chemicals that are noxious to infecting organisms. They fight organisms by literally trying to engulf or swallow them, and then releasing onto the organisms the chemicals contained in the granules, thus destroying them.

The second type are called lymphocytes. These are small white blood cells that are derived from lymph nodes, the spleen, and an organ called the thymus which is found in the center of the chest, next to the heart. Lymphocytes are further divided into two types: T-cells, which originate from the thymus gland, and B-cells, which come from the bone marrow. They both fight infections, but B-cells produce antibodies and the T-cells play a supporting and influencing role.

Antibodies are a type of protein. They circulate in the blood and attack and, with the help of other substances, destroy infecting organisms. They are only produced after the infecting organism has been present in the body for several days, or if the person has already been exposed to the same or a similar infection. So we tend not to get German measles or chicken pox twice because we have built up antibodies to the German measles or chicken pox viruses. There are different types of antibodies (also known as immunoglobulins) called immunoglobulins-G, -A and -M. The T-cells do not themselves produce antibodies, but modify the B-cells either by helping or by suppressing them.

So there are two types of white cells, one that produces an immediate response to an infection and another that produces a delayed response remembering a past infection to which the individual is now immune.

The cells of the immune system, both the granulocytes and the lymphocytes, are sensitive to changes in the nutritional state. While it is fairly obvious that severe malnutrition will substantially reduce an individual's resistance to infection, lesser deficiencies in individual vitamins and minerals are now recognized as an important, if less obvious, cause of impaired resistance to infection, and thus a significant cause of chronic or recurrent infections in otherwise healthy people.

Nutrients and Immunity

Vitamins B6, B5, C, E, and folic acid and essential fatty acids are vital for normal immune function. Iron, zinc and certain other minerals are crucial too. To be able to resist infections the body also needs an adequate supply of calories and protein.

DIETARY AND OTHER SUPPRESSORS OF IMMUNITY

While nutritional deficiencies undoubtedly make recurrent infections more likely, so can excesses of certain dietary agents, as well as other substances, reduce resistance to infection.

An important and remarkable effect is that of refined carbohydrates such as glucose and sucrose. These, together with fruit sugar (fructose), have a depressant effect upon the immune system within one hour of eating them. Fasting for thirty-six to sixty hours improves immune function.

The role of dietary fats in impairing resistance to infection is uncertain. It is possible that a high-animal-fat diet might not be advantageous.

Alcohol, because it depletes the body of B vitamins and zinc, may, if taken in significant amounts, have an indirectly suppressant effect upon immunity. Cigarette smokers tend to have an increased number of white cells in the blood. This might suggest that they have an improved resistance to infection, but the high level of white cells is in fact a sign of a mild, chronic chest infection (smokers are particularly prone to chest infections such as bronchitis and pneumonia). Smokers do not respond as well as non-smokers when immunized against influenza.

On the positive side, certain foods can actually improve one's resistance to infection. Live yogurt contains a "friendly" bacterium *lactobacillus acidophilus* which may have some activity against harmful bacteria. Garlic contains agents which appear to have both anti-bacterial and antifungal activity. It is quite possible that raw vegetables contain naturally occurring antifungal agents which prevent them becoming moldy, and that consuming relatively large quantities of raw or lightly cooked foods may benefit people with chronic gastrointestinal infections.

The first thing you should do if you suffer from repeated infections is to have a thorough examination from your family doctor.

He or she may then want to perform the following tests:

- Collect specimens to identify the infecting organism. This could mean taking a swab from an infected boil or a urine test in the case of cystitis.
- A blood test for anemia, a full blood count, and to check the level of white blood cells.
- A blood test to measure levels of IgG, IgA, and IgM.
- A blood test to measure levels of iron in the body—to look for iron deficiency even if you are not anemic.
- X-rays such as a chest X-ray, a sinus X-ray, or a dental X-ray in the case of chronic infection in these areas.
- A urine test for sugar to check for diabetes. Diabetics are especially prone to repeated infections.

Tests for specific nutritional deficiencies are not performed routinely. If a severe zinc deficiency is suspected, a test of the patient's serum zinc, taken after they have fasted overnight, can be of value, but milder forms of zinc deficiency will not be detected by a simple blood test.

While these tests are under way the person involved or the parent, in the case of a child, can make some simple changes in diet which are bound to help:

- Completely avoid refined carbohydrates, glucose and sucrose. Limit your intake of fructose (fruit sugar).
- Ensure that you eat a well-balanced diet (see Appendix 1).
- Avoid potentially harmful dietary agents including tobacco, alcohol and excesses of tea and coffee.
- Take a multivitamin supplement, particularly one containing vitamins C and B in a good dosage.
- Take a trace-element supplement providing 5–10 mg of zinc for children and 20–30 mg of zinc per day for adults. **(Iron**

deficiency should be corrected by the use of iron tablets from your doctor. Iron and zinc supplements should not be taken at the same time—they are best separated.)

- Think about possible food allergens: if symptoms such as migraine, rhinitis, eczema, bowel complaints, tiredness or aches and pains are unresponsive to the above regime, then it makes sense to think of a food allergy (see page 154).
- Ensure that you get plenty of fresh air, sunlight and exercise. This can only do you good. Remember that a good diet, fresh air, and sunlight was the main treatment for tuberculosis before the discovery of antibiotics.

Advice for Specific Infections

The above advice applies to the majority of people with recurrent infections. Here is some more specific advice on individual infections.

RECURRENT THRUSH (see also page 346)

- Avoid antibiotics
- Detect and correct diabetes, if present.
- Detect and correct iron and zinc deficiencies.
- Reduce your intake of refined carbohydrates and increase your intake of complex carbohydrates, raw or lightly cooked vegetables, fruits and grains.
- Take live, plain yogurt by mouth and vaginally.
- Women with recurrent vaginal thrush should take antifungal agents both by pessary and by mouth. Prolonged treatment for six weeks may be necessary.
- Treat your sexual partner who may be a carrier of thrush.

HERPES SIMPLEX INFECTION

There are two types of herpes virus: Type I produces infection of the mouth, lips, gums, skin on the face (cold sores) and sometimes widespread and serious infections can occur. Type II herpes simplex virus is the cause of genital herpes, a condition that can be very resistant to treatment. Simple treatment for either infection involves:

- Taking vitamin C, 600–1000 mg, together with bioflavonoids, 600–1000 mg, each daily.

- Taking the amino acid lysine, 300–1200 mg daily, together with a diet low in its contrasting amino acid arginine (avoid peanuts, chocolate, seeds and cereals). Lysine and arginine are two essential amino acids. Lysine appears to inhibit and arginine to favor growth of the herpes simplex virus.
- Using a local application of ointment containing 8% lithium and 0.05% zinc sulphate, together with a smaller quantity of vitamin E, may also be of value for Type I infections.
- Using a local application of iodine ointment for Type I infections. Iodine is known to have powerful antiviral activity.

All of these are suitable DIY measures. It also makes sense to avoid precipitating factors such as stress and exposure to sunlight. Needless to say, you should correct any nutritional deficiencies and follow a healthy diet. Immunization against flu has been shown to help patients with recurrent herpes.

GLANDULAR FEVER (INFECTIOUS MONONUCLEOSIS) AND POST-VIRAL SYNDROME

Glandular fever is caused by an infection with the Epstein-Barr virus, a close relative to the herpes viruses. Infection usually occurs in teenagers and young adults who complain of a severe sore throat, enlargement of the lymph glands in the neck, and varying degrees of malaise. Some people recover very slowly from such an infection and the malaise can be very persistent. Recently, a number of abnormalities, including the induction of food allergies, changes in the immune system and in cell metabolism, as well as persistence of the virus, have been shown to occur after such infections. Some such youngsters are dismissed as neurotic or as malingerers, yet they often feel very ill. No treatment is yet of proven value. However, in our experience, undetected nutritional deficiencies (particularly of zinc and iron and perhaps of vitamin B) are not infrequent. Try taking the following. We have found them to be helpful.

- Zinc: 30–40 mg daily
- B complex: 20–30 mg daily
- Vitamin C: 1 g or more daily
- Evening primrose oil: 500 mg 2–6 capsules a day

Talk to your doctor about the possibility of a food allergy and hidden iron deficiency with or without anemia.

An exclusion diet under medical supervision, along with nutritional supplements, can sometimes speed up recovery from glandular fever and similar infections.

Post-viral malaise

Neville, a fifty-year-old car dealer, had had a severe bout of glandular fever eighteen months previously. Since then he had had recurring episodes of malaise and enlarged glands in his neck, for which no cause could be found, except that it was a residual effect of his original episode of glandular fever. He had also experienced weight loss, depression, loss of taste and headaches. Investigations showed him to have a normal level of zinc in his blood, but a very depressed level of zinc in his sweat, 107 parts per billion (normal range 360–680). Within a week of taking supplements of zinc, 50 mg per day, and multivitamins, his sense of taste returned and his malaise improved. Over the following three months there was an almost complete return of his energy level and disappearance of the enlarged glands. He was able to return to his work, which had suffered considerably because of his continuing ill-health. Deficiencies of zinc, iron, and vitamin B6, are relatively common, and important causes of poor resistance to or poor recovery from infection. Sometimes zinc deficiency can be present even though blood levels of zinc are normal, and a trial of zinc therapy, together with multivitamins and a healthy diet, is certainly worthwhile.

COLDS, COUGHS, SINUSITIS AND BRONCHITIS

Minor infections of the upper respiratory tract are very common and are usually caused by a viral infection. If they are caused by bacteria, antibiotics may be valuable. High doses of vitamin C have been advocated, but results are not convincing and the response is very variable. However, short-term, high-dose vitamin C (3–5 g per day) may be worth a try. Recently, the use of zinc lozenges was shown by a group of doctors from Texas to shorten the duration of symptoms in patients with the common cold.

CYSTITIS

Repeated infections of the bladder are not uncommon, particularly in women. Cystitis produces symptoms such as pain and burning on passing urine, with an increased desire to pass water. Abdominal cramps and fever can also occur. The infecting organism, a bacterium, has usually spread from the anus. The response to antibiotics is usually dramatic, but this doesn't prevent a recurrence of the infection. Any woman with recurrent cystitis should see her doctor. If no infection can be found, it may be that the problem is caused by chronic candidiasis (page 346) or food intolerance (page 154). There are, however, simple measures that can be undertaken to reduce the likelihood of infection:

- Drink lots of fluid, 2–3 quarts per day.
- Eat a healthy diet, low in sugar, alcohol and animal fat.
- Pay attention to personal hygiene. After opening your bowels, the anus should be cleaned in a front-to-back direction, so as not to carry germs towards the external opening of the bladder.
- Don't use soaps, detergents and perfumed toiletries when washing the vaginal and anal areas.
- Don't wear nylon underwear, tights or trousers.
- It is not uncommon in recurrent cystitis for no bacteria to be found in the urine, and the response to antibiotic treatment to be poor. We have found two frequent causes—food allergy and/or candida problems. Addressing these two conditions can result in a cure.

Those with recurrent infections, particularly the elderly, are likely to have hidden nutritional deficiencies. Many studies have demonstrated the use of nutritional supplements and dietary change in improving resistance to infection.

AIDS

- Acquired Immune Deficiency Syndrome—AIDS—is now thought to be caused by a virus and is particularly likely to occur among male homosexuals and residents of the central African country, Rwanda, as well as intravenous drug users, Haitian immigrants who are not homosexual and are not drug abusers, those receiving blood transfusions or blood products (such as hemophiliacs), and women.

  The victim often has a history of recurrent infections of either a viral, bacterial, fungal or parasitic nature, and may have a history of weight loss and lymph node enlargement. Only a small percentage of those infected with the virus go on to develop a severe deficiency in the immune system, characterized by low levels of certain types of white cells. They are then open to infections of all kinds and to certain rare types of cancer. The mortality rate can be as high as forty percent.

Some nutrients are known to stimulate the immune system and could, in theory, be useful. B vitamins, vitamin C and zinc are all worth considering. Studies using nutritional supplements as a possible treatment for patients with AIDS, or those who are at risk of developing AIDS, have not yet been performed but could produce interesting results.

How to Boost Your Immune System

- Eat a good, healthy, basic diet.
- Cut out smoking.
- Drink no more than one or two units of alcohol per day.
- Correct any nutritional deficiencies and ensure nutritional adequacy of zinc, vitamin A and vitamin C and essential fatty acids.
- Get regular fresh air and exercise and get adequate rest.
- Handle any excessive stress in your life.
- Treat any underlying infections (especially chronic candidiasis if present) or underlying medical conditions.
- Deal with any food intolerances.
- Assume a positive approach to life.

CANDIDIASIS

Candida albicans is a yeast which was for some time considered to be totally harmless, but has for many years now been recognized as an important disease-producing micro-organism. It is well recognized as the cause of oral and vaginal thrush, as well as an important cause of death for people who are very severely ill and have extremely poor immune function.

In our opinion, on the basis of published reports and our own experience of a large number of patients, an overgrowth of candida albicans is a significant contributing factor to a wide range of different disorders.

Those Who are Most at Risk from Chronic Candidiasis

It appears that the normal, healthy body can resist infection from this yeast, but that as soon as the immune system weakens, the infection takes a hold. The major factors that predispose to chronic candidiasis are either a compromised immune system, or altered microflora on the mucus membranes of the body, caused by the use of antibiotics.

Changes to the microflora of the mucus membranes happen particularly to people who have been on long-term antibiotic therapy (e.g. for acne or rheumatic heart disease), or those who have had repeated courses of antibiotics for recurrent infections. In the latter case, it is worth seeking an underlying cause for the infection, such as zinc deficiency, food allergy or diabetes.

Oral contraceptives also predispose to candida infections and should be suspected in any woman whose symptoms first occur after she has been on oral contraceptives for some time. Anti-inflammatory drugs such as prednisone and hydrocortisone also predispose to candida problems.

Immune suppression and incompetence occur as a result of certain common nutrient deficiencies. The most common of these are perhaps iron and zinc deficiencies, especially in women and vegetarians. This is discussed in the preceding section.

Various normal physiological changes predispose to candida infection. These start with infancy, when the immune system is immature. A baby may become inoculated with candida during birth if its mother's vagina is infected. Pregnancy, like the use of oral contraceptives, predisposes to candida overgrowth, and a woman's symptoms may very well date back to the first time that she was pregnant or shortly after. Old age, like infancy, is associated with reduced functioning of the immune system, possibly because old people eat insufficient nutrients in their diet, or because they can no longer efficiently absorb the nutrients that they eat.

Deficiency of immunoglobulin A (an important antibody), too little gastric acid, and other conditions can predispose to chronic candidiasis, and other illnesses should always be borne in mind by a doctor treating someone for candidiasis. Acquired immune deficiency syndrome (AIDS) can start off with oral candidiasis (but if you have oral candidiasis it does *not* mean that AIDS is likely.)

Clues that Should Make You Think of Chronic Candidiasis

Chronic candidiasis can show up with a whole range of different symptoms, affecting almost any system of the body. However, it appears that women are more susceptible to the condition than men and many women can have neuropsychiatric symptoms due to candida.

The following symptoms, many of which can be long-term, may indicate chronic candidiasis:

- Fatigue, lethargy, irritability, headaches, migraines.
- Joint pains with or without swelling; muscle pains.
- Nettle rash and hives.
- Irritable bowel syndrome.
- A history of oral thrush.
- Upper abdominal discomfort or burning.
- Worsening of symptoms after eating refined carbohydrates and heavily yeasted foods.
- Sensitivity to chemicals (gasoline fumes, paint, cigarette smoke, etc.).
- Craving for refined carbohydrates and/or alcohol, and alcohol intolerance (see page 164).
- Recurrent vaginal thrush/vulval itching.
- Anal itching.
- Recurrent cystitis with negative bacterial cultures.
- Fungal nail or skin infections (athlete's foot, etc.).
- Iron or zinc deficiency.
- Onset of problems during, or shortly after, pregnancy.
- Sexual partner had candida problems.
- Symptoms precipitated by antibiotics (or a history of excessive, repeated or long-term use of antibiotics).
- Symptoms worse in low or damp places, or near new-mown lawns, raked-up leaves or on days when the atmosphere is damp and dank (all symptoms of mold allergy).

The Treatment of Chronic Candidiasis

As with many of the subjects covered in this book, treatment is holistic, not just drug-based.

There are four basic aspects of treatment:

- Diet (see below).
- Avoidance, where possible, of drugs that promote the growth of candida and other yeasts or fungi; these include antibiotics, the birth-control pill, anti-inflammatory drugs such as cortisone and prednisone, and immunosuppressive drugs such as Imuran.

- Correction of nutrient deficiencies. Deficiencies of vitamin A, certain of the B vitamins, vitamin C, zinc, iron, magnesium and other nutrients predispose to candidiasis.
- The use of anti-candida drugs such as nystatin.

THE DIET

The diet is based on the principle that refined carbohydrates act as "food" for candida in the intestines, leading in some cases to increased bloating, flatulence, soreness, itching, disturbed bowel function, and a general worsening of symptoms. Clinical experience shows that the avoidance of yeasty foods can contribute significantly to clinical improvement.

The basic diet rules

- Eat no *refined* carbohydrates: this means no white flour, no white or brown sugar, or foods or drinks containing these. This is essential for someone on the anti-candida treatment program.
- Avoid yeasted foods (see yeast list, page 437), frozen or concentrated orange juice, cheese, bread made with yeast, alcoholic drinks, grapes and grape juice, unpeeled fruits, raisins, sultanas, food that has been "lying around" for a long time, and B vitamins, unless specifically stated on the label that they are yeast-free.
- Some foods, especially garlic, other herbs and spices and *fresh,* green, leafy vegetables, may contain natural antifungal agents, so eat plenty of these.
- Restrict total daily carbohydrate intake to 60–80 grams. Books giving the carbohydrate values of foods are readily available from many booksellers.

IMPORTANT NOTE

Those who are underweight at the start of the diet should ensure they do not lose any more than one or two pounds on the diet. Any problems should be discussed with your doctor.

NYSTATIN

Nystatin is an anti-yeast preparation, isolated in 1950 from the fungus *Streptomyces noursei*. It is poorly absorbed from the gastrointestinal tract, and is remarkably nontoxic when taken orally.

It is extremely useful in dealing with oral and gastrointestinal candida infections, as well as with vaginal infections. There is no evidence that it is unsafe to use in pregnancy, though if it can be avoided during pregnancy this is obviously preferable. At very high doses it can cause nausea and vomiting, but this is unusual. Normally, nystatin acts only locally in the intestines when taken by mouth. Vaginal pessaries and creams are available to treat specific non-bowel infections.

It must be borne in mind that the conditions outlined in this section are not invariably responsive to nystatin therapy and can be caused by things other than candida.

Nystatin therapy is not a panacea for all ills, but there is published evidence accumulating to suggest that it may be worth trying in a number of situations where other approaches have failed, or where the medical history suggests it is highly likely that candida is a major factor in the development of the symptoms.

Nystatin is one of the least toxic medications available. However, sometimes symptoms can develop if the yeast is being destroyed by the nystatin too rapidly. These are symptoms of toxicity, not from the nystatin itself, but presumably from the absorption of toxins from the candida that are being destroyed by the nystatin. These are sometimes called "die-off" symptoms. If they do occur, you can assume that you are on the right track. How to deal with this reaction is discussed below.

As yet, there is no satisfactory, generally available laboratory test to help a doctor decide whether or not a person will benefit from nystatin therapy. This is a highly unsatisfactory state of affairs, because the doctor has to make the diagnosis on the basis of the patient's history and the response to the anti-candida treatment program.

How to take nystatin

Nystatin is only available on prescription. The nystatin that we use is currently provided in a pure powder form; powder is cheaper and produces fewer unwanted reactions than does the tablet form. It should be taken dissolved in water; the taste is pretty awful, but this is a small price to pay if it results in an increase in well-being and a partial or complete resolution of your symptoms. If your doctor prescribes tablets he'll tell you how to take them.

Women on nystatin should also use vaginal pessaries, one or two at night every night for twenty-one nights, even during menstruation. This applies even to those women who have no history of vaginal thrush. When the pessaries dissolve, a discharge sometimes occurs, which, though inconvenient, is perfectly normal and nothing to worry about.

The sexual partner of a woman with symptoms of vaginal candidiasis (discharge, itching and soreness of the vagina or vulva) should also receive treatment. The vaginal symptoms mentioned can be caused by infections other than candida. If they persist despite the anti-candida treatment, a vaginal swab should be taken, the infection identified and the appropriate treatment instigated.

How long to go on for

This will depend on the length of time it takes for improvement to occur, and varies from individual to individual. Generally, treatment will last for AT LEAST eight weeks. The earliest changes you'll notice are an increase in energy, a lifting of depression, clearance of headaches and improved bowel function. A small percentage of people have to be on the program for up to twelve weeks before they can recognize an improvement in their condition. However, most notice an improvement within the first two to six weeks.

It has been found that nystatin inactivates several of the B vitamins, especially vitamins B2 and B6. It seems sensible, therefore, for those on an anti-candida treatment program who are taking both nystatin and vitamin and mineral supplements to separate the times that they take the nystatin and other supplements.

The best way to take nystatin is away from meal times and we now tell patients to take their nystatin between meals or at least one hour before meals. If you do this and ensure that you take the vitamin B supplements around meal times, the degree to which the nystatin will inactivate the B vitamins will be minimized.

Diet for two weeks before starting with nystatin

"Die-off" reactions which can occur at the start of nystatin treatment can be minimized by starting the anti-candida diet two weeks before starting the nystatin therapy; this reduces the number and severity of reactions. Once on nystatin treatment, the diet should be continued until a marked improvement in symptoms occurs. At this point you can "loosen up" a little on the diet, but the strict *no refined carbohydrates* rule still applies. If, after "loosening up" on the diet, there is a worsening of symptoms, however slight, the strict diet should be resumed.

OTHER STEPS TO REDUCE CANDIDA

Fresh, live yogurt and specialized preparations of *lactobacillus* can help restore the normal intestinal bacterial content. Some food items can help in that these have natural anti-yeast and antifungal activity; these include fresh, raw vegetables, some spices and plant oils, such as garlic, sunflower seed oil, olive oil and cold-pressed linseed oil (*not* linseed oil BP).

PERSISTENT VAGINAL THRUSH

Rosalinde Hurley, professor of Microbiology at Queen Charlotte's Hospital for Women, London, reports that the number of new cases of genital candidiasis *doubled* between 1971 and 1975. She feels that the complacency with which the treatment of the condition has been regarded until recently has resulted in substantial suffering in countless uncured, or partially cured, women with long-standing thrush. She also points out that some women can plunge into a "well of despair" and that the above treatment "proves successful in most cases."

If you have very persistent thrush, here are some guidelines on how to cope:

- If necessary, get a second opinion to discover if it really is thrush.
- Take zinc and iron tablets to remedy any deficiency you might have.
- Try the low-yeast, low-refined-carbohydrate diet for two to four weeks and see if there is any improvement.
- Try vitamin C, yeast-free B vitamins and essential fatty acids (see page 113).
- Follow the nystatin regime outlined above.

For some years, women with troublesome thrush have been advised to use yogurt douches once or twice daily. The theory behind this practice is quite sound. If you use a yogurt it must be the fresh, live, *plain* yogurt. This can be combined with acid preparations such as ACI-Jel (a preparation of acetic acid 0.92% which inhibits candida growth).

N.B. It is possible for women to have symptoms from chronic intestinal candidiasis or candida allergy without having symptomatic vaginal thrush.

DISORDERS OF THE CENTRAL NERVOUS SYSTEM

Conditions affecting the central nervous system which are covered elsewhere include Down's syndrome (page 369), senile dementia (page 375), mental problems (page 377) and mental retardation.

Multiple Sclerosis

Multiple sclerosis is a condition affecting the nervous system whereby the myelin sheath of peripheral nerves becomes interrupted; in certain individuals brain damage can occur. The disease itself can be a mild condition lasting over many years, even decades, with a fluctuating degree of severity. At the other end of the spectrum it can be a "galloping" unremitting condition, resulting in death.

As yet there is no formally recognized definite treatment for multiple sclerosis, but ACTH injections are sometimes used in acute exacerbations of the condition, and trials with immunosuppressive drugs are under way.

In our experience, early multiple sclerosis can be benefited by looking at nutritional status as regards amino acids, essential fatty acids, essential minerals, especially zinc and magnesium, and B vitamins, including B12 and folic acid.

Additionally, food intolerance can play a part in the development of symptoms, and many multiple sclerosis patients have found that by excluding certain foods their symptoms become very much better.

It has also been found that evening primrose oil and even fish oil has benefited some individuals. Under such circumstances, it is important to ensure that one actually takes sufficient dosage—for an adult, 500 mgs, 3 capsules of evening primrose oil three times a day, along with a multivitamin and mineral supplement as found in the Appendices, page 422. Ideally, individual nutritional profiling should be done so that a supplement program, tailor-made for the individual, can be developed.

Toxic metals, especially mercury, can mimic multiple sclerosis. Thus it is our opinion that any patient with multiple sclerosis should be screened for mercury toxicity. The best way to do this is to perform hair mineral analysis and a urine mercury test.

Some patients have been advised in lay publications to have their mercury amalgam fillings removed. While this may be an entirely appropriate thing to do, it is important to bear in mind that a rubber dam should be used by the dentist to prevent the patient from swallowing the dust derived from drilling out the mercury amalgam. The dentist should also use wet, high-powered suction.

Multiple sclerosis

Susan was a twenty-nine-year-old mother of two who had developed blurred vision, pins and needles, loss of balance, and numbness in the legs and one hand. She had been diagnosed as having multiple sclerosis. Full history-taking revealed that she almost certainly had chronic yeast (candida) problems (see page 346). Nutritional assessment showed multiple nutrient deficiencies, despite a sensible "well-balanced" diet, suggesting a problem with absorption of nutrients. She also had tell-tale signs of food allergy (intestinal symptoms, eczema in childhood, migraine). Treating her for chronic candidiasis, treating her food allergies (page 154) and correcting her nutritional deficiencies, including vitamin B12 injections (as she was found to be functionally deficient in it), resulted in a marked improvement, to the point that she became symptom-free within a month of commencing treatment. While spontaneous remissions are quite common in multiple sclerosis, this case is probably a demonstration of how, after removing certain "loads" (deficiencies, candida, food allergy), the body is better able to heal itself. One and a half years later Susan is still symptom-free, with no evidence of any recurrence according to her sixth-monthly check-ups with a neurologist. Furthermore, she feels more fit than at any time during her adult life. **In some situations, anti-candida treatment with nystatin can cause an acute exacerbation of the condition, so one should progress very cautiously in multiple sclerosis.**

Polyneuritis

This is a group of conditions characterized by a failure of or abnormal nerve conduction which may cause weakness, numbness, pins and needles, loss of sensation or position sense. There are a number of different types and as many different causes, including: vitamin B6 toxicity; lead, mercury, pesticide and chemical toxicities; vitamin B12 deficiency; vitamin E deficiency; diabetes and infections. Polyneuritis can sometimes be improved by correcting nutritional deficiencies, boosting the immune system with vitamin B6 complex, B12 injections and essential fatty acids from sunflower and safflower seed oils, and attention to food intolerances. Frequent vitamin B12 injections can be helpful. Diabetic polyneuritis may respond to high-dose vitamin B and supplements of evening primrose oil.

Epilepsy (fits)

These can occur as a result of serious medical conditions and should always be checked out by your doctor. Once the medical diagnosis has been made, sensible nutritional treatment may be of considerable benefit. Hypoglycemia, manganese, calcium, zinc, magnesium and other deficiencies and food intolerances can all contribute to epileptic seizures. **Evening primrose oil should only be given under medical supervision as certain susceptible individuals with epilepsy can have more frequent or more severe fits.**

Myalgic Encephalomyelitis

This condition, also known as Royal Free Disease after an epidemic which occurred at that hospital in the 1950s, is characterized by depression, tiredness and muscle weakness and fatigue. It is believed to be due to a virus and could constitute a part of the post-viral wipeout syndrome. Patients usually have an acute virus-like infection from which they do not seem to recover. The condition may go on for years. There is often associated thyroid gland suppression, nutrient deficiencies, especially of the B vitamins, zinc and magnesium, as well as food intolerances and chronic candidiasis. Approaching it in these ways can often result in considerable benefit. Most people who have it become frustrated and depressed because their doctor tends to dismiss them as neurotic.

MIGRAINE AND RELATED HEADACHES

Many people suffer from migraine. They complain of one-sided headache, often with nausea, vomiting and a dislike of light, and frequently preceded by a number of warning symptoms. These include fluid retention, mood swings, food craving or tiredness, which may be followed by visual disturbances such as flashing lights just prior to the onset of the headache. The headache may last anything from a few hours to two or three days and often forces the sufferer to lie down in a darkened room. It quite often improves or disappears entirely with rest or sleep.

Many drugs recommended for the treatment, as well as the prevention, of migraine are helpful but do not address the *cause* of the migraine.

Researchers have discovered that the blood platelets of migraine patients spontaneously clump and stick together more than normal between attacks. Drugs which apparently reduce platelet aggregation, such as aspirin, may be used as preventives, but we prefer to use specific non-drug items (see below).

Recent studies have reported a high incidence of food allergy as a major factor in childhood migraine. The researchers found that ninety-three percent of eighty-eight children with severe, frequent migraine recovered on a highly restricted diet. A number of causative foods were identified by their careful reintroduction, one at a time.

It may well be that mechanisms other than the usual allergy ones are involved in a percentage of people with migraine and that the triggering of platelet stickiness as a result of eating a particular food may lead to the precipitation of an attack. Once these platelets have stuck together they may release powerful chemicals which in turn produce a migraine headache. In practical terms, it is useful to try to identify and exclude those foods and environmental agents which appear to precipitate a migraine attack. The following advice excludes the major foods that have, from a number of studies, been associated with migraine.

AN EXCLUSION DIET FOR MIGRAINE

Cut out the following:

- Smoking.
- The Pill.
- Tea, coffee and other caffeine containing foods such as cola drinks, cocoa and chocolate.
- Alcohol, especially red wine.
- Sugar.

The above may be all that is necessary in a significant percentage of patients. If not, then the following should also be avoided:

- Foods containing tyramine, such as chocolate, yeast extracts and yeast products, liver, sausages, broad beans, pickled herrings and cheese.
- Foods containing histamine such as cheese, sauerkraut, salami and sausage meat.
- Foods containing other natural chemicals likely to precipitate migraine, such as oranges and bananas.
- Food additives—tartrazine, benzoate, butylated hydroxytoluene, monosodium glutamate.
- Wheat.
- Milk.

These are the major foods associated with migraine and this diet, preferably in whole, should be followed for four weeks or at least for long enough to be able to judge whether there is a clinical response in the frequency or severity of migraine attacks.

If you find you do not have migraines while on this program, then introduce individual foods at three to seven day intervals to see if you can determine which foods on the list trigger your attacks. If a migraine headache is triggered, it is pointless to try a further food in the next three or four days as platelet abnormalities may not be apparent during this period, and the precipitation of migraine, even if you are eating another causative food, will be most unlikely.

If you fail to improve on such a program, a more severe, modified exclusion diet which only allows some ten to fifteen foods can be tried. **This ought to be done under the supervision of a doctor** (see page 429).

Alternatively, or in addition, you can try taking supplements which are known to prevent platelet clumping. This approach has the added advantage that you don't have to restrict your diet so severely. Nutritional substances with known, powerful anti-platelet aggregatory effects include vitamin B6, vitamin C, vitamin E, essential fatty acids (such as linseed oil, evening primrose oil, or MaxEPA) and certain foods such as ginger. The above diet, together with a yeast-free multivitamin supplement (as recommended in the Appendix on page 422), may produce a substantial improvement. Women with contraceptive-induced or aggravated migraine could try vitamin B6. Estrogens increase vitamin B6 needs—and vitamin B6 doses of 50 mg per day have powerful platelet anti-clumping effects.

Other factors in the precipitation of migraine are environmental chemicals (e.g. cigarette smoke and perfumes), watching excessive television, stress, tiredness, vertebral misalignments (often correctable by osteopathic or chiropractic manipulation), and hypoglycemia. Missing a meal can often precipitate a migraine. It is important to eat regularly.

Migraine and milk intolerance in a fifteen-year-old boy

John was an intelligent, chirpy sort of chap who was evidently very concerned about the fact that he was losing up to three days a week at school from severe migraine. The family doctor thought that he was malingering, as did his teachers, so he was referred to the school psychiatrist who also thought that he was malingering. However, his parents knew him better than that, and realized that something was amiss. They insisted on referral to a neurologist, who did a number of different tests and diagnosed migraine. The drug treatment that he was given was relatively ineffective, but the amount of time he missed from school because of migraine was reduced to approximately two days a week. When they brought him to see me it was evident from his history that as an infant he had tended to avoid cows' milk, but that this gradually became less of an issue when he was about six years old and started to accept milk without objection. At this point he developed catarrh. He was put on a milk-free diet and although he wasn't actually cured, the length and the severity of the migraines were reduced slightly, so that he would only miss one to two days a week instead of two or more. I thought, therefore, that some other food had to be a problem and put him on a much stricter diet, excluding grains and colorings, etc. This was quite early on in my career as a nutritionally orientated doctor, so I sent him to another doctor who had had considerably more experience than I. He instantly realized that John was using margarine with whey in it, and instructed his mother to buy a margarine that was whey-free. From that point onwards John has been able to attend school without being plagued by migraine. This case illustrates that there are some people who are exquisitely sensitive to a given food item, and it is only when you exclude it totally from the diet that you can see an alleviation of symptoms.

Migrainous Neuralgia (Cluster Headache)

This type of headache is similar to migraine but has certain distinguishing features. The headaches usually occur in adults and more commonly in men. They "cluster," with one or two attacks per day for several days in a row for a few weeks. The sufferer is then symptom-free for a few months until a further "cluster" of headaches occurs. The pain is usually centered around one eye, which may water, and there may also be a watery nasal discharge and stuffiness on the same side.

Such headaches are often caused by the same things as migraine. It may be worthwhile excluding major potential sensitizing foods such as tea, coffee, sugar, alcohol and tobacco and it makes sense to keep a food diary. Alternatively, if a batch of headaches appear, write down all the foods you have eaten or drunk within the preceding twenty-four hours and then perhaps start a modified exclusion diet, based on these notes, together with a number of nutrients to reduce platelet stickiness.

Other types of headaches can be caused by:

- high blood pressure
- food allergy
- nervous tension
- tea and coffee excess or withdrawal
- excess alcohol
- missed meals

A case of migraine with coffee and tea

Fifty-year-old Mrs. R. had a thirty-year-old history of severe migraine resulting in vomiting, a pounding head, aversion to lights, and feeling ghastly for a twenty-four hour period after the disappearance of these symptoms. The migraines tended to occur in periods of stress, and were really quite incapacitating. She consumed a significant amount of tea and coffee, and simple exclusion of these and chocolate resulted in a total alleviation of her migraine. She can now experience stressful situations which would previously have precipitated migraine, but no longer do so.

- premenstrual syndrome
- sinus problems
- drug side-effects
- eye problems (need new glasses?)
- spinal problems
- other medical conditions requiring a full check-up

If your migraine or headache persists consult your doctor for a medical check-up.

CHILDREN'S PROBLEMS

This section deals with those problems of childhood that are quite common and which often have a substantial nutritional component.

Hyperactivity, Behavior and Learning Disorders

Behavior and learning problems are very common. While a disrupted or unhappy home can contribute to or cause these problems, there are often several nutritional changes that can bring about a remarkable improvement in a child's condition.

The term "hyperactive" is very often applied to a child who demonstrates a range of different problems. Other terms meaning the same thing are hyperkinesis, minimal brain dysfunction, or overactivity. The symptoms include head-banging, rocking, restlessness, overactivity, being always on the move, excitability and impulsiveness. Such a child disturbs other children, fails to finish things, has a short attention span, is very demanding and easily frustrated, cries often and easily, has temper tantrums, explosive and unpredictable behavior, is clumsy and compulsively touches people and things. Hyperactive children may refuse to go to sleep, or may wake up many times during the night; they tend to walk on tiptoes. Boys, especially those with blue eyes and blond hair, are affected much more often than are girls. Such a child may have a normal or high IQ yet do badly at school. He or she may also be dyslexic. Not all of these symptoms need be present in the same child for nutritional intervention to be effective.

Obviously, such a child is difficult to handle and can cause frustration and unhappiness in the family.

Infants who fall into this category are always crying, sleep very little, may not be pacified easily with cuddles, and often have bowel disturbances and bloated stomachs, frequent infections and bad diaper rashes.

It is this sort of baby that can drive his or her parents to frustration and despair. **Child abuse becomes a very real possibility and if you find yourself in this situation, discuss it with your doctor immediately.** Such infants and children may have other features which should lead you to suspect that food or nutritional status may have something to do with their behavior. These include recurrent headaches; dry, patchy skin; eczema or skin rashes; asthma; hay fever; epilepsy; bedwetting; aching legs; dry, cracked lips; dandruff or bad cradle cap; colic; difficulty feeding; fussy eating; excessive dribbling or sweating. The child may be very thirsty; suffer a constant stuffy or runny nose and frequent infections; crave sweets, chocolate or sugary foods; have abdominal bloating, constipation or diarrhea and episodes of inappropriate fatigue.

There is often a history in one or both parents of migraine, asthma, eczema, hives, hay fever, or food allergy, but not always. The mother may have quite bad premenstrual syndrome, quite bad nausea and vomiting in early pregnancy, or postnatal depression. Many mothers of such children say that the baby was very active in the womb.

Unsurprisingly, mothers of children with these symptoms tend to become very frazzled, tired, distraught and weepy, so when they go to their doctor, all too often the doctor puts the blame on the mother, thinking that she is neurotic and inadequate, which makes the problem even worse. Doctors seldom address the underlying causes of the problem.

WHAT ARE THE CAUSES OF HYPERACTIVITY, BEHAVIOR AND LEARNING DISORDERS?

It is becoming clear that food allergy is a major contributing factor. Also, nutrient deficiencies and excessive refined carbohydrates (sugary things), food colorings and preservatives contribute too. Colorings used in prescription drugs (pills, capsules and syrups) are also often a problem. Many such children drink a lot of milk, eat a lot of junk foods and drink sweet, colored drinks.

Food allergy

The means of finding out if food allergy is a problem is discussed on page 154, and there is an allergy diet for children on page 431 (Appendix 3). Cows' milk and cows' milk products, food preservatives and colorings, wheat, chocolate, eggs, citrus fruits and foods containing salicylates (see page 432) are among the most common offending foods in children.

We see many families in which much misery is caused by behaviorally disturbed children, and in whom a dramatic "cure" occurs with the elimination of offending foods. We consider that opponents of this approach have never actually witnessed the remarkable effects that we and many others have seen.

Food additives. It has been shown in animal studies that certain food colorings can spectacularly increase the spontaneous release of certain brain chemicals. Studies with children have shown that a small percentage react dramatically with behavior problems and impaired learning performance when challenged with food colorings.

Salicylates. A group of foods that seem to affect a significant proportion of these children are those containing this naturally occurring group of chemicals which are rather like aspirin. A list of such foods appears on page 432. Some hyperactive children should not eat these foods.

Chemical exposure

Considerable research suggests that exposure to certain types of chemicals, including organic solvents, can influence the behavior of a child. We have repeatedly seen children whose behavior has been changed quite dramatically when they are no longer exposed to the solvents contained in such things as aerosol sprays, colored felt-tip pens and cleaning fluids.

Nutrient deficiencies

Deficiencies of vital nutrients can give rise to childhood problems. These deficiencies are not uncommon, because of the increased requirements during rapid growth, and inadequate dietary supply.

Iron (page 58). Deficiencies of iron (with or without anemia) can cause abnormalities of electrical activity in the brain (EEG) and an impairment of learning. Quite severe iron deficiency can be present without any of the changes in red blood cells usually associated with iron-deficiency anemia, and can produce apathy, irritability, poor appetite, ice-craving and decreased exercise tolerance.

Zinc (page 62). This is more common than is generally realized, especially among hyperactive children. A lack of zinc influences behavior, it is common in growth retardation and is associated with white spots on the fingernails. Zinc deficiency can cause sleep disturbances too.

Vitamins B1 and B6 (pages 10 and 19). Children on a high junk-food diet have a very poor intake of these vitamins, leading to neurotic symptoms, sleep disturbances, restlessness, night terrors, personality changes, fatigue, night sweats, loss of appetite, depression and learning problems.

Magnesium (page 53). Magnesium deficiency is quite common, especially in children who drink a lot of milk, and can cause a whole range of disturbances such as poor appetite, nervousness, muscle cramps, insomnia, weakness, tiredness and behavior disturbances.

Essential fatty acids (page 107). Studies from the Hyperactive Childrens' Support Group suggest that many hyperactive children do well on supplements of evening primrose oil, boys more so than girls. (Evening primrose oil 500 mg, 1–3 capsules two or three times per day.) This has been our experience too.

Toxic metal overload. This can arise with such commonly occurring substances as lead, cadmium and aluminum. Hair mineral analysis is quite a good screening test for this.

Lead poisoning and zinc deficiency

Anstey was an eight-year-old boy who was a bit of a tearaway at school. He came from a broken home and tended to be rather disruptive socially. One day, at break-time, there was panic in the playground when Anstey tried to hang himself by his tie on the climbing frame. His father was called, and he was taken home. The following day we arranged a mineral screen. It was found that his lead levels were twice the upper acceptable level, and his zinc level was one third the lower limit of normal. It was also evident that he was eating a lot of refined carbohydrates and junk food, and drinking a lot of colas. Here you have a situation of multiple nutrient deficiencies on the one hand, a high level of a toxic metal and lots of artificial food additives on the other, in association with a presumably stressful domestic situation culminating in self-destructive behavior. I spoke at length to Anstey and his father, and Anstey was given a multivitamin and mineral supplement with extra zinc and vitamin C, to correct the deficiencies and promote the excretion of lead. He had acquired the lead, presumably, when he had been living in the Middle East with his father. Anstey became a much more manageable boy, seemed to enjoy life more, and subsequently did better at school.

Lead (page 90). It is now recognized that children who are heavily exposed to lead from car exhausts and pollution often suffer from learning and/or behavioral problems. Some hyperactive children, treated to remove lead from their bodies, improve. Children in inner city regions and heavily industrialized areas are particularly at risk. Children who are deficient in magnesium, iron, vitamin D, calcium or zinc are affected by lead more than those whose nutritional status is good. The same applies to cadmium. Severe poisoning with these toxic metals is a medical emergency requiring treatment in hospital.

Aluminum (page 94). Aluminum is now implicated as being neuro-toxic and there are several studies which show that behaviorally disturbed children have a higher than normal body burden of aluminum, as judged by blood and/or hair aluminum levels.

Skipped meals and hypoglycemia

It has long been recognized that children who skip their meals tend to be more cranky, disobedient and likely to have tantrums, and that this soon settles down when they are given something to eat. This is presumably due to hypoglycemia (low blood sugar) or food allergy. This should be borne in mind if your child tends to be hyperactive or has learning problems. Children who perform poorly at school or who have behavior problems are often found to have skipped breakfast. In coping with any behavior or learning disorder, remember that breakfast is very important. Junk food, sweets and food allergies can cause hypoglycemia too.

Over-tiredness

It seems obvious that a child who is over-tired is more likely to be badly behaved, but this is often overlooked in the management of childhood behavior and learning problems by parents and doctors alike.

Drug reactions

Many children react badly to medications, resulting in learning impairment and behavior and sleep disorders. These may be due to a direct action of the drugs themselves, or to the colorings in the tablets, capsules or syrups. If you notice your child reacting badly to any medication, discuss it with your doctor. If the doctor doesn't think that it is likely to be the drug, ask him to prescribe a form of the medication that contains *no* coloring for your child. If in doubt, ask the pharmacist if a coloring-free form of the drug exists.

A brain-injured child reacting to colorings in anti-convulsant drugs

Little Sara was quite severely handicapped and had been a very difficult child to manage. At five years she would throw food and drinks all over the kitchen and would scream and scream and scream; this was finally resolved by eliminating artificial colorings and additives from her diet, which resulted in a considerable improvement in her behavior and made her much more manageable. She would take medications on a regular basis to stop her epilepsy, and this seemed to be very effective. However, the manufacturers of the drugs decided that they wanted to make their brand line into a nice color of purple and, accordingly, put a purple coloring into the children's syrup preparation as well as the adult table preparation. Additionally, the labels and boxes for these medications had a similar color of purple on them. Sara became totally crazy on a continuous basis for three days, screaming, shrieking, not sleeping, "going up the wall." Her mother, having supervised the coloring-free diet previously, realized that it was the change in the packaging of the anti-convulsant drug that was most likely responsible for the sudden and dramatic change in her child's behavior. Until coloring-free preparations were available, Sara's mom had to wash the coloring off the tablets (she gave Sara tablets crushed up, because Sara would just spit out the syrup!). After the removal of the coloring Sara gradually settled back down to normal over a forty-eight-hour period. Her mother subsequently tested it again, just to make very sure, and found that, yes, Sara was reacting to the coloring.

Ante-natal effects

Interestingly, it has been found that ante-natal conditions can influence the behavior and learning abilities of infants and older children. Circumstances which appear to predispose to hyperactivity and other nervous system problems include ante-natal oxygen lack; maternal consumption of alcohol during pregnancy; toxemia in pregnancy, and maternal smoking. Some mothers with hyperactive children say that they were aware the baby was overactive even when it was in the womb. This can be a good pointer to the future behavior of the child.

Candida (page 346)

If giving nutritional supplements, and excluding offending foods, colorings and chemicals has not helped your child, then it may be that he or she has an overgrowth or allergy to the yeast, *candida albicans*. This is especially likely if he or she has had repeated courses of antibiotics in the past, or has had oral thrush or a candida rash treated successfully with a drug called nystatin, or if a sore, itchy vulva or anus is a problem. Treatment of the underlying candida problem can dramatically improve behavior and health problems in some children.

Incontinent bowel movements in a five-year-old

Young Jeremy had been unable to control his bowel movements, which had lead to difficulty and upset at kindergarten. This had been going on ever since the family had been on vacation in Greece, four weeks after his sister was born. He had an episode of diarrhea when he was away, and on returning to England the problem persisted. His parents took him to their family doctor who said that it was an attention-seeking mechanism due to jealousy of his sister. His parents considered this was not so and requested a referral to a pediatrician, who confirmed the family doctor's views and referred him to a child psychiatrist. Family therapy was undertaken, with some reluctance on the part of the parents. The problem did not resolve, so the parents asked to be referred. On looking more closely at what had actually happened when he was away, it was discovered that he had had a stomach bug the year before, which was treated with antibiotics, and which didn't really clear up. Ever since then he had had a red, sore anus and, it emerged, he had also had a history of oral thrush on several occasions but had never had any problem with his bowel function. Treatment with nystatin resulted in his regaining control of his bowel movements within three days, and the problem never recurred. The nutritional relevance of this point is that he was found to be zinc and iron deficient, and these two factors predisposed to the development of candida.

Physical illness

Underlying medical disorders may be a cause of the problems. **If there has been a sudden change in your child's personality, discuss it with your doctor.**

Television
Some children behave much better if the amount of TV they watch is kept to a minimum. It's worth a try.

Psychosocial
An unhappy or disrupted home environment, quarreling parents, unpleasant teachers or neighbors, or bullies at school can be factors, too, in upsetting your child and causing him to behave badly. Discuss this with your doctor or teachers at the school.

TREATMENT OF THE HYPERACTIVE BEHAVIOR OR LEARNING PROBLEM CHILD

No prolonged diets should be embarked upon without the advice of your doctor or a dietitian. Growing children have special nutritional needs which have to be met.

- Ensure that no underlying medical condition is present.
- Try the Modified Exclusion Diet for Children (page 431) *and* exclude salicylates (page 432).
- If there is no improvement after three weeks, then discontinue.

If your child has been on a poor diet or is underweight, do *not* put him or her on any elimination diet except one that is free of colorings and preservatives, salicylates, and refined carbohydrates, without first using a nutritional supplement and improving the diet.

Other Childhood Problems

BEDWETTING (ENURESIS)

Some children continue to wet the bed beyond the age of four or five, or it may start in a child who was previously dry at night. The matter is usually taken to the doctor if the child is between the ages of four and seven. There are many causes other than emotional problems, but if no obvious diagnosis can be made by your doctor and the problem continues, it is worthwhile thinking of a food or chemical intolerance or allergy. Try your child on the exclusion diet on page 431. If this doesn't work, take your child to an osteopath or chiropractor as vertebral misalignment can be a cause.

DELINQUENCY

Crime among teenagers is increasing, but there are now nutritional approaches to reducing such antisocial behavior. Very often, such teenagers are on a very poor junk-food diet, rich in refined carbohydrates and poor in vitamins and minerals. They may be addicted to milk drinks, cola drinks, excessive tea, coffee and alcohol, and may have vitamin and mineral deficiencies and addictive food allergies or hypoglycemia. Cutting out or down on these foods and drinks, improving the diet and giving nutritional supplements, can often work wonders—as has been shown in several clinical trials.

DYSLEXIA

Dyslexia is a condition in which a child (or an adult) has difficulty reading or writing, gets letters the wrong way round in words, confuses right and left, and yet may have a normal or high IQ. Such children often have allergies as well as many of the symptoms listed in the hyperactivity section (see page 360). Many of these children are zinc deficient too. Correction of nutrient deficiencies and food allergies, as well as special tuition, can often improve their dyslexia.

SLEEP DISTURBANCES

Food intolerance can cause sleep disturbances, as can a deficiency of zinc—which is quite common in young children (see page 69). Hyperactive children very often sleep badly, and while stress and upsets within the family or at school or with friends can disturb the sleep pattern, it is important to bear in mind that there are many other causes such as food intolerances, candida problems and nutrient deficiencies.

Insomnia in a child

Beth was three years old and her mother was driven to despair by the fact that she tended to wake up several times during the night. Beth's mother had tried several diets that she had read in women's magazines—all to no avail. She was then advised to give the child some zinc (1 mg of zinc per kilogram of body weight) and within two weeks Beth was sleeping through the night as peacefully as a lamb. Clinical studies have shown that a zinc and manganese supplement can help sleep disturbance in children, though it is not always successful.

ABDOMINAL PAIN IN CHILDHOOD

Abdominal pain can be a sign of food intolerance, worms and intestinal parasites, migraine, constipation, infective diarrhea, chronic candidiasis, emotional stress, or some other underlying condition requiring medical investigation.

LEG ACHES

Aching legs, especially on walking, can be a sign of food intolerance. Certain types of leg aches can be associated with deficiencies of calcium, magnesium, zinc and manganese. Colored, immigrant children sometimes have rickets due to a calcium and/or vitamin D deficiency, and these can cause leg aches.

FOOD ADDICTION

Food addiction can occur in children and should be thought of as a sign of food intolerance. Addiction to, or compulsion to eat only one, two or three foods should alert both parents and physician that they are dealing with a food-allergic child. Naturally, it is important to seek other signs of food intolerance before making such a diagnosis (see page 154).

POOR GROWTH

Poor growth can be caused by deficient diet. Zinc is the trace element most likely to be involved in growth retardation. However, there are other problems related to serious growth retardation and any child who isn't growing properly should be thoroughly investigated by a specialist.

MENTAL RETARDATION

Behavior problems very often accompany mental retardation, and these may be amenable to the nutritional supplementation and food allergy approaches. Just because it is known that the child has brain damage or Down's Syndrome (mongolism), there is no reason not to try supplements and the food allergy approach. In such cases a broad spectrum multivitamin and mineral can be helpful.

NUTRITION IN OLD AGE

The elderly, along with children, have a disproportionately heavy burden of health problems, which is reflected in the cost and percentage of health services apportioned to them. Not only are there specific nutritional problems in this age group, but nutritional factors may well be important in the process of aging. Accordingly, we may well be able to modify some of the features of aging by careful attention to our nutrition.

There has been considerable debate as to whether man has a built-in lifespan which cannot be exceeded, or whether aging is due to a number of outside factors. It may be that some families, because of their genetic background, are predisposed to longevity, just as others are predisposed to heart disease, thyroid disease or cancer.

The role of external factors has also been investigated and a number of interesting animal studies, dating back to the 1930s, have shown that restricting calorie intake when young produces an increased lifespan in a number of different animal species. It may well be that limiting our dietary intake of calories could be an important factor in promoting longevity. Of course, we would have to find a careful balance, particularly as nutritional deficiencies are so frequent in the elderly. An individual of seventy or more who is of normal weight would gain no benefit by trying to reduce his or her weight. Restricting calorie intake at this stage would simply increase the chances of developing nutritional deficiencies. If anyone is to benefit, it would be the obese forty or fifty year old, who, by losing weight at this stage, might influence his health and perhaps his lifespan in the coming years.

Nutritional States in the Elderly

A study performed by doctors in Yorkshire, England, showed the frequency with which nutritional deficiencies are found in ill, geriatric patients. The majority of the patients were aged seventy or more and *all* were found to have at least one, and usually several, nutritional deficiencies. The most common deficiencies in these acutely ill patients were of vitamin C, vitamin E, carotene (plant-derived vitamin A), vitamin B3, iron, folic acid, and vitamin A. Occasionally, evidence of a vitamin B2 or vitamin B1 deficiency was also found. Measurements of trace minerals such as zinc, copper, chromium and selenium were not performed, but it is likely that deficiencies of these would also have been found in many of the patients, particularly for zinc.

In otherwise healthy old people, nutritional deficiencies are obviously found less frequently. They are, however, still common. A survey in 1972 revealed that about three percent of the elderly population of the UK was malnourished. In particular, such people had poor intakes of protein, calories, iron and certain vitamins. A number of things contribute to a poor nutritional state in the elderly:

- *Ignorance*. The elderly widower who has never had to fend for himself in the kitchen may be incapable of preparing a balanced meal following the death of his wife.
- *Social isolation*. Dietary intake of nutrients is high in those individuals with a large number of outside interests. Eating in company is a considerable stimulus to the preparing of a meal as well as its actual consumption.
- *Physical disabilities*. Strokes, arthritis, and poor vision influence an individual's ability to obtain, prepare and consume food.
- *Mental disturbance*. Depression, confusion or senile dementia all influence such things as shopping, and the preparation and consumption of food.
- *Certain dietary recommendations*. Some of these may be inappropriate for the elderly (e.g. taking bran for constipation may impair the absorption of calcium and zinc, or low-fiber diets for peptic ulcers may be deficient in vitamin C).
- *Poverty.* This is an overwhelming factor in certain areas of Britain. The reliance upon cheaper, easy-to-prepare packaged foods instead of fresh produce, particularly when fruit and vegetables are out of season, results in a considerable impairment of nutritional intake.
- *Impairment of appetite*. A poor appetite occurs as part of the normal aging process, but can also be caused by many illnesses, smoking and certain nutritional deficiencies (e.g. zinc may produce a loss of appetite, resulting in a vicious circle).
- *Poor chewing*. Poor dental health influences an old person's ability to chew and thus to digest food. Those with bad teeth, dentures, or no dentures, tend to avoid foods such as meat which need a lot of chewing. Meat is a major dietary source of iron, zinc and vitamin B and while we hear a lot about the disadvantages of animal protein, moderate quantities of good, lean meat can be a very important part of the diet, particularly for the elderly. Ill-fitting dentures (often caused by gum shrinkage) also make chewing difficult.
- *Malabsorption*. Changes occur in the gastrointestinal tract with aging which can impair the absorption of nutrients.
- *Alcohol and drugs*. The more well-to-do elderly are particularly at risk from a high, or moderately high, alcohol intake

which may have particularly damaging effects upon the metabolism of the B vitamins, magnesium and zinc. The effect of drugs upon nutrients is discussed on page 142.

- *Diseases*. Certain conditions, common in the elderly, such as diabetes, thyroid disease, kidney failure, and gastrointestinal diseases, significantly alter nutritional requirements.
- *Increased requirements*. It may well be that as a part of the aging process there are increased requirements for certain nutrients in order to maintain the level found in healthy, younger adults. In particular, requirements for vitamin C have been thought by some researchers to be increased in the elderly.

All of the things in this list can influence the nutritional state of the elderly.

It is important to be able to identify old people who are at particular risk. It may be helpful for doctors, health visitors, social workers, wardens, concerned relatives and those who supervise the elderly in a professional or voluntary capacity to have a list of risk factors in mind. The main risk factors are:

- those who are over 70
- men
- those who are losing weight
- those who consume little or no fresh produce, including fresh fruit, fresh vegetables, and fresh meat or fish
- those on long-term drugs or who consume alcohol regularly
- those who find it difficult or impossible to go shopping or to cook for physical or social reasons

Medical Problems of the Elderly, Related to Nutrition

There are certain medical and nutritional problems that are more likely to occur in the elderly.

ACUTE ILLNESS

Almost any acute illness in the elderly is accompanied by a loss of appetite before, during and after the illness. Recovery times in the elderly are longer too.

Because nutritional deficiencies appear in *all* acutely ill geriatric patients (see above), we feel they should be given significant multivitamin/multi-mineral supplements as a routine. We cannot emphasize this enough.

OSTEOMALACIA (vitamin D deficiency)

This condition is primarily due to a deficiency of vitamin D. Lack of sunlight, poor diet and a deficiency of calcium are also influences. It is considered in detail on page 37.

OSTEOPOROSIS

This is different from osteomalacia and is due to a thinning rather than a softening of the bones. The main problem is a loss of calcium rather than a lack of vitamin D. Minor degrees of osteoporosis are not infrequent in the elderly who complain of a loss of weight, increased curvature of the spine, and a predisposition to fractures such as those of the hip.

PERNICIOUS ANEMIA

A deficiency of vitamin B12 is not infrequent in the elderly and causes anemia as well as neurological changes including poor memory and dementia. This is usually the result of a poor absorption of vitamin B12 (see page 22).

ANEMIA

Significant anemia has been reported as occurring in as many as seven percent of the elderly population and it is often the result of deficiencies of iron, folic acid or vitamin B12.

HEART FAILURE (see index for references)

DIABETES

Elderly people with diabetes tend not to require insulin and can manage with a special diet. However, many such elderly people are unwilling, or unable, to follow a diet rigidly and may have to take oral antidiabetic drugs. Chromium deficiency is common in such people and supplements can be particularly beneficial (see page 78), especially when combined with a diabetic diet.

PRESSURE SORES AND LEG ULCERS

Leg ulcers or pressure sores that don't heal are fairly common in the elderly. Supplements of zinc and vitamin C are of proven value and are more likely to be successful if the person has a poor diet. Vitamin C, 1–3 g, and 23–50 mg of elemental zinc per day are valuable.

THYROID DISEASE

An overactive thyroid gland shows up as weight loss, mental confusion, palpitation or heart failure. An underactive thyroid gland can show up as voice changes, dry skin, mental confusion, and weight gain. The onset of either is usually slow and is easily missed, even by a doctor, unless specifically tested for. Those with an overactive thyroid often have increased demands for certain nutrients, particularly for the B vitamins and trace minerals. A multivitamin/multi-mineral supplement is recommended.

SEVERE DROP IN BODY TEMPERATURE (hypothermia)

This is a major risk for the elderly, particularly those who are poor, living on their own and without central heating, those who are immobile and those who have impaired social and survival skills. It is a good policy for such old people to take a nutritional supplement.

DRUG MEDICATION (see page 142)

A high proportion of old people receive long-term drug medication for such conditions as high blood pressure, diabetes, minor psychiatric complaints, insomnia and arthritis. The risks of drug therapy rise with increasing numbers of drugs, and with age. It has been estimated that up to ten percent of geriatric admissions to the hospital are the result of the drug they are receiving.

The elderly are particularly at risk from drug side-effects because of their impaired nutritional state. Mild deficiencies of vitamin C can have adverse effects upon the function of certain liver enzymes that are involved in drug metabolism. Vitamin B6, vitamin E and selenium all seem to be of some relevance, too. So an elderly person who has a deficiency of these and other nutrients may be unable to metabolize drugs normally, and an ordinary dose of the drug means that it accumulates with the production of toxic side-effects.

CANCER

Cancer in the elderly is often very slow-growing and may not even be the essential cause of death. Many old people die for other reasons and happen to have a cancer as well. The slower metabolic rate of the elderly is perhaps an advantage in this situation.

GASTROINTESTINAL CONDITIONS (see page 194)

There is a considerable number of gastrointestinal conditions that are particularly likely to occur in the elderly. These include gastric ulcer, the aftermath of gastric surgery, pancreatic insufficiency, celiac disease and a poor blood supply to the intestines. All of these can produce an impairment of nutrients absorption. Such people require the advice of an experienced dietician.

SENILE DEMENTIA (see page 390)

Dementia is a term applied to any deterioration in mental function. We all expect at least some mental deterioration as a normal part of aging. This deterioration, if it occurs before the age of sixty, is called pre-senile dementia.

In senile dementia, subtle changes in behavior occur. These include an increased forgetfulness for minor things (particularly recent occurrences rather than ones from the distant past). "Losing" household items, forgetting things on a shopping list and forgetting appointments can all be early signs. Sometimes depression is a feature of the disease and it can be difficult to decide whether minor changes in mental function are caused by depression or by a definite deterioration in brain function. The old person often becomes socially withdrawn, argumentative, irritable and finally apathetic. Sometimes, however, they may be effusive, apparently cheerful and laughing, but be unable to perform the simplest of mental tasks. These mental changes are almost always noticed more by relatives than by the individuals themselves, who rarely appreciate their change in mental state. Causes include thyroid disease, vitamin B12 deficiency, high blood pressure and Alzheimer's disease.

In someone with pre-senile dementia (Alzheimer's disease), these mental changes occur at a younger age—before sixty-five—and the treatment is often difficult. A number of causes have been suggested, particularly a slow virus infection, genetic factors, and aluminum toxicity. High levels of aluminum have been found in some of those people with the condition and aluminum, which is neuro-toxic, produces changes in brain structure similar to those seen in Alzheimer's disease itself. Sometimes Alzheimer's disease runs in families.

The assessment of aluminum status in those with Alzheimer's disease is advisable. If aluminum is elevated, the old person should throw away her aluminum cookware and replace it with glass or stainless steel. Supplements of vitamin C, calcium and magnesium inhibit aluminum absorption from food and may help reduce aluminum accumulation in the body.

The following recommendations for a nutritional program are made, not because of their proven value, but because of the theoretical support for such a program. It would be appropriate for someone who had pre-senile dementia, or senile dementia at a relatively early age, for which no cause can be found.

Dementia and nutritional deficiencies

Hilda was a rather dotty, but very sweet, eighty-two-year-old lady who was beginning to have increasing difficulty looking after her eighty-four-year-old husband who had recently suffered a disabling stroke. Hilda thought that little was wrong with her, but speaking to her daughter gave a very different picture. She had become increasingly confused and forgetful. Caring for the home and cooking meals for her disabled husband, which were previously routine tasks, were now only performed with difficulty, and her daughter was rightly becoming very worried. General physical examination found her to be in good health for her years, though her memory was rather poor. Routine blood investigations showed no sign of anemia, kidney, liver or thyroid disease, but she did have a low level of an enzyme called alkaline phosphatase. Low levels of this enzyme can be caused by zinc deficiency, and a blood zinc level showed her value to be two thirds of normal! This was almost certainly due to her increasingly poor diet and lack of meat, which is a major source of zinc. She had supplements of zinc—Solvazinc, one a day—together with multivitamins, as it seemed likely she would have other unidentified nutritional deficiencies. This was followed by a marked improvement in her mental function and her ability to cope at home. With the support of her daughter she was able, once again, to look after her husband, and noticed, herself, how much less confused and more mentally alert she was. Deficiencies of zinc, vitamin B, vitamin C, iron and magnesium can all affect mental function at any age, and are particularly likely to occur in the elderly. An elderly patient who has decreasing memory and mental function should have a full physical examination and assessment of his or her nutritional state. Trial of a multivitamin/multi-mineral supplement is undoubtedly worthwhile in most cases.

Recommendations

- Eat a basic healthy diet (see page 398).
- Take supplements including:
  (a) a multivitamin supplement providing vitamin C, 1000 mg per day and vitamins B1, B2, B6, together with B12 and folic acid at doses of approximately 20–50 mg per day
  (b) a zinc salt providing 30 mg of elemental zinc per day
  (c) essential fatty acid supplements—evening primrose oil and fish oils should also be considered.
- Get your doctor to give you an injection of 1 mg of vitamin B12, intramuscularly, once a week.
- Get more physical exercise.
- Use your mental functions and activities.

These recommendations will vary from case to case. Certainly, any deficiency of the above nutrients which is found on testing should be treated.

NUTRITIONAL PSYCHIATRY

Nutritional psychiatry can be defined as those areas of mental disturbance that are amenable to nutritional treatment. Since brain function depends on the correct balance of nutrients reaching it, it is hardly surprising that diet and dietary supplements can markedly affect a wide range of mental conditions.

While there is still a lot to be learned in nutritional psychiatry and especially about how chemical transmitters work in the brain, there already is a wealth of information which has not yet found its way into day-to-day psychiatric practice, often to the detriment of people who find themselves placed in the general "psychiatric" category. This section tries to outline the major areas of therapeutic intervention that can bring about an improvement in an individual's ability to adapt to his environment, like a resulting reduction in or disappearance of his psychiatric symptoms.

Factors That Can Cause Psychiatric Illness

The physical causes of mental disturbances can often easily be overlooked by doctors and psychiatrists. These include thyroid gland problems and other hormonal imbalances, diabetes, epilepsy, high blood pressure, hardening of the arteries, drug toxicity (medical and illegal), alcoholism, liver and kidney disease, metabolic disorders, lead poisoning, chronic painful conditions, hidden infections, and a wide variety of nutritional deficiencies.

Anyone with a serious psychiatric condition should have a thorough physical and neurological examination by a sympathetic and well-informed physician, including extensive laboratory investigations. These should include, as a minimum:

- Hematology screen—to check for anemia, infection etc.
- Biochemistry screen—to test for liver and kidney disease and the common metabolic imbalances.
- Thyroid function tests.
- Urine test for diabetes, infection and kidney disease.
- Laboratory assessment of nutritional state—including zinc, iron, vitamins B1, B6, B12, folic acid and other specific nutrients as indicated by the patient's condition. These are discussed in this chapter.

Other factors relevant to the development of mental problems include genetic influences, antenatal development, parents and family, development and education, infections and parasites, toxic overload, cancers, trauma, inadequate light, exercise, oxygen and rest.

This section, however, deals primarily with nutritional factors. Nutrient imbalances and deficiencies, allergies and food intolerance can cause psychiatric symptoms which can be manipulated without necessarily having to resort to drug therapy.

Central Nervous System Neurotransmitters and Mental Function

It is currently thought that all mental and other activity in the brain occurs as a result of very specific chemical messengers (neurotransmitters) acting at particular sites. These neurotransmitters are vital to brain function. In recent years it has become apparent that all kinds of things can alter these chemicals and this has opened a new door to the whole subject of psychiatric illness and treatments.

Both the public and the medical profession have been brought up to think that the absorptive capacity of the intestines and the regulatory control mechanisms of the body protect the brain from varying levels of substances in the blood except in extreme illness, for example in diabetic coma or severe liver disease. However, one of the most exciting things to emerge from research over the last decade or so is that the amino acid content of foods can potently influence brain neurotransmitter activity.

Most drugs that modify behavior do so by changing the amounts of activity of particular neurotransmitters present within the brain. If a single food constituent is shown to cause similar changes in the release or reactions of one of these neurotransmitters, there is every reason to expect that the nutrient will also be able to influence behavior or to modify other processes controlled by the brain. This has now been shown to be the case and the subject is being intensively researched.

There are known to be numerous neurotransmitters at work within the brain. Let's just look at a single key one—serotonin—because it exemplifies many of the interesting things about neurotransmitters.

Serotonin is produced from the essential amino acid tryptophan. Treatments that raise or lower brain tryptophan levels can rapidly alter the rate at which it produces serotonin. A high-carbohydrate, protein-poor meal raises brain tryptophan, thus accelerating serotonin production. The way this is brought about is that a carbohydrate-rich meal triggers the pancreas to secrete insulin, which results in a lowering of the plasma levels of certain amino acids but has little effect on plasma tryptophan. This means that plasma tryptophan does not have to compete with these amino acids for uptake by the brain and more is available for use.

Conversely, a protein-rich meal depresses the uptake of tryptophan by the brain. The nerve cells in the brain which react to serotonin inform the rest of the brain about the proportion of proteins and carbohydrate in the most recent meal.

The idea that food balance and composition could have had such a profound effect on brain function would have seemed like a fairy tale fifty years ago. It has now been shown that it is possible to increase the release of serotonin from brain cells by eating pure tryptophan, especially when taken with a carbohydrate-rich meal.

People suffering from certain types of depression have been shown to have low levels of serotonin. By taking tryptophan, serotonin levels are increased and their depressive symptoms diminished.

Having looked, albeit briefly, at just one amino acid and its effect on the brain, let's now look in more detail at various other dietary components.

Vitamins and Psychiatric Disorders

VITAMIN B1 (thiamin) (see also page 10)

Vitamin B1 deficiency is a well-recognized factor in the development of the profound brain changes and mental illnesses associated with alcoholism. But this is the very severe end of the spectrum. Well before such gross deficiencies occur, a lack of vitamin B1 can cause clinical problems.

One study from Cleveland, Ohio, followed up twenty patients who had symptoms that were apparently neurotic but who had blood changes indicating vitamin B1 insufficiency. In many of the cases the cause of the thiamin deficiency appeared to be a heavy consumption of junk foods, which included refined carbohydrates, carbonated or sweet drinks and sweets, though this was not so in all of them.

The interesting thing about this study is that the subjects had a wide range of symptoms, as follows (in order of frequency): abdominal and/or chest pains; sleep disturbance, restlessness, talking, walking, night terrors; personality change; insomnia; recurrent fever of unknown cause; intermittent diarrhea, often alternating with constipation; chronic fatigue; night sweats; loss of appetite; headache; nausea and/or vomiting; depression; nasal congestion and/or cough; difficulty with talking; dizziness; recurrent frightening dreams; recurrent blurred vision; recurrent sore throat.

Evidence such as this must make doctors seriously suspect thiamin deficiency in people suffering from these conditions. The Ohio study found that 150–300 mg of thiamin per day was needed to improve the symptoms. It is certainly worth trying this dose for a few weeks to see if it improves matters.

It is our opinion that if you are going to take this dosage, part of it should be in the form of a supplement of B-complex vitamins and not vitamin B1 alone.

VITAMIN B2 (riboflavin) (see also page 14)

There is very little evidence to suggest that riboflavin deficiency has any great effect on mental function, though drugs such as Largactil and Depixol, which are used for mental problems, may induce vitamin B2 deficiency (see page 147).

VITAMIN B3 (niacin or nicotinic acid) (see also page 15)

Nicotinic acid, tryptophan and essential fatty acid metabolism

Mental irritability and vitamin B deficiency

Mrs. V., a sixty-five-year-old lady, asked her general practitioner if she could see somebody about diet. A few years previously she had an overactive thyroid which had resulted in her becoming very nervous and anxious. This had been treated, but her symptoms had recently returned. She was irritable and jumpy if the phone rang or a door slammed. She had episodes of palpitations, and her own general practitioner had repeated her thyroid function tests, which were normal. At the time of consultation she was most angry and irritable indeed, not the least because she had been kept waiting an extra forty-five minutes! Her husband told me that this was typical of her behavior and was most unlike how she had been in the past. Her very anxious state and history of irritability and palpitations would make most doctors think of an overactive thyroid, but this had already been ruled out. Her diet was well balanced and she did not drink excessively. However, she drank six cups of tea and three to four cups of coffee per day, and undoubtedly the high caffeine intake was aggravating her anxiety symptoms. I asked her to stop these completely, and also asked her to take a dosage of vitamin B1, thiamin, 100 mg twice a day, together with some multivitamins. She took her first dose that afternoon and, when I saw her two weeks later, her husband commented that, by the same evening, there had been a remarkable improvement in her mental state. She had ceased to be so irritable and jumpy and, indeed, apologized for her behavior and mental state at her next consultation! Such a dramatic response would almost certainly point to a marked vitamin B deficiency. This can, at times, be corrected within hours of administering high dose vitamin B. Cases are, however, recorded in the literature, of improvement taking several weeks. The cause for her vitamin B1 deficiency was never fully ascertained, but it appears that some otherwise normal individuals may have increased requirements for certain vitamins and minerals, and this may come to light with increasing age.

are interlinked in the development of psychiatric disease, especially in some forms of schizophrenia.

The first double-blind experiment in psychiatry, in 1952, compared the effects of a placebo, nicotinamide and nicotinic acid (both forms of vitamin B3) in thirty acute schizophrenics.

The results showed that those given vitamin B3 together with standard schizophrenia treatments (mainly electroconvulsive therapy) fared better than those simply given a placebo.

On several occasions we have found surprisingly beneficial results of using the vitamin in doses of 0.5–2 g per day.

VITAMIN B6 (pyridoxine) (see also page 19)

Vitamin B6 deficiency is much more common than previously thought and can produce anxiety, depression and personality change. Some fifteen percent of "normal" women of childbearing age are deficient in this vitamin.

Depression is a very common part of the premenstrual syndrome (see page 301), and as a result of taking the combined oral contraceptive (see page 309). This can often be alleviated by taking vitamin B6 supplements.

VITAMIN B12 AND FOLIC ACID (see also pages 22 and 25)

A severe deficiency of vitamin B12 can cause pernicious anemia, but it can first show up as severe psychological disturbance without there being any of the obvious blood or nerve problems that are usually part of the diagnosis of pernicious anemia. A vitamin B12 deficiency does not *have* to manifest itself as a dramatic mental illness, it may just cause depression.

One very extensive study of mentally ill patients screened them for serum folate and serum B12 status. The results illustrated two points. First, that vitamin B12 and folate insufficiencies may very frequently be present in a psychiatric population (and some of their psychological symptoms may be improved by supplementation with these nutrients) and second, the importance of screening such people routinely, rather than relying on finding abnormal blood cell types characteristic of true pernicious anemia or folate deficiency anemia.

VITAMIN C (ascorbic acid) (see also page 28)

Vitamin C deficiency is associated with depression, lethargy, hysteria and hypochondriasis. Supplementation should be considered in people with these symptoms.

Researchers from Dundee, Scotland, have studied the effects of vitamin C supplementation in manic-depressive psychosis. Both manic and depressed patients were significantly better following a single 3 g dose of vitamin C daily.

ESSENTIAL FATTY ACIDS AND MANIC DEPRESSION *(see also page 107)*

People with manic depression may benefit from an EFA supplement such as evening primrose oil during the depressive phase, but it may worsen matters during the manic phase. **Thus, supplements of evening primrose oil should only be given to manic-depressives under close medical supervision.**

Minerals and Psychiatric Disorders

The role that trace elements play in psychiatric illness has been researched in some depth.

Brain metabolism involves a highly complex interplay of different factors, all of which are modulated by enzyme systems both within and outside the brain. The basic working materials for these systems are derived primarily from the diet. Vitamin and mineral metabolism plays an important role in the production of appropriate neurotransmitters and the transport of active factors from the blood to the brain. Though there is considerable knowledge on the area, there is far more yet to be unraveled. Maintaining an awareness of trace and toxic elements in the management of psychiatric conditions can lead to effective, nontoxic therapeutic intervention in some instances.

ZINC *(see also page 68)*

Zinc is involved in over 100 different enzyme systems. Specific zinc deficiency signs can include sullenness, schizoid behavior, depression, irritability, mood swings, and tearfulness. In certain cases, especially with high copper (see below), there can be severe mental disturbance.

In view of the fact that zinc requirements are increased quite dramatically (approximately doubled) during pregnancy and lactation, it would be interesting to look at the zinc status and the response to therapeutic zinc supplements of women with postnatal depression. Though hormonal changes are implicated, hormone function is in part dependent upon appropriate zinc/copper ratios. A severe imbalance of these may well make a woman more susceptible to a failure to adapt to the dramatic hormonal changes that occur at and around birth.

Women on the Pill have elevated copper levels, which could be associated with an actual or relative zinc deficiency which in turn influences brain metabolism. Therefore, any woman who has psychiatric symptoms and is on the Pill, should be taken off it and her zinc and copper status evaluated and dealt with accordingly, along with possible increased requirements of vitamin B6.

It has been suggested that zinc deficiency may be a cause of senile dementia.

POTASSIUM (see also page 50)

Potassium depletion is common and is often produced as a result of increased urine production either from the use of diuretics (water tablets), alcohol, excessive tea and coffee drinking or diabetes mellitus or diabetes insipidus. Mental symptoms of potassium deficiency include depression, mental apathy, fatigue and lethargy.

MAGNESIUM (see also page 53)

Magnesium deficiency can cause a whole range of psychiatric disturbances, yet is often forgotten as a contributory factor in psychiatric patients. Mental symptoms include: loss of appetite, apathy, weakness, tiredness, anxiety, insomnia, hyperactivity, depression. Low levels of magnesium are often found in women with premenstrual syndrome.

CALCIUM (see also page 44)

The importance of calcium in mental illness has generally been underestimated, and everyone with psychiatric problems should have their calcium status investigated—too much or too little calcium can cause mental disturbances.

MANGANESE (see also page 81)

Low manganese has been found in people with brain seizures, and another report, albeit anecdotal, suggested that schizophrenics tended to be low in zinc and manganese and that their condition improved when the levels of these two minerals were normalized.

IRON (see also page 58)

The role of iron deficiency in mental symptoms is very common and often overlooked, primarily because we have come to think of iron solely in terms of what it does in the blood. However, one can have an iron deficiency without blood changes. Mental symptoms that have been linked to iron deficiency include poor learning in children, weakness, tiredness and lassitude, depression and anxiety.

CHROMIUM (see also page 78)

Chromium deficiency can lead to impaired glucose tolerance and a resultant increased tendency to hypoglycemia (see page 292) and diabetes mellitus (see page 286) with an increased possibility of the mental changes that are associated with these conditions (fatigue, depression, anxiety, etc.).

COPPER (see also page 72)

High copper levels have been associated with dementia, irritability, emotional lability and schizophrenia. The effects of copper excess are worse in the presence of a zinc deficiency.

VANADIUM (see also page 75)

Research has suggested that an excess of vanadium may play a part in the cause of manic-depressive illness, and that a low-vanadium diet plus a high dose of vitamin C can help such patients.

Toxic Metals and Psychiatric Disorders

ALUMINUM (see also page 94)

Aluminum has been implicated in the development of Alzheimer's (pre-senile) dementia and the mental deterioration seen in kidney patients on dialysis. It has also been implicated in childhood hyperactivity, learning disorders and behavioral problems.

LEAD (see also page 90)

Lead is a potent neuro-toxin and is ubiquitous in our environment. There are provable and well-documented psychological effects on children following long-term, low-level lead exposure from exhaust fumes, tap water and so on, as well as the "classical," if rare, lead encephalopathy (poisoning of the brain with lead).

MERCURY (see also page 95)

Mercury has very definitely been associated with impairment of mental function. Dentists and dental nurses are two professional groups who are occupationally exposed to mercury and can have neuropsychological impairment.

There is now a growing medical literature on the long-term toxicity of mercury from dental fillings (amalgam) and a whole range of symptoms have been cured by removing old amalgams, especially if they were present in the mouth with other metals such as gold. A few of the conditions that are now thought to be caused by long-term ingestion of mercury from fillings include: sleep disturbances, headaches, migraines, fatigue, irritability, depression, mood swings, and mania as well as physical symptoms such as heart problems, arthritis, burning sensations in the mouth, mouth ulcers, kidney disorders and even skin problems and asthma.

Depression

The causes of depression are legion. Its degree can vary from feeling a bit low to severe debilitating depression with suicidal tendencies. **If depression is very severe, do not delay in seeking medical help.** Depression may be caused by an underactive thyroid gland or some other physical condition, but much more commonly it is precipitated by stress, such as marital problems, unemployment or bereavement.

However, there are a number of nutritional approaches that can help the situation, in addition to the basic steps outlined on pages 391–394.

As mentioned previously, the amino acid tryptophan can be taken, 500 mg three times a day, with some carbohydrate, between meals, and this can be tried for two or three weeks. If the depression is associated with insomnia, taking 1500 mg of tryptophan once a day, half an hour or so before bedtime, can be a help for some. However, see tryptophan warning on page 106 before use. If this is unsuccessful, other amino acids in similar doses can be tried; these include 1-phenylalanine or tyrosine.

Deficiencies of B vitamins, zinc, vitamin C, iron, magnesium or potassium can all give rise to depression, as can food intolerances, hypoglycemia or chronic candidiasis. Depression in women occurring in the seven to fourteen days prior to a period can be responsive to B6 100–150 mg per day and magnesium 200–400 mg per day. Depression associated with the Pill may be responsive to 50–150 mg of vitamin B6 daily.

We have found wheat to be one of the most common causes of food intolerances associated with depression in adults. Depression after childbirth may also be amenable to nutritional intervention. Vitamin C deficiency can show up as depression, hysteria and hypochondriasis. Depression is often also associated with fatigue, lassitude and anxiety and as the depression lifts, so too do these associated symptoms.

Anxiety, Insomnia and Panic Attacks

These symptoms, together or singly, often respond to the basic recommendations listed on page 398. Excessive tea and coffee drinking, hypoglycemia, food intolerance and hyperventilation can also cause or contribute to these situations and are discussed in the relevant sections of this book. Drugs such as Diazepam, Mogadon and Lorazepam have been used in treating these conditions and, in our experience, withdrawal from them can be associated with a temporary but quite severe increase in symptoms, which eventually pass. Taking calcium, 1000–1500 mg, with magnesium, 200–500 mg, per day can also have a tranquilizing effect, and we recommend that you should try taking these supplements and avoid Ativan if possible.

Insomnia, especially if associated with depression, can be helped by taking tryptophan, 1000–1500 mg before bed. However, see tryptophan warning on page 106 before use. Taking B vitamins late in the day may cause insomnia. Insomnia or night waking associated with hypoglycemia can be helped by taking nicotinamide at bedtime (but see page 296 for warning).

Schizophrenia

This can be a debilitating condition and a terrible burden for the sufferer to bear. Psychiatric drugs may be particularly helpful and sudden withdrawal from such drugs can be associated with a relapse. **For this reason nutritional intervention should take place under medical supervision. Withdrawal from drug treatment should only be undertaken once the person has corrected any nutritional problems and should be done slowly and cautiously (again only under medical supervision).**

Nutrient deficiencies, especially of the B vitamins, zinc, magnesium, chromium, manganese and vitamin C, and food intolerance are common in many schizophrenics. Essential fatty acid supplements can also be very helpful (e.g. evening primrose oil, 500 mg, three capsules two or three times a day, or concentrated fish oil (MaxEPA) 300 mg, two or three capsules twice a day).

Family support is an almost essential component for the recovery of a person suffering from schizophrenia.

A case of schizophrenia

Alf flipped at college when he was nineteen years old. He heard voices telling him to destroy every lamppost in his town, and this became his passion in life. He was admitted to the hospital where he stayed for seven months under heavy drug therapy. He was finally discharged home on heavy anti-psychotic medication—injections every two weeks, drugs to prevent or minimize the side-effects of the injections, tranquilizers to keep him calm, and sleeping pills to help him sleep. He had tried cutting down the dose and frequency of his injections, but his old symptoms would return and his parents always managed to persuade him to have the usual dose. He remained depressed and withdrawn on his drugs, but that was considered better than his outrageous psychotic behavior before.

Nutritional assessment at this stage showed profoundly low zinc levels and chromium levels, inadequate vitamin C and vitamins B1 and B6, disturbances in calcium/magnesium balance, thyroid gland function at the lower end of the normal range, and indications of food allergy and hypoglycemia.

His drug dosage was not reduced initially. He was put on a tailor-made nutritional supplement program, using a broad spectrum multivitamin and mineral as a basis, with extra zinc, calcium and magnesium, chromium, vitamin C and B vitamins as well as some amino acid supplements. Offending foods were excluded from the diet. A small dose of thyroid hormone was added later.

He also agreed to take regular outdoor exercise in the form of a daily walk.

Over a two-year period his drugs were gradually reduced and eliminated completely and he stayed on an even keel for two years.

It is important that the anti-psychotic medication that schizophrenics are almost always put on is not discontinued suddenly, as a relapse in psychotic behavior almost always occurs.

Correction of the underlying nutrient imbalances, food allergies and hormone shortages, along with family support to help restore self-esteem can, but not always, result in being able to gradually withdraw, in a controlled way, the anti-psychotic medication without relapse of the schizophrenia.

Manic Depression

This is a condition characterized by phases of extreme physical and mental activity followed by quite deep depression. It is most commonly treated by psychiatrists using lithium carbonate. Nutritional intervention can sometimes be of help, but caution

Manic depression and wheat allergy?

Marion, a thirty-two-year-old art teacher, had been experiencing severe mood swings for the preceding ten years. This had been diagnosed by her psychiatrist as severe manic depression, and she had been treated with the drug Lithium. While this controlled the severe swings in mood, she still felt very depressed and lethargic. Investigations of her nutritional state had shown only a mild zinc and magnesium deficiency. Treatment with supplements of these had made little difference to her mental state. She was, therefore, asked to try an exclusion diet. She started on a diet composed entirely of fruit, vegetables, rice, meat and fish. All dairy products, grains, refined carbohydrates, tea and coffee, as well as food additives, were avoided. Response was not dramatic but, after a month, she felt distinctly less depressed and had few swings in mood. After two months she had increased her work from two days a week to four, and her friends and colleagues had noticed a remarkable improvement in her moods and in her previously glum appearance. Some well-meaning friends told her that food allergy could not affect mood. Indeed, there are no reports, to the authors' knowledge, of food allergy or intolerance being associated with manic depression. However, she became severely depressed three days after eating bread. She had to stop work for six weeks and nearly lost her job. Despite going back on to the exclusion diet, it took six or eight weeks for her to return to anything like her previously good mental state. Both she and her consultant psychiatrist agreed that she should stay on the diet and not try out any more foods. This case illustrates how, sometimes, food allergy or intolerance can present purely mental symptoms. In the authors' experience depression, anxiety, agoraphobia, premenstrual syndrome and, occasionally, manic depression, can be influenced by dietary factors.

should be exercised in supplementation with essential fatty acids as these may sometimes worsen the mania. Some success has been found in treating the condition with high-dose vitamin C (1–2 g per day) and a low-vanadium diet.

Dementia

This condition, which most commonly affects old people, is characterized by memory impairment, a lack of orientation, failure to look after oneself and so on. While it can be caused by a hardening and a furring up of the arteries in the brain, there may be associated deficiencies of the B vitamins, zinc, magnesium and vitamin C. By prescribing 100–150 mg daily of the B vitamins, 50 mg per day of zinc and 1–3 g per day of vitamin C, as well as improving the diet, we have seen a number of elderly demented people improve. Sometimes vitamin B12 injections (1000 mcg intramuscularly once or twice weekly) can be helpful where appropriate, even in the absence of any obvious vitamin B12 deficiency.

Similarly, oral supplementation with 1–2 g daily of nicotinamide is sometimes helpful. It is vital to bear in mind the possibility that side-effects from the drugs the patient is taking may be contributing to the dementia.

Anorexia Nervosa

Anorexia nervosa is a psychological and physiological disorder which is mainly seen in adolescent girls. The mortality rate can reach as much as twenty percent. The main causes of death include starvation, infections, disorders of heart rhythm and even suicide. **For all these reasons it is a very serious condition and must be treated seriously.**

While no one really knows what causes anorexia nervosa it is generally considered that social stresses cause girls to avoid food and independently produce changes in the personality, rather than that a particular type of personality produces anorexia.

A typical case is that of a depressed, weepy, hostile and often agitated teenage girl who tends to wear heavy clothing to hide her thin frame and to keep warm. She complains of severe constipation and a loss of periods and breasts.

Psychological features include depression, anxiety, occasional obsessive thoughts, lowered self-esteem and a history of high motivation to succeed.

Anorexics are preoccupied with avoiding food, sometimes eating only for this to be followed by vomiting and purging; they are hyperactive; and obsessed by exercise. They have a decreased interest in sex, a disturbed body image, distorted hunger awareness, a denial of fatigue, a sense of ineffectiveness and a feeling of being controlled by their environment.

It has been suggested that zinc deficiency may play a role in anorexia nervosa and that the features of zinc deficiency are similar to those of anorexia nervosa. Teenage girls are a group who are particularly at risk of developing zinc deficiency for three reasons. First, zinc intake is often marginal in this group because so many are slimming or eating poorly; second, because they may be taking oral contraceptives which enhance zinc excretion; and third, because zinc requirements are increased during rapid growth phases such as adolescence. As soon as a teenage girl starts dieting, for cosmetic reasons, a true zinc deficiency may develop which in itself causes a loss of appetite. Then a vicious circle sets in.

A supplement of zinc is worth considering for people with anorexia nervosa.

Things You Can Do to Help Recovery from Mental Disturbances

It is very important to bear in mind that some mental conditions are actually acute medical emergencies and should be dealt with by your doctor and/or specialist. This section should not be thought of as being a substitute for the personal care and attention of a competent physician.

However, there are certain things you can do to help yourself.

1. *Cut out all sugar, refined carbohydrates and junk food*
   This can improve the metabolism and make mental symptoms less likely to occur, or less severe. It will also go a long way to correcting the overload on the pancreas to produce more insulin that can result in a low blood sugar.

2. *Cut out tea, coffee, chocolate, cola drinks and caffeine-containing medications.*
   Caffeine can produce a whole range of symptoms on its own (see page 131) and the avoidance of caffeine can result in a considerable improvement in a proportion of individuals. It is important to remember that giving up caffeine, especially in coffee, can result in withdrawal headaches and lethargy for about twenty-four to seventy-two hours.

3. *Cut out alcohol*
While alcohol can have a relaxing effect, if you habitually consume large amounts, the effect on both metabolism and mental health, as well as your nutritional status, can be quite devastating. Withdrawal from alcohol can be helped by taking supplements of calcium and magnesium, B vitamins, zinc and vitamin C. Naturally you should avoid completely any illegal drugs.
4. *Have regular meals*
Eating regularly can prevent falls in blood sugar (see page 292) and this is even more true if you also avoid refined carbohydrate, as mentioned above. Eating regularly is important for maintaining health. Many people with severe mental symptoms go through a phase of not eating anything, or of eating poorly for a time, and such a phase may well precede an acute psychiatric episode.
5. *Nutritional supplementation (adult dosages)*
Calcium: 500–1000 mg per day.
Magnesium: 250–500 mg per day.
Vitamin B complex: 50–100 mg of the main B vitamins.
Zinc: 10–20 mg of zinc in the form of zinc gluconate, zinc sulphate, zinc aminochelate or zinc orotate.
Vitamin C: 500–1500 mg or more per day.

This nutritional supplementation program is unlikely to mask any severe underlying conditions unless it makes you delay in seeking medical advice from your doctor. It is extremely unlikely, especially if you are run down, that your family doctor will object to your taking such supplements. A number of people with psychiatric symptoms improve quite substantially after at least a week or two on such a supplementation program. **Starting such a supplementation program should not put you off seeking professional advice if symptoms are becoming severe.** A nutritionally orientated psychiatrist or doctor would probably tailor the above supplement program to your own needs.

6. *Adequate sleep*
If you have difficulty sleeping, despite the withdrawal of caffeine, bear in mind that taking high doses of vitamin B complex shortly before bedtime can act as a stimulant and worsen insomnia. Supplements which may help you sleep include calcium, magnesium, vitamin B6 and zinc, as mentioned above. Furthermore, tryptophan, 1500 mg at night, can also act as an aid in getting to sleep, especially in those

who are depressed. This dosage should not be exceeded in an adult and, if there is no discernible improvement, should not be followed for more than a couple of weeks.

7. *Food intolerance*
   This can cause a whole range of mental symptoms in susceptible individuals which can diminish or disappear if offending foods are excluded from the diet. Thus the exclusion diet on page 429 can provide a remarkable degree of relief in some people.

   People who are obsessive, are severely introverted, or those with a major psychosis should not go on an exclusion diet without proper medical supervision. It is important to read the section on page 425 before contemplating an exclusion diet.

8. *Lifestyle tips*
   (a) Keep away from television or newspapers. These generally carry bad news and can be depressing even to the most stable person. Additionally, the mental effect of being bombarded with news and stories can be detrimental for many in a delicate state of mind. It is better to read a book, do a jigsaw puzzle or follow one of your interests or hobbies.
   (b) Get regular daily exercise. This can bring about an increased sense of well-being, both physical and mental. The usual precautions about not overdoing exercise if you are not used to it should be observed.
   (c) Go for a walk for half an hour once or twice a day. This is especially good for those with insomnia and exhaustion in the absence of physical illness and those who don't spend much time outdoors.
   (d) Tidy up your home and/or work environment. This can have a remarkable therapeutic effect.
   (e) Complete unfinished things that need to be done, e.g. pay bills, answer outstanding letters etc. Having your attention caught up by uncompleted tasks and unfulfilled responsibilities is a source of mental stress. Take one thing at a time, completing it before starting the next. Work your way through them one by one and don't be put off by how much is still to be done.

9. *Be productive*
   Set yourself achievable targets at home, at work, socially and also for your interests and hobbies. A sense of achieve-

ment, however small, can be of great value in resolving mental problems. Production is the basis of good morale.

10. *Religious solace*
    Some people find comfort in discussing their problems with a minister of religion or in prayer or contemplation. If this seems right for you, follow it through.
11. *See your doctor*
    If none of the above seems to have helped, it is important not to delay seeking professional help.
12. *Hope*
    Remember you have not always been depressed, mentally disturbed or whatever. Man's powers to overcome adversity are formidable and you could be well again much sooner than you think.

APPENDICES

HOW TO USE THE APPENDICES

The Appendix is the reference section of the book. It contains much useful information that is not contained elsewhere in the book. It gives details on the recognition of nutritional deficiencies and where supplements can be obtained. Basic advice on diet, the use of supplements, and for healthy living, are also given, as well as specialized diets for food allergy sufferers. It may be very useful, indeed essential, to read parts of the Appendix before beginning any type of diet or using supplements as detailed in the other sections of the book. This will help you to get the most out of any nutritional program that you follow. If you feel there have been any significant omissions from the Appendix, or other parts of the book, we will be delighted to hear from you, so that any other helpful information can be included in further editions.

APPENDIX ONE
Living Healthily

BASIC RECOMMENDATIONS FOR A HEALTHY DIET

The following recommendations are made on the basis of a substantial amount of scientific and medical data. It is suggested that they are followed by:
(a) anyone who wishes to improve their resistance to some of the major degenerative diseases of Western society.
(b) anyone who is on a nutritional program to improve their health.
(c) anyone who has completed a nutritional program, e.g. an exclusion diet, and is now able to eat a more balanced diet.

1. Sugar and refined carbohydrates: Intake should be minimal or none. This includes sucrose, table sugar, white, brown or other sugars, glucose, honey and sorbitol. Many foods, such as sweets, cakes, chocolates, biscuits, puddings, jam, ice cream, soft drinks and other sweet-tasting foods contain large amounts of sucrose or other refined carbohydrates. White, refined flour has a lower content of vitamins and minerals than unrefined flour, and again should only be consumed in small quantities.

2. Animal and vegetable fats: Intake should be moderated. On average, most people in Western societies are advised to reduce their fat consumption to about seventy-five percent of current levels. In particular, avoid relatively poor quality foods that have a high fat content, such as fried foods, pies, sausages, preserved and canned meats. Dairy products are also high in fat and low-fat forms should be preferred, or they should be taken sparingly.

3. Ensure a good daily intake of vegetables, especially green leafy ones. Such foods are rich in the vitamins and minerals that are most commonly found to be lacking in many ill or elderly people. Furthermore, ensuring a good intake of raw or lightly cooked green vegetables or salad may help protect against some of the more common and more serious diseases in Western society.

4. Ensure a good intake of fiber. This may help with many minor conditions, such as constipation, as well as having long-term health benefits. High-fiber foods include beans, fruits, vegetables and cereals, e.g. wheat, oats, barley, rye, corn and rice. Do not rely too heavily on one type of food, e.g. wheat or bran, for your source of fiber.

5. Eat a varied and interesting diet. Eating a limited range of foods may make it difficult to obtain adequate amounts of all the nutrients required. Eating should also be a pleasure, and is an important social event. So take pleasure and interest in your food and eating.

6. Alcohol consumption should be moderate. A maximum of one or two drinks per day is a safe recommendation. (One drink = 8 oz. of beer or lager = one shot of spirits = one glass of wine.) Women who are pregnant or trying to become pregnant, and men or women with liver disease should not consume any alcohol.

7. Limit your intake of salt in cooking and in foods. Excessive salt consumption may well be a cause of high blood pressure for many people and should be avoided.

8. Eat fresh foods and avoid foods containing additives whenever possible. Additives such as coloring agents, preservatives, emulsifiers, texturizers and flavorings may have both short- and long-term adverse effects, and fresh foods, free of these, are best consumed in their place.

9. Ensure a good but not excessive intake of protein-rich foods. Lean meats, fish, eggs, poultry (without the skin), nuts, seeds, peas, beans, lentils, sprouted beans and whole grains are all rich in protein, vitamins and minerals.

10. Avoid being or becoming obese by not eating excessively, especially fatty foods and foods high in refined carbohydrates. Being significantly overweight reduces life expectancy and aggravates many conditions such as gout, high blood pressure and arthritis. Lose weight if you are overweight. Try eating foods rich in fiber and essential nutrients, rather than those rich in fat and sugar.

RULES FOR HEALTHY LIVING

Eating a good diet is not the only necessary step to good health. There are other essential physical and psychological factors.

1. **Do not smoke.** Tobacco has many harmful effects and, fortunately, many people have reduced their consumption or given up.
2. **Do not take illegal drugs.** Considerable harm and tragedy is caused by the illicit use of drugs. The dangers far outweigh any possible benefits that might result from their use.
3. **Take medical drugs only if essential.** Indiscriminate or excessive use of medical drugs, obtained either on prescription or directly from the pharmacy or supermarket, can lead to serious physical ill-health, as well as mental impairment. **Drugs** are **drugs,** and are not essential to health unless there is a defined medical problem.
4. **Get regular physical exercise.** In order to maintain good physical health, regular exercise is necessary, ideally three to four episodes of moderately strenuous exercise for forty to sixty minutes per week. Walking, jogging, swimming, cycling, or a sporting activity are all suitable. It is important you enjoy the type of exercise you do, as well as the type of food you eat.
5. **Take regular mental exercise.** Yes, you have a mind as well as a body, and if you do not want to lose it, use it. The mind undoubtedly affects the body in many ways, and mental health is often necessary in order to achieve physical health. Mental activities such as reading, writing, the creative arts, or any hobby in which you have an interest, can be stimulating to the mind. Do not rely upon others to entertain you, but create your own entertainment. Watching excessive amounts of television or videos does not allow you to exercise your own creativity, and can sometimes have an almost hypnotic effect on some people. Children may be particularly hypnotized by television and videos.
6. **Have and follow a goal and purpose in life.** It is important that you have a goal in life that you are interested in and genuinely wish to achieve. This may be via your job or home life, or by being a member of a local or national society. Without an interest in wanting to achieve something, life often becomes dull and meaningless.

7. Maintain a wide range of interests and activities. Man does not survive just by being interested in one activity, so it is important to have a varied range of interests and activities. Life can be divided into certain areas, such as your own personal interest, your family, your friends, work and groups or societies that you belong to. Also, you can consider your relationship to your fellow humans, animals, plants and environment as well as the physical and spiritual aspects of your own life, as all being areas for your interest and activity.

8. Complete any responsibilities that you have taken. Make sure that if you have agreed to do something, that you do take responsibility. A considerable amount of stress is caused by a failure to take responsibility for those things that one knows one should do.

9. Do not allow your home or work environment to become untidy or dirty. It may be difficult to feel relaxed and calm in surroundings that are chaotic or dirty, so do keep your home and work environment clean and tidy.

10. Remember to enjoy life. Even when you are unwell or under stress, there is much enjoyment to be had. Do not dwell upon your physical complaints unduly. You create your own future, and your enjoyment of it will depend on having a positive attitude.

DIETARY ADVICE FOR VEGETARIANS

"Vegetarian" is loosely used to describe someone who does not eat meat. More properly, the term vegan is used to describe those who only consume vegetable produce, and thus do not eat any meat, fish, poultry, eggs or even dairy products. Most vegetarians consume milk, and may be known as lacto-vegetarians. An omnivore is someone who eats all types of food, vegetable and animal. Many vegetarians or vegans have not been educated on how to eat a good, healthy, vegetarian diet. The following may be helpful points of advice:

1. Avoid refined carbohydrates. Refined carbohydrates are low in essential minerals and vitamins, and should not be consumed in any substantial quantities.

2. Ensure an adequate balance of protein in your diet. No single vegetable protein contains all the appropriate nutrients required for a suitable protein intake, and thus you must always combine different types of vegetable proteins in any vegetarian dish. Protein-rich foods include nuts, seeds, peas, beans, lentils, whole grains, brown rice, sprouted beans and soybean preparations. Vegetarians should not rely heavily upon any one single source of vegetable protein, including soya. The following combinations should be used:

Rice with legumes, sesame or cheese.
Wheat with legumes or peanuts and milk, or sesame and soybeans.
Corn with legumes.
Peanuts with sunflower seeds.
Sesame seeds with:
(i) beans or peanuts and soybeans; or
(ii) peanuts and soybeans; or
(iii) wheat and soybeans.

The addition of *any* first-class protein (including milk, cheese, and particularly eggs), to a vegetarian dish will enhance its nutrient value. If you are not a vegan, we recommend that you eat one or more eggs per day to ensure good intake of protein and other nutrients.

Cooking and digesting beans. Beans are a particularly good source of nutrients for many vegetarians. Particularly nutritious beans include mung beans, red kidney beans, haricot beans, butter beans, chick peas, red pigeon beans, lentils, peas and split peas. Sprouted beans may be more appetizing and more digestible. Soaking beans for twenty-four hours, and de-husking them, may reduce the problem of flatulence which affects some people.

3. Avoid foods that block mineral absorption. A number of foods may block the absorption of bulk and trace minerals, including calcium, magnesium and zinc. Such foods include bran and unleavened wheat, particularly wholegrain wheat, as in pastry, biscuits, and sauces thickened with wholewheat flour. You should be careful not to eat too much of these foods. Furthermore, tea and coffee may have powerful inhibiting effects upon the absorption of iron, and to a lesser extent, zinc. Consuming tea with meals is particularly inadvisable, especially for women, who have increased need for iron.

4. Eat fruit and vegetables daily. These foods are high in minerals and vitamin C in particular. Consuming green vegetables or salads with midday and evening meals will ensure a good intake of vitamin C. This will increase the absorption of iron from vegetarian foods.

5. Vegetarians in special situations

Infants and children. Infants being weaned, and children up to the age of two years, should *not* be placed on a strict vegetarian/vegan diet. This may result in considerable ill-health. Good sources of protein and minerals, including eggs and dairy products, are usually required.

Pregnant and breast-feeding women. The nutritional requirements for such women must be met, and a good, balanced vegetarian diet is essential for both mother and baby. Your doctor should consider giving supplements of iron, zinc and vitamin B12.

The elderly. Some old people have a declining food intake, and it is essential to ensure good intake of nutrient-rich foods. If it is difficult to consume adequate quantities of vegetarian proteins, consuming one or two eggs per day should be considered.

The ill. Vegetarian diets certainly do not suit everyone. Some people's metabolism may not fully acclimatize to a vegetarian diet. Some people can trace their ill-health back to a time after they started a vegetarian diet, especially if they have not been careful to ensure adequate intake of essential nutrients. Hidden nutritional deficiencies may be particularly likely. Sometimes, some people are just better off eating meat.

Food allergies and intolerance in vegetarians. Unfortunately, such foods as cows' milk, wheat and yeast, are very common culprits in causing food allergy. For those who are intolerant of such foods, it may be impossible to devise a nutritious vegetarian diet, and such individuals will be well advised to include eggs, fish, or meat in their diet, either in the short- or long-term.

6. Nutritional supplements. Many vegetarians are aware of the fact that their diets can be low in vitamin B12. Deficiency only rarely develops, however. Vitamin B12 may be found in small quantities in eggs, brewers' yeast and dairy products. Strict vegans may be at particular risk, especially pregnant and breast-feeding mothers, who should take vitamin B12 supplements routinely. If deficiency of vitamin B12 occurs in a vegetarian, it should not be assumed to be due to dietary inadequacy; other causes should also be considered.

APPENDIX TWO
Nutritional Deficiencies and Supplements

HOW TO RECOGNIZE A NUTRITIONAL DEFICIENCY

This is a brief summary of some of the physical signs that can be indications of nutritional deficiencies. It should be borne in mind, however that all of the signs or symptoms below can be caused by other medical conditions. In particular, symptoms marked with an asterisk (*) can be caused by a yeast or fungal infection. **If you have any of these physical signs, we urge you to consult your own medical practitioner before undertaking any self-help therapy.**

SIGN OR SYMPTOM	CAN BE CAUSED BY DEFICIENCIES OF
Cracking at the corners of the mouth*	iron, vitamins B2, B6, folic acid
Recurrent mouth ulcers	iron, folic acid, vitamin B12
Dry, cracked lips	vitamin B2
Smooth (sore) tongue*	iron, vitamins B2, B12, folic acid
Fissured tongue	vitamin B3
Enlargement/prominence of taste buds at the tip of the tongue (red, sore)	vitamins B2 or B6

Bruising or enlargement of veins under the tongue	vitamin C
Red, greasy skin on face, especially sides of nose	vitamins B2, B6, zinc or essential fatty acids
Rough, sometimes red, pimply skin on upper arms and thighs	vitamin B complex, vitamin E or essential fatty acids
Scrotal and vulval dermatitis*	vitamin B2, zinc
Skin conditions such as eczema, dry, rough, cracked, peeling skin	zinc, essential fatty acids
Poor hair growth	iron or zinc
Dandruff	vitamin C, vitamin B6, zinc, essential fatty acids
Bloodshot, gritty, sensitive eyes	vitamins A or B2
Night blindness	vitamin A or zinc
Dry eyes	vitamin A, essential fatty acids
Brittle or split nails	iron, zinc or essential fatty acids
White spots on nails	zinc
Pale appearance due to anemia	iron, vitamin B12, folic acid (**essential to consult your doctor**)

For many nutrients there may be no reliable physical signs of nutritional deficiency. This is particularly true for vitamin D, vitamin E, vitamin K, some of the minor B vitamins, calcium, magnesium, chromium, selenium, copper, potassium and sodium. These deficiencies are usually suspected by a doctor from the patient's complaints or knowledge of their diet.

WHAT TO EXPECT WHEN YOU START A NUTRITIONAL PROGRAM

When you start a nutritional program (***ideally, under the guidance of your doctor***) a number of changes are likely to occur. It is important to consider different component parts of such a program. This is best divided into the following headings: drugs, diet, supplements, exercise, and lifestyle changes.

DRUGS

If you are on medication from your practitioner or a specialist continue with this. **Do not stop any drug medication without first consulting with your doctor.** It is best to take the drugs at a different time from your nutritional supplements if at all possible.

DIET

Changing your diet can have a profound effect upon metabolism. If you are on an exclusion diet there can be a worsening of your symptoms for the first few days. This usually passes and will be helped by resting, eating regularly and not over-stressing yourself. It is advisable, before beginning the diet, to go shopping and plan your menus for the first week, at least, so that you do not start the diet unprepared. This is particularly true for exclusion diets. If you find the dietary changes too hard to make, then try gradually introducing new changes over a week or two.

SUPPLEMENTS

It is not commonly appreciated that there can be adverse reactions to vitamin or mineral supplements. This may be particularly likely to occur if large doses of multivitamins or individual nutrients are taken by someone who is not accustomed to taking nutritional supplements. It is advisable to take them with or after meals, rather than on an empty stomach, unless otherwise specified by your doctor. Minor symptoms such as abdominal discomfort, skin irritation or a worsening of symptoms can occur. If this happens, then reduce the dose to the smallest quantity and try again, taking the supplements after a meal. By gradually increasing the dosage, you may well be able to tolerate the supplements advised. If a reaction occurs a second time, then cease completely.

After one to three weeks of taking supplements, toxic reactions can sometimes be experienced. These may include loss of appetite, nausea, headaches, and even swollen lymph glands. The cause of this is unknown, but it usually settles down by itself. It may be necessary to stop, or reduce, the supplements for a few days and then restart again. Do, also, ensure a good fluid intake.

EXERCISE

Exercise may be of considerable benefit for a number of conditions, including obesity, depression, insomnia and certain types of heart disease. **In this last case, the exercises should always be taken under appropriate supervision.** Muscle stiffness, aches and tiredness can occur, certainly in the first few days of starting an exercise program, and this is quite normal. It is better to do a little gentle exercise every day rather than try to push yourself too hard. Remember exercise should be enjoyable.

LIFESTYLE CHANGES

Changes in lifestyle, such as stress-reduction and increasing or reducing your responsibilities at work or at home, may be a necessary part of a health-care program. When introducing such changes into your life, a certain amount of disruption may occur, which might be temporarily disturbing to yourself or others. A change in your schedule or activities may require you to give some explanation to others, such as your friends, family or workmates. It is important that you see the sense of any recommended lifestyle changes before making them. Further details are given in "Rules for healthy living," page 400.

An important part of the healing process is for you, yourself, to maintain a positive attitude. The first steps to getting better are to recognize that there is something wrong with either your physical or mental health, and to be willing to experience an improvement in it. The more you can do for yourself, the greater the likelihood of a successful outcome. If you have many symptoms, it is very easy to forget that three or four previously troublesome symptoms have now disappeared because you may be preoccupied with the remaining ones.

If, despite following the program recommended by your doctor, your symptoms fail to improve, this may be due to incorrect diagnosis, and consequently incorrect treatment, or correct diagnosis, but incorrect treatment. Only careful review by your doctor will be able to decide which. What he or she requires from you is that you report your symptoms accurately, without overplaying or underplaying them. Furthermore, if something else is wrong, such as an unexpressed, unresolved stressful situation, or a continuing heavy consumption of alcohol, or use of legal or illegal drugs without your doctor's knowledge, then it may be impossible for any program, no matter how appropriate, to result in improvement. It is important that you take responsibility for your illness, and by so doing you, with the aid of your medical practitioner and medical science, will rise above it.

It may be helpful to remember some of these principles if you are experiencing temporary adverse reactions. Such symptoms as abdominal discomfort, flatulence, bloating, change in bowel habit, insomnia, lethargy, muscle aches and pains, headaches, feelings of malaise, may temporarily worsen. Such changes usually do not persist for more than seven to ten days. Changes in menstrual cycle can quite easily occur and it may take two or three months before this settles back to normal. **Always mention such changes to your medical practitioner.**

WHERE TO OBTAIN NUTRITIONAL SUPPLEMENTS

Nutritional supplements can be obtained from a number of sources. Three major ones are health food stores, pharmacies and specialist suppliers. The latter normally supply by mail order on request either from a doctor, or direct from a patient. Quite a number of nutritional preparations are available over the counter in pharmacies, without a doctor's prescription. Prices of these may be easily comparable with those in health food stores.

As a rule, health food stores tend to carry a more substantial range of nutritional supplements, in particular those of higher strength. If your doctor advises you to take a particular supplement that he cannot prescribe, then this will have to be obtained either over the counter in a pharmacy, or from a health food store. Some of the rare supplements, such as certain trace minerals, amino acids, and unusual combinations, have to be obtained from specialist suppliers.

NOTE

The authors do not personally endorse any one particular type of nutritional supplement or company supplying nutritional supplements.

List of nutritional supplements

Key: P = PHARMACY HFS = HEALTHFOOD STORE SS = SPECIALIST SUPPLIER Pr. = BY PRESCRIPTION

NUTRIENT	PREPARATIONS	STRENGTH PER TABLET	DAILY DOSAGE	SUPPLIER	NOTES
Vitamin A	Many, e.g. cod or halibut liver oil also contain vitamin D	4–10,000 IUs (capsule)	Up to 10,000 IUs	**P/HFS/Pr. for dose**	Doses above 20,000 IUs per day may be toxic.
	Halibut liver oil capsules BP	4,000 IUs		**Pr.**	
Beta-carotene (water soluble vitamin A)	Few only	10–25,000 IUs	Up to 25,000 IUs per day	**SS/HFS**	Rarely needed supplement.
B vitamins					
B1 (thiamin)	Many	2–500 mg	Usually up to 50 mg	**Pr./P/HFS**	Usually as vitamin B complex or multivitamins.
B2 (riboflavin)	Many	2–500 mg	Usually up to 50 mg	**Pr./P/HFS**	

Key: P = PHARMACY HFS = HEALTHFOOD STORE SS = SPECIALIST SUPPLIER Pr. = BY PRESCRIPTION

NUTRIENT	PREPARATIONS	STRENGTH PER TABLET	DAILY DOSAGE	SUPPLIER	NOTES
B3 (nicotinamide)	Many	5–500 mg	Variable	**Pr./P/HFS/SS**	High doses under medical supervision.
B3 (nicotinic acid)	Many	5–500 mg	Usually up to 50 mg	**P/HFS/Pr./SS**	High doses (several grams) need medical supervision.
B6 (pyridoxine)	Many, some slow	10–500 mg	Up to 200 mg	**P/HFS/SS**	Toxicity possible; above 200 mg should be under medical supervision.
B complex	Many	Variable, 2–100 mg of B1, B2, B3, B6 and other B vitamins	As directed, often just 1 per day	**P/HFS/Pr./SS**	Many indications.
	Parenterovite Pabrinex	Injections	As directed	**Pr.**	For severely ill patients, e.g. alcoholics under medical supervision.
Folic acid	Many Folic acid BP	10–400 mcg 100 mcg–5 mg	10–400 mcg Up to 15 mg	**HFS/SS/Pr.**	Should be under medical supervision for proven deficiency only.

B12	Several	100–1000 mcg (tablets)	100 mcg	**HFS**	Tablets only needed for strict vegans.
	Cytacon	50 mcg tablets	As directed	**Pr.**	
	Neocytamen	1000 mcg injection	As directed	**Pr.**	For medical use only to correct deficiencies and as a therapeutic agent.
Biotin	Few	200–600 mcg	Not known 200–1000 mcg	**SS/Pr.**	Rarely used supplement.
B5 (pantothenic acid)	Few	50–1000 mg	Up to 500 mg	**SS/Pr.**	Rarely used supplement.
Choline	Few	250–500 mg	500 mg–several grams per day	**SS**	Rarely used. High doses under medical supervision.
Inositol	Few	250–750 mg	Variable	**SS**	Rarely used. High doses under medical supervision.
PABA (para amino benzoic acid)	Few	50–500 mg	500 mg	**SS**	
	Potaba	500 mg–3g	Up to 12 g	**Pr.**	High doses under medical supervision only. May cause hypoglycemia.

Key: P = PHARMACY HFS = HEALTHFOOD STORE SS = SPECIALIST SUPPLIER Pr. = BY PRESCRIPTION

NUTRIENT	PREPARATIONS	STRENGTH PER TABLET	DAILY DOSAGE	SUPPLIER	NOTES
Vitamin C (ascorbic acid)	Innumerable variety: powder, tablets, buffered preparations, sodium and calcium ascorbates	10–1000 mg	50 mg–10 g or more daily	**HFS/P** **SS** for some preparations	Doses up to several grams per day are usually harmless.
	Ascorbic acid BP	25, 50, 100, 200, 250 mg tablets	Variable	**Pr.**	High doses and intravenous administration under medical supervision.
	Vitamin C with bioflavonoids			**HFS/SS**	
Bioflavonoids (a variety of plant derived compounds)	Few	100–1000 mg	Variable	**HFS/SS**	True indication unknown. May enhance vitamin C activity.
Oxerutins (a type of bioflavonoid)	Paroven	250 mg	3–4 daily	**Pr.**	For varicose veins and related problems only.

Vitamin D	Cod or halibut liver oil capsules vitamin D	400 IUs	1 per day	**HFS/P**	Dangerous to exceed dose unless medically supervised.
	Cod liver oil	400 IUs per 5ml	5 ml	**HFS/P**	Also contains vitamin A.
	Calciferol tablets: high strength BP 1980 vitamin D	10,000 IUs	Variable	**Pr.**	
	Calciferol tablets: strong BP 1973	50,000 IUs		**Pr.**	Medical supervision only.
	Other specialized vitamin D preparations			**Pr.**	
Vitamin E	Many	10–600 IUs	Up to 600 IUs	**HFS/P**	Toxicity extremely rare.
Synthetic (1 mg = IU approx.)	Ephynal	3, 10, 50 and 200 mg capsules	600 mg	**P/Pr.**	
	Vita E preparations (several)	75–400 IUs	Up to 600 IUs	**P/Pr.**	Doses above 20 IUs per day should not be given to patients on anticoagulants without medical supervision.

Key: P = PHARMACY HFS = HEALTHFOOD STORE SS = SPECIALIST SUPPLIER Pr. = BY PRESCRIPTION

NUTRIENT	PREPARATIONS	STRENGTH PER TABLET	DAILY DOSAGE	SUPPLIER	NOTES
Natural (36% more effective than synthetic; 1 mg = 1.36 IU approx.)	Many	10–600 IUs	600 IUs	**HFS/SS**	
Vitamin K	Konakion or Synkavit	10 or 50 mg per ampoule or 10 mg per tablet	1 ampoule 1 tablet	**Pr.**	Rarely used.
Calcium	Calcium gluconate	600 mg	Up to 20 tablets (approx.)	**P/Pr.**	Only one tenth of tablet is calcium.
	Calcium lactate	300–600 mg	10–20 tablets	**P/Pr.**	Only one fifth of tablet is calcium.
	Sandocal calcium salts	3 g	Up to 5 tablets	**Pr.**	400 mg calcium per tablet.
	Ossopan (bone-derived calcium)	800 mg or powder	4–8 or equivalent in powder	**Pr.**	Expensive.

	Dolomite	Variable 250–500 mg	3–20	**HFS**	Cheap, but effectiveness uncertain.
	Calcium orotate Chelate	Variable	Up to 1000 mg of calcium	**HFS/SS/ Pr.**	
Calcium and vitamin D	Calcium with vitamin D tablets	Calcium 30 mg of element (approx.) with vitamin D 500 IUs	1–2	**Pr.**	Rarely used. Not indicated for osteoporosis or osteoarthritis.
Magnesium	Magnesium	Approx. content of magnesium:	1–2 tablespoons	**P/Pr.**	Cheap but messy and awkward. Dissolve or mix with lemon juice or vinegar.
	Hydroxide	40%			
	Oxide	60%			
	Carbonate (white powders)	10–25%			
	Magnesium orotate	Variable	Equivalent to 400 mg magnesium	**HFS/SS/ Pr.**	Easy to take effective supplement.
	Magnesium chelates	200 mg		**HFS/SS/ Pr.**	
Iron	Many, e.g. ferrous sulphate, ferrous gluconate, ferrous fumerate, etc.	2–300 mg	1–3	**Pr.**	Used for treatment of iron deficiency. Iron best taken with vitamin C, 50–100 mg.

Key: P = PHARMACY HFS = HEALTHFOOD STORE SS = SPECIALIST SUPPLIER Pr. = BY PRESCRIPTION

NUTRIENT	PREPARATIONS	STRENGTH PER TABLET	DAILY DOSAGE	SUPPLIER	NOTES
Iron	Sometimes with folic acid, vitamins or zinc		Variable	**Pr.**	Must not be taken with tea or coffee.
	Other iron preparations: Fumarate, gluconate or chelate	30–60 mg of elemental iron	1–3	**HFS/SS/P**	Must not be taken with tea or coffee.
Zinc	Solvazinc zinc sulphate/citrate	200 mg (45 mg zinc)	1–3	**P/Pr.**	More than one a day needs medical supervision.
	Zincomed zinc sulphate	200 mg	1–3	**Pr.**	Can cause nausea.
	Z-span spansules	61.8 mg (22.5 mg zinc)		**P/Pr.**	
	Zinc gluconate, orotate, chelate	10–100 mg (15% is elemental zinc)	1–3 = 50 mg of elemental zinc	**HFS/SS**	

Chromium	Brewers' yeast	300 mg tablets	Up to 30	**HFS/P**	High doses needed but may cause nausea and indigestion.
	Chromic chloride solution (Cr.Cl3) (made up by pharmacist)	70 mg of Cr.Cl3 in 500 ml of water	5 ml	**Pr.**	Very nontoxic. Medical supervision required in diabetics.
	Chromium GTF	200 mcg	1	**SS/HFS**	
Selenium	Seleno-methionine or sodium selenite	50–500 mcg	Up to 200 mcg	**SS/HFS**	**Do not exceed 200 mcg per day**, except under medical supervision.
Iodine	Kelp	Variable	1–3	**HFS**	Excess doses can be toxic.
Manganese	Manganese gluconate, chelate and orotates	Variable. 10–20% of preparation is elemental manganese	5–25 mg of element	**HFS/SS**	Doses above need medical supervision.
Copper	Copper amino acid chelate	3 mg of elemental copper	1	**SS**	Proven copper deficiency must be demonstrated prior to supplementation.

Key: P = PHARMACY HFS = HEALTHFOOD STORE SS = SPECIALIST SUPPLIER Pr. = BY PRESCRIPTION

NUTRIENT	PREPARATIONS	STRENGTH PER TABLET	DAILY DOSAGE	SUPPLIER	NOTES
Potassium	Potassium chloride Several other preparations, some combined with diuretics	Slow-K 600 mg potassium chloride	1–6 after meals	**Pr.**	For patients with proven deficiency or at risk of deficiency. May cause nausea and abdominal pain.
	Potassium gluconate		1–6 after meals	**Pr.**	
	Potassium aspartate and others	300 mg (65 mg potassium)	1–3		Higher doses under medical supervision.
	Salt substitutes high in potassium Selora Ruthmol		Up to 6	**Pr./P/HFS**	May be indicated for those unable to do without ordinary table salt.
Essential fatty acids	Marine Lipids MaxEPA	EPA 18–20% DHA 12–14%	1–4	**HFS/SS/P**	Specialized supplement with specific indications. Higher doses need medical supervision.

	Evening primrose oil (EPO), e.g. Efamol	250–500 mg capsules 8–9% gamma-linoleic acid per capsule	2–8 capsules of 500 mg strength	**HFS/SS/P**	Available on prescription.
	Other sources of essential fatty acids, e.g. blackcurrant seed oil and borage seed oil are unevaluated as to clinical efficacy at present				
Combined EFA supplements	Efamol marine naudicelle plus (EPO and marine lipid mixture)		1–6	**HFS/SS/P**	Available on prescription.
Amino acids	L-tryptophan (Pacitron or Optimax)	500 mg	Up to 6	**Pr./HFS/SS**	Used in depressive illness and insomnia.
	Tyrosine, DL-phenylalanine, L-lysine, taurine and others	Variable	Variable	**SS**	Specialized uses.

Key: P = PHARMACY HFS = HEALTHFOOD STORE SS = SPECIALIST SUPPLIER Pr. = BY PRESCRIPTION

NUTRIENT	PREPARATIONS	STRENGTH PER TABLET	DAILY DOSAGE	SUPPLIER	NOTES
Digestive aids	Stomach enzymes and acids: Acidol pepsin	97 mg pepsin, 388 mg betaine hydrochloride	1–3 tablets dissolved in water with each meal	**Pr.**	Drink via a straw.
	Muripsin	55 mg pepsin 500 g glutamic acid hydrochloride	1–2 tablets with each meal	**P/Pr.**	
	Pancreatic enzymes: Combizym, Combizym Compositum, Cotazym, Creon, Nutrizym, Pancrex V Forte	Variable	Variable	**Pr.**	For pancreatic insufficiency only.
	Bile supplements: Opobyl, Veracolate, ox bile	Variable	Variable	**Pr.**	For biliary insufficiency only.

Fiber	Celevac, Cellucon (methyl-cellulose), Fybogel, Isogel, Metamucil, Regulan, Vi-Siblin (Ispaghula) Fibranta, Proctofibre, Trifyba (cereal), Normacol Special (Sterculia)	Variable	Variable	**Pr.**	For correction of constipation due to lack of fiber. Cereal-based fiber supplements are contraindicated in people with celiac disease and wheat or gluten sensitivity.
	Bran and other cereal fibers, e.g. oats, soya bran, rice bran, etc.		1–2 tablespoons	**HFS/P**	Widely available, also found in grocery stores, etc.
Gallstone preparations	Chendol, Chenocedon, Chenofalk, Destolit, Roachol, Ursofalk	Variable	Variable	**Pr.**	For specific types of gallstones. Only under medical supervision.

SUPPLEMENTS FOR ADULTS AND THE ELDERLY

The following is the contents we suggest for a broad spectrum multivitamin, multimineral supplement suitable for adults and old people. The ranges given are for one tablet, and dosage could vary from one to six tablets per day, as appropriate.

Such a supplement should be free from yeast, wheat, gluten, milk, corn, soya, artificial colorants and preservatives.

CONTENTS PER TABLET	
Vitamin A	*500–1200 IUs*
Vitamin D3	*20–100 IUs*
Vitamin B1	*2–10 mg*
Vitamin B2	*2–10 mg*
Vitamin B6	*2–15 mg*
Vitamin B12	*10–25 mcg*
Vitamin C	*25–150 mg*
Vitamin E d-Alpha	*10–50 IUs*
Biotin	*20–50 mcg*
Calcium Pantothenate (B5)	*30–60 mg*
Choline	*5–15 mg*
Bioflavonoids	*5–25 mg*
Folic acid	*50–100 mcg*
Nicotinic acid	*5–10 mg*
Nicotinamide	*10–20 mg*
P.A.B.A.	*5–10 mg*
Beta-carotene	*2–5 mg*
Iodine from kelp	*10–25 mcg*
Calcium (element)	*50–150 mg*
Chromium	*20–30 mcg*
Iron (element)	*2–3 mg*
Magnesium (element)	*20–60 mg*
Selenium (element)	*10–25 mcg*
Zinc (element)	*2–4 mg*

Such a supplement may be particularly appropriate for the severely ill, or the elderly who are ill, when multiple nutritional deficiencies are likely to occur.

NUTRITIONAL SUPPLEMENTS FOR CHILDREN

Nutritional supplements, such as the one described above, should not be given to children without first consulting with your medical practitioner. Specialized supplements for children, available in a liquid form or as a chewable tablet, are often preferred.

RECOVERING FROM THE PILL

This is the daily supplement program we would recommend to women when they stop taking the Pill. It should be continued for two or three months.

Vitamin B1	*10–50 mg*
Vitamin B2	*10–50 mg*
Vitamin B3	*10–50 mg*
Vitamin B5	*50–100 mg*
Vitamin B6	*50–100 mg*
Vitamin B12	*200–400 mcg*
Folic acid	*400 mcg–2 mg*
Inositol	*50–75 mg*
Choline	*50–75 mg*
Vitamin A	*not needed usually*
Vitamin C	*250–2000 mg (or more)*
Vitamin E	*50–200 IUs*
Magnesium	*100–200 mg (or more)*
Zinc	*5–15 mg (or more)*
Manganese	*3–5 mg*
Copper	*contraindicated, usually*
Iron	*? nil (depends on individual's iron status)*

PRECONCEPTION SUPPLEMENT PROGRAM FOR WOMEN

Women who are on the Pill should go onto the "Recovering from the Pill" program (page 314) for two or three months before embarking on the program outlined below for one or two months.

This supplement would be suitable to ensure, as far as possible, good vitamin and mineral status in a woman even if she has a medical condition, e.g. diabetes, that might adversely influence her nutritional state.

Ideally, individual nutritional assessment should precede such a program, but we recognize that this may not always be possible. Any woman who has previously had a baby with a birth defect, herself has a significant medical condition, or has had serious problems in a previous pregnancy, should get a thorough individual medical assessment before conception. This is the kind of supplement your doctor may wish to prescribe.

	DAILY
Vitamin E	*100–200 IUs*
Vitamin A	*2500–5000 IUs*
Vitamin C	*100–500 mg*
Vitamin B1, B2, B3, B6	*2–20 mg*
Vitamin B12	*200–300 mcg*
Choline	*10–20 mg*
Inositol	*10–20 mg*
Folic acid	*400–800 mcg*
Zinc	*10–20 mg*
Manganese	*5–10 mg*
Chromium	*50–100 mcg*
Magnesium	*200–400 mg*
Calcium	*400–800 mg*
Copper	*0.5–1 mg*
Iron	*10–20 mg*
Selenium	*25–50 mcg*

APPENDIX THREE

Exclusion Diets and Food Lists

Many conditions may be caused or aggravated by an allergy or adverse reaction to various foods. Details of this are given in the section on allergies (page 154). Such conditions include asthma, rhinitis, eczema, urticaria (nettle rash), some types of arthritis, migraine, hyperactivity in children, episodes of abdominal pain, bloating and diarrhea or constipation. It is often impossible to determine which food(s) are causing symptoms in an individual patient without their undergoing some kind of exclusion diet. There are several types of such diets:

(a) Five-day fast.
(b) Lamb and pears diet.
(c) Modified exclusion diet for adults or children.
(d) Exclusion diets for specific conditions, such as migraine or hyperactivity in children.

Which diet is the most suitable depends on the nature and severity of the symptoms. **Such diets are best followed under the guidance of someone with experience in this field, e.g. a doctor, dietitian or nutritionist, who is aware of the problems and pitfalls that can occur.**

An exclusion diet is primarily performed for diagnostic purposes, not therapeutic, to find out if your symptoms are caused or affected by the foods you eat. If they subside after you have followed the diet for the appropriate length of time, the foods will be added back one by one to see if a reaction is provoked. Foods are added back singly at one or two day intervals. Common and important high-risk foods such as wheat, oats, barley and rye, cheese, milk, yeast and eggs are best added back singly for a test period of two or three days each.

Before starting an exclusion diet, it is well worth being aware of the following:

GENERAL POINTS ABOUT EXCLUSION DIETS

(a) Symptoms (e.g. headache or exacerbation of asthma) may become worse in the first few days of the diet.
(b) Improvement may only become apparent after anything from two days to two or even three weeks on the diet.
(c) Adverse reactions to foods may be more likely to occur if you have certain nutritional deficiencies, problems with digestive or intestinal function or if you are consuming excessive amounts of some other foods, e.g. salt, sugar, alcohol or if you are a smoker. Such factors must also be taken into account.
(d) Anyone embarking on a dietary exclusion program should be given advice to make sure that his or her diet contains adequate quantities of nutrients, and if not, that appropriate supplements are given. Don't take vitamins or mineral supplements unless they have been approved as part of your program. Some contain coloring agents, or you may be sensitive to some of their constituents, e.g. yeast.
(e) An exclusion diet is used for diagnosis *not* treatment. An exclusion diet is best performed carefully, and thoroughly; a partially followed one may be impossible to interpret, and be useless.
(f) Do not continue the diet indefinitely. It can be most unhealthy. Such diets are intended to be followed for a limited period only, and should not be considered to be nutritionally complete in the long-term.
(g) Do not embark on an exclusion program if you will be unable to adhere to it for the allotted time. Events such as Christmas, weddings and holidays may disrupt the dietary schedule, and an allowance of up to eight weeks should be made for those following the more rigid diets.
(h) When on the diet, follow your doctor's advice. If you have sensitivities to inhalants such as house dust, animal fur or chemical fumes, then you will also have to take appropriate steps to avoid them as well.
(i) Do not smoke. (An exclusion diet is a good opportunity to give up smoking.)

(j) Prepare for the diet by first going shopping for those foods allowed on your diet. It may be useful to start your diet on a Thursday or Friday so that any initial problems that arise will probably do so over the weekend when you will not be at work, or have so many commitments.

(k) Under most circumstances better results are obtained if medical drugs are avoided for the duration of the exclusion diet. **Check with your doctor before coming off drugs.**

YOUR PROGRESS ON AN EXCLUSION DIET

If your symptoms are due to a food reaction, then there should have been some improvement or even complete disappearance of your symptoms while following the appropriate diet. It is now important to reintroduce foods, and by so doing, determine which foods, if any, are responsible for your symptoms. It is important to bear in mind the following points:

(a) On introducing foods, reactions can occur within minutes, hours, or several days of consuming a new food. The speed with which symptoms occur depends to some degree upon the type of symptoms. Nettle rash or facial swelling due to food allergy can occur within minutes or hours; symptoms such as muscle aches and pains, or even arthritis, can sometimes take three or four days to appear.

(b) If the reaction occurs, stop consuming the food that you have just introduced, and wait for the reaction to settle down before reintroducing another food. This may take two or three days.

(c) If your symptoms are severe, particularly if it is a migraine, you may try taking a drink of two teaspoonfuls of bicarbonate of soda dissolved in water. Also, breathing with a paper bag over your nose and mouth may help abort a migraine attack. Such measures can be useful in reducing the severity of a reaction.

(d) If you only consume a small amount of the test food, a positive reaction may be missed. It is important that you consume a normal-sized portion, not an excessive amount, of the food in question.

(e) If you are uncertain whether there has been a reaction or not, it is usually advisable to leave the food off, assuming that a positive reaction has occurred. It can be tested later. If, however, you are on a very restricted diet, it may be unwise to do this.

(f) If you are on a very restricted diet, it is usually advisable to reintroduce relatively safe foods, i.e. further vegetables, meat, and fruits early on. It is often better to leave common, high-risk foods, such as wheat and dairy products, until later in the diet.

Remember that an exclusion diet is done to determine whether or not you have a food sensitivity. Only by reintroducing foods can this be determined. It is very often the case that a considerable amount of weight is lost on such a diet. It is important that this amount is not excessive, and that before starting an exclusion diet, you do not have any physical signs or symptoms attributable to nutritional deficiencies. If so, your doctor will advise you to take appropriate supplements for several weeks before commencing the diet.

In the long run, reactions to various foods may be diminished by avoiding excessive consumption of salt, sugar and alcohol, even if you are not sensitive to these. Factors such as cigarette smoking, that interfere with normal digestive processes, can be a contributory factor. Long-term avoidance of those foods to which you react may sometimes result in a reduction of the sensitivity to them. It is not uncommon that those who were previously sensitive to a food can, after several months of appropriate dietary management, tolerate small quantities of the foods to which they reacted previously.

FIVE-DAY FAST

Nothing is consumed except bottled water for a period of five days. **This is a severe program and should only be undertaken under medical supervision.** People are particularly likely to feel unwell, weak, or have a worsening of symptoms on such a program during the first two or three days. By the end of five days there should be very definite evidence of improvement of overall symptoms; you should not smoke, or take medical drugs or be exposed to excessive amounts of chemicals, including car fumes, household chemicals and cleaning fluids etc., during this fast, as reactions to these things can mask true improvements from withdrawal of offending foods. **Do not come off medical**

drugs without medical supervision. A written record of daily weight and symptom scoring should be kept throughout the fast and throughout the reintroduction of foods.

Foods can be introduced at the rate of one or two new foods a day and responses noted in writing.

This diet is only used rarely.

LAMB AND PEARS DIET

This is probably the most successful exclusion diet. Only the following foods are consumed:

(a) Lamb, including lambs' offal, kidney, liver and sweetbreads.
(b) Pears—without the skins.
(c) Bottled mineral water.

The lamb may be roasted, grilled or casseroled with pear slices. Make sure the pears are not over-ripe or moldy. An alternative to lamb is turkey and turkey livers if preferred. Follow this diet for five to seven days only.

MODIFIED EXCLUSION DIET FOR ADULTS

This diet is based on considerable work in the USA and the UK, especially at the Hospital for Sick Children, Great Ormond Street, London, and at Addenbrooke's Hospital, Cambridge. It is the easiest to follow and the one most often recommended.

	EXCLUDED	INCLUDED
Meat	*Beef, pork, preserved meats, bacon, sausages.*	*Lamb, turkey, rabbit, game, always lean cuts, cooked plainly.*
Fish	*All smoked fish, shellfish.*	*White fish (except for patients with eczema).*
Vegetables	*Potatoes, onions, sweetcorn, soya.*	*Spinach, celery, lettuce, leeks, peas, lentils, all beans,* except *broad and green beans, brussels*

	EXCLUDED	INCLUDED
		sprouts and cabbage. Patients with bowel symptoms are not allowed any beans, lentils, brussels sprouts or cabbages.
Fruit	*All fruits except five (see opposite). Tomatoes are excluded.*	*Five fruits: bananas, peeled pears, mangoes, pomegranates.*
Cereals	*Wheat, oats, barley, rye, corn.*	*Rice, ground rice, rice flakes, rice flour, sago, Rice Krispies, tapioca, millet, buckwheat, rice cakes.*
Cooking oils	*Corn oil, soya oil, vegetable oil, nut, especially peanut.*	*Sunflower oil, safflower oil, olive oil, linseed oil.*
Dairy products	*Cows' milk, butter, most margarines, cows' milk yogurt and cheese. All goats', sheep's and soya milk products, eggs and chicken.*	*Margarine. (Some margarines contain colorings, wheatgerm and cows' milk derivatives, etc., and should be avoided.)*
Beverages	*Tea, coffee (beans, instant and decaffeinated), fruit squashes, orange juice, grapefruit juice, alcohol, tap-water.*	*Herbal teas, e.g. camomile, mineral, distilled, deionized or filtered water. Use a water filter.*
Miscellaneous	*Chocolate, yeast, preservatives. All food additives (see separate list). Herbs, spices, sugar, honey.*	*Sea salt.*

MODIFIED EXCLUSION DIET FOR CHILDREN

Eliminate totally from the diet the following foods for a period of up to three weeks to establish whether or not your child's condition responds. **For any longer than this you should seek professional advice.**

This diet is especially useful for recurrent ear infections, asthma, eczema, bedwetting, hyperactivity and bowel disturbances. Most children respond before three weeks are up. Once you know that your child is better on this diet, you should seek professional advice to make sure your child does not become malnourished.

EXCLUDED	INCLUDED
All carbonated and colored drinks	*Plain potato crisps*
All colorings and preservatives	*Fish (except in cases of eczema)*
All sugar, sweets and chocolates	*Pork*
Tea, coffee and cocoa, tap water	*Lamb*
Eggs, and foods containing eggs	*Poultry*
All dairy products (cows', goats' and sheep's milk products)	*Rabbit*
All wheat, oats, rye and corn products	*Lentils*
Beef	*Rice, millet*
Citrus fruits (oranges, lemons, grapefruits, etc.)	*Lettuce, cauliflower*
Apple juice	*Bananas, peeled pears, mangoes*
Salicylate-containing foods (see below) if your child is hyperactive or has hives or asthma.	*Duck eggs*
	Filtered or bottled water
	Soya milk (see N.B. below)

N.B. If your child has been drinking soya milk because of a suspected cows' milk allergy, then soya should be eliminated too.

Supplements and drugs

Take none unless specifically approved by your doctor. They may contain coloring agents and additives.

Labels

Read *all* labels on packaged food, to see what is in the food.

LOW-SALICYLATE DIET

Many foods contain natural salicylates, which are very similar to ordinary aspirin. Some people can be sensitive or allergic to aspirin, and also react to foods containing salicylates. It may be advisable for patients with the conditions below to try a low-salicylate diet, especially if their condition has been made worse by aspirin or aspirin-containing drugs.

It should be remembered that not all patients with the conditions below will respond to this diet, and those that respond only partially may have other causes for their conditions, or have additional sensitivities, e.g. to coloring agents.

CONDITIONS THAT CAN RESPOND TO A LOW-SALICYLATE DIET

1. Urticaria (nettle rash), acute or chronic.
2. Asthma (if aspirin-sensitive).
3. Hyperactivity in children.
4. Ulcerative colitis (occasionally).

Nasal stuffiness due to nasal polyps might respond to a low-salicylate diet if the sufferer also has aspirin-sensitive asthma. The simplest test is—if aspirin makes your symptoms worse, try the low-salicylate diet.

LOW-SALICYLATE FOODS

Fruits
Bananas, mangoes, peeled pears, pomegranates.

Vegetables
All beans (except broad beans and green beans), beansprouts, brussels sprouts, cabbage, celery, leeks, lentils, lettuce, peas, peeled potatoes, fermented soy products (e.g. soy sauce).

All condiments, spices and herbs should be avoided.

Beverages
Gin and vodka.

Cereals
Wheat, oats, barley, rye, rice have no, or minimal, salicylate content.

Nuts and seeds
All are allowed except the following: almonds, brazils, coconut, macadamia nuts, peanuts, pine nuts, pistachio nuts, sesame seeds, walnuts, waterchestnuts.

Miscellaneous
The following contain substantial amounts of salicylate and should be avoided: honey, licorice, peppermint sweets, and yeast-containing produce.

Many processed, canned or packaged foods can be high in salicylates, due to the foods or spices used in their composition.

Meat etc.
All meats, fish, shellfish, dairy products and eggs are low in salicylates.

HIGH-SALICYLATE FOODS

Fruits
Apples, apricots, avocadoes, all berry fruits, melons, cherries, currants, grapes, raisins, dates, figs, guavas, grapefruit, lemons, lychees, mandarins, nectarines, peaches, plums, prunes, oranges, passion fruit, pears with skins, persimmons, pineapples, rhubarb.

Vegetables
Alfalfa, asparagus, broad and green beans, beetroot, broccoli, carrots, chicory, cucumber, eggplant, endive, marrow, mushrooms, okra, olives, onions, parsnips, peppers, chilies, potatoes in their skins, radishes, spinach, sweetcorn, sweet potatoes, tomatoes, turnips, watercress, zucchini.

Condiments (spices and herbs)
Many condiments are extremely high in salicylates. Those with particularly high levels include: aniseed, cayenne, celery seed, cinnamon, cumin, curry, dill, fenugreek, five-spice powder, mace, mustard, oregano, paprika, rosemary, sage, tarragon, turmeric, thyme.

Beverages
Coca-cola, coffee, tea, peppermint tea, most fruit juices and alcoholic drinks.

Cereals
Sweetcorn.

Nuts and seeds
Almonds, brazil nuts, coconut, macadamia nuts, peanuts, pine nuts, pistachio nuts, sesame seeds, walnuts, waterchestnuts.

Miscellaneous
Honey, licorice, peppermint sweets and yeast-containing produce all contain appreciable amounts of salicylates. Many processed, canned or packaged foods may be high in salicylates, due to the foods or spices used in their composition.

PISCINE-VEGAN DIET

This is a strict dietary regime which allows only vegetables, fruit and fish. It is intended for the treatment of people with serious cardiovascular disease or severe cholesterol problems. Many of its components have been observed to have beneficial effects on some of the aspects of heart disease and blood cholesterol problems.

This diet should be followed under medical supervision only. Care has been taken to ensure adequacy of many of the major dietary components, but this diet should not be considered to be perfectly balanced for all people, and appropriate supplementation or further dietary advice may be required.

EXCLUDED

All meat—beef, pork, lamb, vension and rabbit
All poultry—chicken, turkey and game
Eggs—or anything containing them
Milk, cream, butter, cheese (cows', goats' or ewes') or anything containing whey, milk solids, caseinate or lactalbumin
Animal fats—lard, suet, dripping
Use only cold-pressed sunflower, safflower or linseed oils.
Margarines—use only high-quality polyunsaturate margarine

INCLUDED

All vegetables
All fruits
All nuts and seeds
All grains—wheat, oats, barley, rye, corn, rice, millet
Other starches, including buckwheat, tapioca, sago, are also allowed
Fish: only the following are allowed—herring, mackerel, salmon, sardine and tuna. Other fish may be occasionally allowed at the discretion of the doctor
Milk substitute—soya milk, 2–4 oz per day

VEGETARIAN FOOD

It is important that vegetarian foods, e.g. rice, beans, nuts, seeds and grains, are balanced—see dietary advice for vegetarians, page 401.

FISH

About 4–6 oz of one of the fish listed is eaten per day. Smoked mackerel may be consumed occasionally (once every one or two weeks) instead of fresh mackerel. Frozen fish is acceptable and canned fish is OK once a week or so. If fish are canned, they should be in tomato sauce or olive oil, and not in any other preservative.

If you have high blood pressure, salt or salted foods, including salted fish, should be avoided.

TEA AND COFFEE

Consumption should be moderate, no greater than a total of two cups per day.

SMOKING

This should cease completely.

ALCOHOL

This can be consumed at a level of one or two drinks per day. Wine in small quantities (one or two glasses may actually be beneficial).

SUGAR AND SWEET FOODS

These should be avoided. This includes honey and foods containing sugar. Sugar substitutes, such as low-calorie sweeteners, can be used.

FOOD LISTS FOR EXCLUSION DIETS

WHEAT, OATS, BARLEY, RYE AND CORN

Many foods contain these grains. Except for corn (maize, corn on the cob), they all contain gluten, and must therefore be absolutely avoided by patients with celiac disease. People who react to wheat can sometimes tolerate oats, barley and rye, but this varies from individual to individual. Foods containing wheat, oats, barley, and rye include biscuits, all types of bread, most breakfast cereals, except cornflakes and rice cereals, cakes, ordinary flour, bran, semolina, all pasta, e.g. spaghetti and macaroni, noodles, pies, pastries, sausage rolls, some sausages, many puddings, many soups, some canned foods, stuffings, some condiments and many other foods.

Look carefully at the labels of all manufactured foods. If the following are included on the label, they should not be consumed: wheat, wheat starch, edible starch, cereal filler, cereal binder or cereal protein. It may be advisable to check with the original manufacturer to determine whether or not such foods contain wheat. Many large pharmacies stock gluten-free products.

MILK AND OTHER DAIRY PRODUCTS

Cows' milk is found in many products. People who react to milk may not react to cheese. However, cheese should be assumed to be a problem unless otherwise determined. The following foods contain cows' milk and cows' milk products—milk, cream, cheese, butter, yogurt, skimmed milk, skimmed milk powder, as well as foods including non-fat milk solids, caseinates, whey, lactalbumen, and possibly some foods containing lactose. Many margarines contain cows' milk derivatives.

Common foods that frequently contain cows' milk include bread, cakes, biscuits, malted drinks, puddings, ice cream, some sausages, thick soups, foods containing thick sauces, some beverages, chocolate. Children or adults who react to cows' milk very often also react to goats' milk and sheep's milk. However, these should be tested separately. It should not be assumed that they are safe, but they are well worth trying. Goats' and sheep's milk cheeses may be tolerated by those who are intolerant of cows' milk cheeses. Some cows' milk sensitive people may not be able to tolerate beef.

EGGS

A number of foods contain hens' eggs, particularly cakes, biscuits, puddings, batter, egg noodles and pasta, some drinks, mayonnaise, and some pre-prepared meals.

Individuals may be intolerant of egg yolk or egg white, and any foods containing these should be avoided. Lecithin should also be avoided. Curiously, some people who are intolerant of eggs can be tolerant of foods containing eggs if they are cooked. Only individual testing will determine this. Some people may also be sensitive to chicken.

YEAST

There are two different major types of yeast, brewers' yeast and bakers' yeast. Brewers' yeast is used in the fermentation of all alcoholic drinks, and thus anyone intolerant of yeast should be assumed to be intolerant of all alcoholic beverages. Filtered alcohol, however, such as gin and vodka, may be tolerated.

The following foods may contain either bakers' or brewers' yeast: all bread, including pita bread (matzos are yeast-free); any foods containing bread, e.g. bread sauce, breadcrumbs used to coat fish sticks, fish cakes and potato croquettes; some buns; cheese; yogurt; buttermilk, sour cream; synthetic cream; yeast extracts; most stock cubes; beef extract; dried fruits; malt; malted drinks; pizza; some meat products and puddings containing bread; vinegar and pickled foods; condiments containing vinegar; over-ripe or moldy fruits; grapes; mushrooms.

Many foods may become contaminated with yeasts, particularly if they are left out for any length of time in warm, moist conditions. Fruit juices (unless freshly squeezed) may contain a significant amount of yeast and should be avoided.

Many vitamin products contain yeast or yeast-derived vitamin B, and hence should be avoided. Reactions to yeast may be made worse by consuming foods that, though they are yeast-free, promote the growth of yeast, such as sugar and other refined carbohydrates. These foods should be avoided as well by those on a low-yeast diet.

SUGAR

There are many different types of sugar. Table sugar is sucrose, a composite of glucose and fructose (fruit sugar). For the most part, those who have been advised not to consume sugar will need to avoid the following foods. However, some people who are sugar sensitive will also need to limit their intake of other types of sugar, including fructose and glucose.

Foods containing sucrose: all types of sugar, golden syrup, molasses, cakes, biscuits, puddings, honey, jam, blancmange, custard, marmalade, sauces, ice cream, soft drinks, fruit squashes, some fruit juices, many packet and processed foods, some breads, fruit pies, meat pies, some fruits, including maple syrup, figs, dates, chocolate and even some drugs and medicines in the form of syrups.

Sucrose is widely distributed. Always read the label. It can be found in savory, as well as sweet-tasting foods.

CORN

Corn (maize), or sweetcorn, is a common food, and is often used in the form of corn syrup or corn starch. Many foods contain corn derivatives such as edible starch, maize oil, vegetable oil, glucose syrup or dextrose and usually these should be avoid if you are sensitive to corn.

The following foods usually, or may, contain corn: baking powders, cakes, biscuits, bottled sauces, puddings, some baked beans, cornflakes, cornflour, custard powder, margarine and vegetable oils that contain corn or maize oil, popcorn, polenta, tortillas and sweets made with corn syrup. Again, it is important to read the label carefully.

SUBSTITUTES FOR EXCLUDED FOODS

Wheat, oats, barley, rye	Potato flour, rice flour, soya flour, cornflour, buckwheat flour. Usually lesser quantities of these are required. Gluten-free products may be suitable.
Bran (wheat)	Soya bran and rice bran.
Cows' milk, etc.	Goats' milk and ewes' milk may be tolerated, or use soya milk. Almond milk may be suitable in some situations. Non-dairy powdered milk substitutes can be used. Canned, evaporated milk may also be tolerated by some people.
Butter	Polyunsaturate-based margarine.
Cows' milk cheese	Goats' or ewes' milk cheese.
Eggs	Duck eggs and other types of eggs can be tried.
Yeast	Baking powder for baking, e.g. to make soda bread.
Sugar	Artificial sweeteners, not honey.
Corn	Other flours, e.g. wheat, oats, soya, rice.
Corn oil	Sunflower seed oil, safflower seed oil, linseed oil.
Chocolate	Carob.
Tea, coffee	Herb tea, chicory.

Vinegar	Lemon juice.
Potato	Sweet potato (yams).

FOOD ADDITIVES

There are many types of food additives. Many food additives are natural, vegetable-derived compounds, or even vitamins, and are perfectly harmless. However, these are not used frequently. The following additives are the ones that can be associated with the exacerbation of certain medical problems:

Azo-dyes
Benzoates
Sulphur dioxide and sulphites
Nitrites and nitrates
Proprionic acid and propionates
Anti-oxidants, BHA & BHT
Monosodium glutamate (MSG) and related compounds

A full list of additives follows below.

ADDITIVES LIST

Curcumin
Riboflavin (lactoflavin)
Riboflavin-5′-phosphate
Tartrazine
Quinoline yellow
Yellow 2G
Sunset yellow FCF (orange yellow S)
Carmine (cochineal)
Carmoisine (azorubine)
Amaranth
Ponceau 4R (cochineal red A)
Erythrosine BS
Red 2G
Patent blue V
Indigo carmine (indigotine)
Brilliant blue FCF
Chlorophyll
Green S (acid brilliant green S or lissamine green)
Caramel
Brilliant black PN
Vegetable carbon (carbon black)
Brown FK
Chocolate brown HT
Alpha-, beta- and gamma-carotene
Annatto, bixin, norbixin
Capsanthin (capsorubin)
Lycopene
Beta-apo-8′-carotenal (C 30)
Ethyl ester of beta-apo-8′-carotenoic acid (C 30)
Flavoxanthin
Lutein
Cryptoxanthin

Additives List (continued)

Copper complexes of chlorophyll & chlorophyllins
Violaxanthin
Rhodoxanthin
Canthaxanthin
Beetroot red (betanin)
Anthocyanins
Calcium carbonate
Titanium dioxide
Iron oxides & hydroxides
Aluminum
Silver
Gold
Pigment rubine (lithol rubine BK)
Sorbic acid
Sodium sorbate
Potassium sorbate
Calcium sorbate
Benzoic acid
Sodium benzoate
Potassium benzoate
Calcium benzoate
Ethyl 4-hydroxy benzoate
Sodium ethyl 4-hydroxy benzoate
Propyl 4-hydroxy benzoate
Sodium methyl 4-hydroxy benzoate
Methyl 4-hydroxy benzoate
Sodium methyl 4-hydroxy benzoate
Sulphur dioxide
Sodium sulphite
Sodium hydrogen sulphite
Sodium metabisulphite
Potassium metabisulphite
Calcium sulphite
Calcium hydrogen sulphite
Biphenyl (diphenyl)
Orthophenylphenol (2-hydroxybiphenyl)
Sodium orthophenylphenate
Rubixanthin
Hexamethylenetetramine (hexamine)
Potassium nitrite
Sodium nitrite
Sodium nitrate
Potassium nitrate
Acetic acid
Potassium acetate
Sodium hydrogren diacetate
Sodium acetate
Calcium acetate
Lactic acid
Propionic acid
Sodium propionate
Calcium propionate
Potassium propionate
Carbon dioxide
DL-malic acid, L-malic acid
Fumaric acid
L-ascorbic acid (vitamin C)
Sodium L-ascorbate
Calcium L-ascorbate
Ascorbyl palmitate (6-0-palmitoyl-L-ascorbic acid)
Natural extracts rich in tocopherols
Synthetic alpha-tocopherol
Synthetic gamma-tocopherol
Synthetic delta-tocopherol
Propyl gallate
Octyl gallate
Dodecyl gallate
Butylated hydroxyanisole (BHA)
Butylated hydroxytoluene (BHT)
Lecithins
Sodium lactate
Potassium lactate
Calcium lactate
Citric acid
Mono-, di- and trisodium

Additives List (continued)

(sodium biphenyl-2-yl oxide)
Thiabendazole (2-thiazol-4-yl benzimidazole)
Nisin
Mono-, di- and tricalcium citrates
L-(+)-tartaric acid
Monosodium L-(+)-tartrate & disodium L-(+)-tartrate
Monopotassium L-(+)-tartrate (cream of tartar) & dipotassium L-(+)-tartrate
Potassium sodium L-(+)-tartrate
Orthophosphoric acid
citrates
Mono- and tripotassium citrates
Sodium dihydrogen orthophosphate
Disodium hydrogen orthophosphate
Trisodium orthophosphate
Potassium dihydrogen orthophosphate
Dipotassium hydrogen orthophosphate
Tripotassium orthophosphate
Calcium tetrahydrogen diorthophophate

Many food allergy associations give details of suppliers of foods suitable for people who suffer from allergies.

Many supermarkets now will provide lists of their products that are free from additives, milk, wheat, eggs, etc. For those who wish to request further details, it is suggested that you contact the customer relations department of the appropriate supermarket chain.

Bibliography

Many journals now regularly feature both review and specialist articles on nutrition. They include the *British Medical Journal,* the *Lancet,* the *New England Journal of Medicine* and the *Journal of the American Medical Association.* A useful review journal that abstracts papers on nutrition from many leading medical journals is the *International Clinical Nutrition Review.* Details are obtainable from PO Box 344, Carlingford, New South Wales, 2118, Australia. For a more detailed review journal, *Nutrition Abstracts and Reviews, Series A: Human and Experimental*—now incorporating *Reviews in Clinical Nutrition*—from Commonwealth Agriculture Bureaux, Farnham Royal, Slough, SL2 3BN, is the most comprehensive abstract publication of relevance to nutritional medicine, covering some 8,000 articles per year. It is published monthly. Also useful, *The Journal of Nutritional Medicine*. A quarterly journal of the British Society for Nutritional Medicine. Available from BSNM, PO Box 3AP, London, W1A 3AP.

INTRODUCTORY READING LIST FOR PRACTITIONERS

These references have been chosen for their information content and ease of reading to enable the busy practitioner to get into the subject.

1. Schroeder, H. A. *Trace Elements and Nutrition—Some Positive and Negative Aspects*. Faber & Faber, London, 1973, 171pp

An excellent book giving an introduction to the basic subject of trace elements and human and mammalian metabolism. It provides very good grounding for further reading.

2. Lesser, M. *Nutrition and Vitamin Therapy.* Thorsons, Wellingborough, 1985, 240pp

A highly readable book by a practicing clinician who has had many years experience in nutritional medicine. It contains some excellent references for further reading.

3. Marks, J. *A Guide to the Vitamins—Their Role in Health and Disease*. MTP, Lancaster, 1975, 208pp
Covers a lot of the basic biochemistry of the vitamins and their clinical significance.

4. Schroeder, H. A. *The Poisons Around Us*. Indiana University Press, Bloomington, 1970, 144pp
Provides the reader with interesting information about the degree to which we have contaminated our environment with certain toxic metals, and the research that has been conducted into the clinical ill-effects of such contamination.

5. Randolph, T. G. and Moss, R. W. *Allergies—Your Hidden Enemy*. Thorsons, Wellingborough, 1981, 268pp
A practical introduction to the subject of food intolerance and environmental allergy that includes case histories. Randolph has been publishing papers on the subject since 1940.

6. Wright, J. V. *Doctor Wright's Book of Nutritional Therapy*. Rodale Press, Pennsylvania, 1979, 520pp
A well-referenced book of case histories which explains the philosophy behind the nutritional medical approach, as well as providing a lot of extremely practical tips on case management.

7. Wright, J. V. *Doctor Wright's Guide to Healing with Nutrition*. Rodale Press, Pennsylvania, 1984, 603pp
Another well-referenced compendium of case histories and discussions providing further useful tips.

8. Wright, J. V. and Gaby, A. *Clinical Applications of Nutritional Biochemistry*. Eighteen-hour taped lecture course from 6931 Fieldcrest Road, Baltimore MD 21215.
Comes with a well-classified set of 1400 references, of which some 350 are abstracted. The most comprehensive training course in nutritional medicine to date which gives excellent access to the literature in a readily assimilable fashion and also provides a wealth of practical tips.

9. Goodhart, R. S. and Shils, M. E. *Modern Nutrition in Health and Disease*. 6th edn. Lea & Febiger, Philadelphia, 1980, 1370pp
The definitive reference book. Multi-authored, it is an invaluable standby.

10. Bland, J. (ed.) *Yearbook of Nutritional Medicine 1984–85*. Keats, New Canaan, Connecticut, 1985, 325pp
Covers a wide range of important aspects of nutritional medicine

in an academic fashion. Well presented, well referenced and highly informative.

11. British Society for Nutritional Medicine, PO Box 3AP, London W1A 3AP.
A society for medical doctors which provides an educational forum for nutritional medicine.

SUBJECT READING LIST

Note

An asterisk next to a reference means that it is suitable for non-medical people as well as doctors and researchers.

INTRODUCTION

1. *Proposals for Nutritional Guidelines for Health Education in Britain,* prepared for the National Advisory Committee on Nutrition Education (NACNE). Health Education Council, London, Sept 1983

2. Cheraskin, E., Ringsdorf, W. M. and Clark, J. W. *Diet and Disease*. Keats, Connecticut, 1968

3. Mount, J. L. *The Food and Health of Western Man*. Charles Knight & Co. Ltd. London & Tonbridge, 1975

*4. Ballentine, R. *Diet and Nutrition—A Holistic Approach*. Himalayan International Institute, Honesdale, Pennsylvania, 1978

5. Rose, J. *Nutrition and Killer Diseases*. Noyes, New Jersey, 1982

*6. Walker, C. and Cannon, G. *The Food Scandal*. 2nd edn. Century, London, 1985

7. Marvon-Davis, A. and Thomas, J. *Diet 2000*. Pan Books, London, 1984

Recommended Daily Allowances

1. *Recommended Intakes of Nutrients for the United Kingdom*. DHSS report on public health and medical subjects No. 120, HMSO, London, 1969

2. *Recommended Daily Amounts of Food Energy and Nutrients for Groups of People in the United Kingdom*. DHSS report on health and social subjects No. 15, HMSO, London, 1979

3. *Recommended Dietary Allowances*. 9th edn. Committee on Dietary Allowances, Food and Nutrition Board, National Research Council, National Academy of Sciences, Washington DC, 1980

4. Trusswell, A. S. "Recommended dietary intakes—introduction," *Nutrition Abstracts and Reviews in Clinical Nutrition Series A*, 53:11 (1983), 940–7

5. Shorland, F. B. "Do recommended daily dietary allowances stand up to scrutiny?" *Nutrition and Health*, 2 (1983), 105–9

Vitamins

1. McLaren, D. S. *Nutrition and Its Disorders*. Churchill Livingstone, London, 1981

2. Ministry of Agriculture, Fisheries and Food. *Manual of Nutrition*. HMSO, London, 1976

3. Goodhart, R. S. and Shils, M. E. *Modern Nutrition in Health and Disease*. 6th edn. Lea & Febiger, Philadelphia, 1980

4. McLaren, D. S. "Vitamins and trace elements" in D. J. Weatherall, J. G. G. Ledingham and D. A. Warrell (eds.) *Textbook of Medicine*. OUP, Oxford, 1983

5. Marks, J. *A Guide to the Vitamins—Their Role in Health and Disease* MTP Press, Lancaster, 1979

*6. Wright, J. V. *Dr. Wright's Book of Nutritional Therapy*. Rodale Press, Pennsylvania, 1979

*7. Wright, J. V. *Dr. Wright's Guide to Healing With Nutrition*. Rodale Press, Pennsylvania, 1984

*8. Davies, A. *Let's Get Well*. Unwin Books, London, 1966

9. Diplock, A. T. *Fat-Soluble Vitamins*. Heinemann, London, 1985

*10. Gaby, A. *A Doctor's Guide to Vitamin B6*. Rodale Press, Pennsylvania, 1984

11. Horwitt, M. K. *Vitamin E—Abstracts for Health Professionals*. Henkel Corporation, USA

*12. Cheraskin, E., Ringsdorf, W. M. and Sisley, E. L. *The Vitamin C Connection*. Harper and Row, New York, 1983

13. Counsell, J. N. and Hornig, D. H. *Vitamin C. Ascorbic Acid*. Applied Science Publishers, London, 1981

14. Brozek, J. "Psychological effects of thiamin restriction and deprivation in normal young men," *American Journal of Clinical Nutrition,* 5 (1951), 109–20

15. Carney, M. W. P., Williams, D. G. and Sheffield, B. F. "Thiamin and pyridoxine status in newly admitted psychiatric patients," *Brit. J. Psychiat.* 135 (1979), 249–54

16. Goodwin, J. S., Goodwin, J. M. and Garry, P. J. "Association between nutritional status and cognitive function in a healthy elderly population," *JAMA,* 249 (1983), 2917–21

17. Hills, O. W., Liebert, E., Steinberg, D. L. and Horwitt, M. K. "Clinical aspects of dietary depletion of riboflavin," *AMA Archives Int. Med. 87* (1951), 682–93

18. Kawai, C. *et al.* "Reappearance of beri beri heart disease in Japan," *American Journal of Medicine,* 69 (1980), 383–6

19. Lonsdale, D. and Shamberger, R. J. "Red cell transketolase as an indicator of nutritional deficiency," *American Journal of Clinical Nutrition,* 33 (1980), 205–11

20. Rivlin, R. "Riboflavin metabolism," *NEJM,* 283 (1970), 463–72

21. Stannus, H. S. "The problems in riboflavin and allied deficiencies," *BMJ,* 2 (1944), 103–5 and 140–4

22. Sishii, M. and Nishiharra, Y. "Pellagra among chronic alcoholics: clinical and pathological study in twenty necropsy cases," *Journal of Neurology, Neurosurgery and Psychiatry,* 44 (1981), 209–15

23. General Practitioner's Research Group, "Calcium pantothenate in arthritis conditions," *Practitioner,* 224 (1980), 208–10

24. Ellis, J. M. *et al.* "Response of vitamin B6 deficiency and the carpal tunnel syndrome to pyridoxine," *Proc. Natl. Acad. Sci.* USA 79 (1982), 7494–8

25. Whitehead, N., Reyner, F. and Lindenbaum, J. "Megaloblastic changes in the cervical epithelium—associated with oral contraceptive therapy and reversal with folic acid," *JAMA,* 226 (1973), 1421–4

26. Ellis, F. R. and Nasser, S. "A pilot study of vitamin B12 in the treatment of tiredness," *Br. J. Nutr.,* 30 (1973), 277–83

27. Matthews, D. M. and Linnell, J. C. "Vitamin B12: an area of darkness," *BMJ,* 2 (1979), 533–5

28. "Vitamin B12," *Merck Service Bulletin,* Merck & Co. (Merck, Sharp and Dohme), Rahway, New Jersey, 1958

29. Milner, G. "Ascorbic acid in chronic psychiatric patients —a controlled trial," *Brit. J. Psychiat.,* 109 (1963), 294–9

30. Acheson, R. M. and Williams, D. R. R. "Does consumption of fruit and vegetables protect against stroke?" *Lancet,* i (1983), 1191–3

31. Cox, B. D. and Butterfield, W. J. H. "Vitamin C supplements and diabetic cutaneous capillary fragility," *BMJ,* 2 (1975), 205

32. Wassertheil-Smoller, S. *et al.* "Dietary vitamins C and uterine cervical dysplasia," *American Journal of Epidemiology,* 114 (1981), 714–24

33. Editorial. "Vitamin C, disease and surgical trauma," *BMJ,* 1 (1979), 437

34. Karlowski, T. R. *et al.* "Ascorbic acid for the common cold: a prophylactic therapeutic trial," *JAMA,* 231 (1975), 1038–42

35. Cooke, W. T., Swan, C. H. J., Asquith, P., Melikian, V. and McFeely, W. E. "Serum alkaline phosphatase and rickets in urban school children," *BMJ,* 1 (1973), 324–7

36. Cooke, W. T., Asquith, P., Ruck, N. D., Melikian, V. and Swan, C. H. J. "Rickets, growth, and alkaline phosphatase in urban adolescents," *BMJ,* 1 (1974), 293–7

37. Brooke, O. G. "Supplementary vitamin D in infancy in childhood," *Archives of Disease in Childhood,* 58 (1983), 573–4

38. Brooke, O. "Vitamin D supplements in pregnancy," *Journal of Maternal and Child Health,* 1 (1981), 18–20

39. Ellis, G., Woodhead, J. S. and Cooke, W. T. "Serum-25-hydroxyvitamin-D concentrations in adolescent boys," *Lancet,* i (1977), 825–8

40. Christiansen, C., Rodbro, P. and Lund, M. "Incidence of anti-convulsant osteomalacia and effects of vitamin D: controlled therapeutic trial," *BMJ,* 4 (1973), 695–701

41. Clements, M. R., Chalmers, T. M. and Fraser, D. R. "Enterohepatic circulation of vitamin D: a reappraisal of the hypothesis," *Lancet,* i (1984), 1376–9

42. Bieri, J. G. "Medical uses of vitamin E," *NEJM,* 308 (1983), 1063–71

43. Chiswick, M. L. *et al.* "Protective effect of vitamin E (DL-alpha-tocopherol) against intraventricular haemorrhage in premature babies," *BMJ,* 2 (1983), 81–4

44. Schnare, D. W., Denk, G., Shields, M. and Brunton, S. "The valuation of detoxification regime for the fat-stored xenobiotics," *Medical Hypotheses,* 9 (1982), 265–82

45. Peto, R., Doll, R., Buckley, J. D. and Spoond, M. D. "Can dietary beta-carotene naturally reduce cancer rates?" *Nature,* 290 (1980), 201–8

Minerals

GENERAL REVIEWS

1. Goodhart, R. S. and Shils, M. E. *Modern Nutrition in Health and Disease*. 6th edn. Lea & Febiger, Philadelphia, 1980

*2. Schroeder, H. A. *The Trace Elements and Nutrition in Man: Some Positive and Negative Aspects*. Faber & Faber, London, 1973

*3. Pfeiffer, C. C. *Zinc and other Micronutrients*. Keats, Connecticut, 1978

4. Underwood, E. J. *Trace Elements in Human and Animal Nutrition*. 4th edn. Academic Press, London, 1977

5. Prasad, A. S. *Trace Elements and Iron in Human Metabolism*. John Wiley & Sons, Chichester, 1978

6. Passwater, R. A. and Cranton, E. M. *Trace Elements, Hair Analysis and Nutrition*. Keats, New Canaan, Connecticut, 1983

7. Seelig, Mildred S. *Magnesium Deficiency in the Pathogenesis of Disease*. Plenum Publishing, New York, 1980

8. Taylor, A. "Trace elements in human disease," *Clinics in Endocrinology and Metabolism,*14:3, (Aug. 1985), W. B. Saunders and Co., Eastbourne

9. Prasad, A. S. "Clinical, biochemical and nutritional aspects of trace elements," *Current Topics in Nutrition and Disease,* Vol. 6. Alan R. Liss, New York, 1982

10. Solomons, N. W. and Rosenberg, I. H. "Absorption and malabsorption of mineral nutrients," *Current Topics in Nutrition and Disease,* Vol. 12. Alan R. Liss, New York, 1984

PAPERS

11. Singh, R. B. and Cameron, A. E. "Relation of myocardial magnesium deficiency to sudden death in ischaemic heart disease," *American Heart Journal* 103:3 (1982), 449–50

12. Juan, D. "Clinical review: the clinical importance of hypomagnesemia," *Surgery,* 91:5 (1982), 510–17

13. Oski, F. A. "Non-haematological manifestations of iron deficiency," *Am. J. Dis. Child,* 133 (1979), 315–22

14. Juswigg, T., Batres, R. and Solomons, N. W. *et al*. "The effect of temporary venous occlusion on trace mineral concentrations in plasma," *Am. J. Clin. Nutr.,* 36 (1982), 354–8

15. Barber, S. A., Bull, N. L. and Buss, B. H. "Low iron intakes among young women in Britain," *BMJ,* 290 (1985), 743–4

16. Pollitt, E. and Leibel, R. L. *Iron Deficiency: Brain Biochemistry and Behaviour,* Raven Press, New York, 1982

17. Morck, T. A., Lynch, S. R. and Cook, J. D. "Inhibition of food iron absorption by coffee," *Am. J. Clin. Nutr.,* 37 (1983), 416–20

18. Disler, P. B., Lynch, S. R. and Charlton, R. W. *et al.* "The effects of tea on iron absorption," *Gut,* 16 (1975), 193–200

19. Simpson, K. M., Morris, E. R. and Cook, J. D. "The inhibitory effect of bran on iron absorption in man," *Am. J. Clin. Nutr.,* 34 (1981), 1469–78

20. Lingam, S. "Severe nutritional iron deficiency and behaviour disorder in an infant," *J. Human Nutr.,* 34 (1980), 41–2

21. Oski, F. A. and Honig, A. S. "The effects of therapy on developmental scores of iron-deficient infants," *J. Paediatrics,* 92:1 (1978), 21–5

22. Hambidge, K. M., Krebs, N. F. and Jacobs, M. A., *et al.* "Zinc nutritional status during pregnancy: a longitudinal study," *Am. J. Clin. Nutr.,* 37 (1983), 429–42

23. Davies, S. "Zinc, nutrition and health—a review," in J. Bland (ed.), *Yearbook of Nutritional Medicine 1984–85* pp. 112–52. Keats, New Canaan, Connecticut, 1985

24. Davies, S. "Effects of oral zinc supplementation on serum, hair and sweat zinc levels in seven subjects," *Science of Total Environment,* 42 (1985), 45–8

25. Davies, S. "Assessment of zinc status," *International Clinical Nutrition Review 1984,* (June), PO Box 344 Carlingford, NSW 2218, Australia

26. Breskin, M. W. *et al.,* "First trimester serum zinc concentrations in human pregnancy," *Am. J. Clin. Nutr.,* 38 (1983), 943–53

27. Jameson, S. *Effects of Zinc Deficiency in Human Reproduction.* Linkoping University Medical Dissertations No. 37, Linkoping University, 1976 (also published as supplement 593 to *Acta Medica Scandinavica*)

28. Beach, R. S., Gershwin, M. E. and Hurley, L. S. "Persistent immunological consequences of gestation zinc deprivation," *Am. J. Clin. Nutr.,* 38 (1983), 579–90

29. Meadows, N. J. *et al.* "Zinc and Small Babies," *Lancet,* ii (1981), 135–7

30. Golub, M. S., Gershwin, M. E., Hurley, L. S. *et al.* "Studies of marginal zinc deprivation in rhesus monkeys II pregnancy outcome," *Am. J. Clin. Nutr.,* 39 (1984), 879–87

31. Golub, M.S., Gershwin, M. E., Hurley, L. S. *et al.* "Studies of marginal zinc deprivation in rhesus monkeys: infant behaviour," *Am. J. Clin. Nutr.*, 42 (1985), 1229–39

32. Burnet, F.M. "A posible role of zinc in the pathology of dementia," *Lancet,* i (1981), 186–8

33. Sorenson, J. R. J., Oberley, L. W., Crouch, R. K. *et al.* "Pharmacologic activities of copper compounds in chronic diseases," *Biological Trace Element Research,* 5 (1983), 257–73

34. Pfeiffer, C. C. and Iliev, V. "A study of zinc deficiency and copper excess in schizophrenics" *International Review of Neurobiology,* Supplement 1, (1972), pp. 141–65. Academic Press, New York

35. Walker, W. R. "The results of a copper bracelet clinical trial and subsequent studies," in J. R. J. Sorenson (ed.), *Inflammatory Diseases and Copper,* pp. 469–82. The Humana Press, 1982

36. Klevay, L. M. "Copper and ischaemic heart disease," *Biological Trace Element Research,* 5 (1983), 245–55

37. Klevay, L. M. "Interactions of copper and zinc in cardiovascular disease," *Annals of the New York Academy of Sciences,* 355 (1980), 140–51

38. Klevay, L. M., Inhyg, S. D., Reck, S. J. and Barcome, D. F. "Evidence of dietary zinc and copper deficiencies," *JAMA,* 241:18 (1979), 1916–18

39. Hambidge, K. M. "Chromium—a review" in F. Bronner, and J. D. Coburn (eds.), *Disorders of Mineral Metabolism, Vol. 1: Trace Minerals,* pp. 272–94. Academic Press, London, 1981

40. Boyle, E., Mondschein, B. and Dash, H. H. "Chromium depletion in the pathogenesis of diabetes and atherosclerosis—a review," *Southern Medical Journal,* 70:12 (1977), 1449–53

41. McCarthy, M. F. "The therapeutic potential of glucose tolerance factor," *Medical Hypotheses,* 6 (1980), 1177–89

42. Riales, R. and Albrink, M. J. "Effect of chromium chloride supplementation on glucose tolerance and serum lipids including high-density lipoprotein of adult men," *Am. J. Clin. Nutr.,* 34 (1981), 2670–8

43. Offenbacher, E. G. and Pi-Sunyer, F. X. "Beneficial effect of chromium-rich yeast on glucose tolerance and blood lipids in elderly subjects," *Diabetes,* 29 (1980), 919–25

44. Mertz, W. "Clinical and public health significance of chromium" in *Clinical Biochemical and Nutritional Aspects of Trace Elements,* pp. 315-23. Alan R. Liss, New York, 1982.

45. Mertz, W. "Chromium deficiency and its effects on diabetes," *Practical Cardiology,* 8:9 (1982), 145–56

46. Hurley, L. S. "Clinical and experimental aspects of manganese in nutrition," in A. Prasad (ed.), *Clinical Biochemical and Nutritional Aspects of Trace Elements*, pp. 369–78. Allen R. Liss, New York, 1982

*47. Passwater, R. A. *Selenium as Food and Medicine*. Keats, Connecticut, 1980, 240pp

48. Passwater, R. A. and Cranton, E. M. *Trace Elements, Hair Analysis and Nutrition*, pp. 200–8. Keats, New Canaan, Connecticut, 1983

49. Dutta, S. K., Miller, P. A., Greenberg, L. B. and Levander, O. A. "Selenium and acute alcoholism," *Am. J. Clin. Nutr.*, 38 (1983), 713–18

50. Miettinen, T. A. *et al*. "Serum selenium concentration related to myocardial infarction and fatty acid content of serum lipids," *BMJ*, 287 (1983), 517–19

51. Salonen, J. K. *et al*. "Association between cardiovascular death and myocardial infarction and serum selenium in a matched pair longitudinal study," *Lancet*, ii (1982), 175–9

52. Editorial. "Selenium in the heart of China," *Lancet*, ii (1979), 889–90

53. Chen, X. S. "Selenium and Keshan disease," *Ann. New York Acad. Sci.*, 393 (1982), 224–5

54. Schrauzer, G. N. "Selenium and cancer: a review," *Bioinorganic Chemistry*, 5 (1976), 275–81

55. Willett, W. C. *et al*. "Pre-diagnostic serum selenium and risk of cancer," *Lancet*, ii (1983), 130–4

56. Levine, S. A. and Parker, J. "Selenium and human chemical hypersensitivities: preliminary findings," *Int. J. Biosocial Res.*, 3 (1982), 44–7

57. Nielsen, F. H. "Possible future implications of nickel, arsenic, silicon, vanadium and other ultra trace elements in human nutrition" in A. S. Prasad (ed.), *Clinical Biochemical and Nutritional Aspects of Trace Elements*, pp. 379–404. Alan R. Liss, New York, 1982

58. Cox, M. and Singer, I. "Lithium—a review" in F. Bronner and J. W. Coburn (eds.), *Disorders of Mineral Metabolism, Vol. 1., Trace Minerals*, pp. 370–439. Academic Press, 1981

59. Hodge, H. C. and Smith, F. A. "Fluoride—a review" in F. Bronner and J. W. Coburn (eds.), *Disorders of Mineral Metabolism, Vol., 1, Trace Minerals*, pp. 440–84. Academic Press, 1981

*60. Waldbott, G. L. *Fluoridation: The Great Dilemma*. Coronado Press, Kansas, 1978, 423pp

*61. Bryce-Smith, D. Hodgkinson *The Zinc Solution*. Century Arrow London, 1986

Toxic Metals

GENERAL REVIEWS

*1. Schroeder, H. A. *Poisons Around Us*. Indiana University Press, 1974

2. Goyer, R. A. and Mehlman, M. A. *Toxicology of Trace Elements. John Wiley & Sons,* Chichester, 1977

3. Davies, S. "Lead and disease," *Nutrition and Health,* 2:3/4 (1983), 135–45

4. Rutter, M. and Russell-Jones, R. (eds.) *Lead versus Health—Sources and Effects of Low-Level Lead Exposure*. John Wiley & Sons, Chichester, 1983

5. Prasad, A. S. *Trace Elements and Iron in Human Metabolism*. John Wiley & Sons, Chichester, 1978

6. *Lead or Health—A Review by the Conservation Society Pollution Working Party.* 2nd ed. 68 Dora Road, London, SW19. 1980

7. *Lead in the Human Environment—A Report Prepared by the Committee on Lead in the Human Environment*. National Research Council, National Academy of Sciences, Washington, DC. 1980

BOOKS AND PAPERS

8. Batuman, V. "The role of lead and gout nephropathy," *New England J. Med.,* 304:9 (1981), 520–3

9. Shaper, A. G., Pacock, S. J., Walker, M. *et al*. "Effects of alcohol and smoking on blood lead in middle-aged British men," *BMJ,* 284 (1982), 299–302

10. Wynn, M. and Wynn, A. *Lead and Human Reproduction*. Clear Charitable Trust, 2 Northdown Street, London N1 9BG. 1982

11. Nixon, G. S., Whittle, C. A. and Woodfin, A. "Mercury levels in dental surgeries and dental personnel," *Brit. Dent. J.,* 151 (1981), 149–54

12. Jones, D. E. "Mercury—a review of the literature," *Brit. Dent. J.,* 151 (1981), 145–8

13. Stortebecker, P. *Mercury Poisoning from Dental Amalgam—A Hazard to the Human Brain*. Stortebecker Foundation for Research, Akerbyvagen 282, S-18335 Taby, Stockholm, Sweden, 220pp

14. Ziff, S. *The Toxic Timebomb—Can the Mercury in your Dental Fillings Poison You?* Thorsons, Wellingborough, 1984

15. Shapiro, I. M., Sumner, A. J., Spitz, L. K. *et al.* "Neurophysiological and neuropsychological function in mercury-exposed dentists," *Lancet,* i (1982), 1147–50

16. Glauser, S. C., Glauser, E. M. and Bello, C. T. "Blood cadmium levels in normotensive and untreated hypertensive humans," *Lancet,* i (1976), 717–18

17. Voors, A. W., Johnson, W. D. and Shuman, M. S. "Additive statistical effects of cadmium and lead on heart-related disease in a North Carolina autopsy series," *Arch. Environmental Health,* 37:2 (1982), 98–102

18. Khera, K., Wibberley, D. G., Edwards, K. W. and Waldron, H. A. "Cadmium and lead levels in blood and urine in a series of cardiovascular and normotensive patients," *Intern J. Environmental Studies,* 14 (1980), 309–12

19. Huel, G., Boudene, Claude C. and Ibrahim, M. A. "Cadmium and lead content of maternal and newborn hair: relationship to parity, birthweight and hypertension," *Arch. Environmental Health,* 36:5 (1981), 221–5

20. Spivey Fox, M. R. and Fry, B. E. "Cadmium toxicity decreased by dietary ascorbic acid supplements," *Science,* 169 (1970), 989–91

21. Passwater, R. A. and Cranton, E. M. "Aluminium—A Review" in *Trace Elements Hair Analysis and Nutrition,* pp. 281–6. Keats, New Canaan, Connecticut, 1983

Proteins and Amino Acids

1. Bender, D. A. *Amino Acid Metabolism.* 2nd edn. J. Wiley & Sons, Chichester, 1985

*2. Chaitow, L. *Amino Acids.* Thorsons, Wellingborough, 1985

*3. Lappe, F. M. *Diet for a Small Planet.* Ballantine Books, New York, 1984

4. Munro, H. N. and Crim, M. C. "The proteins and amino acids" in R. S. Goodhart and M. E. Shils (eds.), *Modern Nutrition in Health and Disease.* 6th edn. pp. 51–98. Lea & Febiger, Philadelphia, 1980

5. Bremer, H. J. *et al. Disturbances of Amino Acid Metabolism: Clinical Chemistry and Diagnosis.* Urban & Schwarzenberg, Baltimore–Munich, 1981

6. Azuma, J. *et al.* "Taurine for treatment of congestive heart failure," *Int. J. Cardiol.,* 2 (1982), 303

7. Madan, B. R. and Khanna, N. K. "Anti-inflammatory activity of L-tryptophan and DL-tryptophan," *Indian J. Med. Res.*, 68 (1978), 708

8. Thomson, J., Rankin, H., Ashcroft, G. W. *et al.* "The treatment of depression in general practice; a comparison of L-tryptophan, amitriptyline, and a combination of L-tryptophan and amitriptyline with placebo," *Psychol. Med.*, 12 (1982), 741

9. Gelenberg, A. J., Wojcik, J. D., Growdon, J. H. *et al.* "Tyrosine treatment of depression," *Am. J. Psychiat.*, 137 (1980), 622

10. Griffith, R. S., De Jong, D. C. and Nelson, J. D. "Relation of arginine–lysine antagonism to herpes simplex growth in tissue culture," *Chemotherapy,* 27 (1981), 209

11. Griffith, R. S., Norins, A. L. and Kagan, C. "A multicentered study of lysine therapy in herpes simplex infection," *Dermatologica,* 156 (1978), 257

12. Jungling, M. L. and Bunger, G. "The treatment of spermatogenic arrest with arginine," *Fert. Ster.* 27 (1976), 282

Essential Fatty Acids

*1. Graham, J. *Evening Primrose Oil.* Thorsons, Wellingborough, 1984

2. Horrobin, D. E. (ed.) *Clinical Uses of Essential Fatty Acids.* Eden Press, Montreal, 1982

3. Davies, S. and Stewart, A. (eds.) *Essential Fatty Acids in Clinical Medicine.* Conference Proceedings, John Wiley & Sons, Chichester, 1987

4. Horrobin, D. F. "Gamma-linolenic acid in medicine" in J. Bland (ed.) *Yearbook of Nutritional Medicine 1984–85,* pp. 23–36. Keats, New Canaan, Connecticut, 1985

5. Rudin, D. O. "Omega-III essential fatty acids in medicine" in J. Bland (ed.) *Yearbook of Nutritional Medicine 1984–85,* pp. 37–54. Keats, New Canaan, Connecticut, 1985

6. Durie, B. (ed.) "Second MaxEPA research conference," *Brit. J. of Clinical Practice,* 38:5 (1984), Symposium Supplement 31, pp. 1–130

Sugar and Carbohydrates

*1. Yudkin, J. *Pure, White and Deadly—A Problem of Sugar.* 2nd edn. Viking, London, 1987

2. Ringsdorf, W. M., Cheraskin, E. and Ramsay, R. R. "Sucrose, neutrophilic phagocytosis and resistance to disease," *Dental Survey,* (1976), 46–8

3. Yudkin, J. "Sugar and disease," *Nature*, 239 (1972), 197–9

4. Cleave, T. L. *The Saccharine Disease*. Wright, Bristol, 1974

5. Gray, G. M. and Fogel, M. R. "Nutritional aspects of dietary carbohydrates" in R. S. Goodhart and M. E. Shils (eds.) *Modern Nutrition in Health and Disease*, 6th edn, pp. 99–112. Lea & Febiger, Philadelphia, 1980

Dietary Fiber

*1. Stanway, A. *Taking the Rough with the Smooth*. Pan Books, London, 1981

2. Royal College of Physicians, *Medical Aspects of Dietary Fibre*. Pitman Medical, 1980

*3. Cleave, T. L. *The Saccharine Disease*. Wright, Bristol, 1974

4. Simpson, K. M., Morris, E. R. and Cook, J. D. "The inhibitory effect of bran on iron absorption in man," *Am. J. Clin. Nutr.*, 34 (1981), 1469–78

*5. Kenton, L. and Kenton, S. *Raw Energy*. Century, London, 1984

6. See also "Wheat, Cows' Milk and Eggs" references.

Wheat, Cows' Milk and Eggs

1. Freed, D. L. J. *Health Hazards of Milk*. Baillière Tindall, London, 1984

*2. Oski, R. A. *Don't Drink your Milk!* Molica Press Ltd., Syracuse, 1983

3. Buisseret, P. D. "Common manifestations of cows' milk allergy in children," *Lancet*, ii (1978), 304–5

4. Jacobson, I. and Lindberg, T. "Cows' milk as a cause of infantile colic in breast-fed infants," *Lancet*, ii (1978), 437–9

5. Corry, D. C. "Milk in diverticula of colon," *BMJ* (6 April 1963), 929–30

6. Sandberg, D. H., Bernstein, C. W., Strauss, J. *et al.* "Severe steroid-responsive nephrosis associated with hypersensitivity," *Lancet*, ii (1977), 388–91

7. Lucas, A., McLaughlan, P. and Coombs, R. R. A. "Latent anaphylactic sensitization of infants of low birth weight to cows' milk proteins," *BMJ*, 289 (1984), 1254–6

8. Paganelli, R., Atherton, D. J. and Levinski, R. J. "Differences between normal and milk allergic subjects in their immune

responses after milk ingestion," *Archives of Diseases in Childhood,* 58 (1983), 201–6

9. Egger, J., Carter, C. M., Wilson, J. *et al.* "Is migraine food allergy?" *Lancet,* ii (1983), 865–9

10. Minford, A. M. B., MacDonald, A. and Littlewood, J. M. "Food intolerance and food allergy in children: a review of sixty-eight cases," *Archives of Disease in Childhood,* 57 (1982), 742–7

11. Alun Jones, V., Shorthouse, M., McLaughlan *et al.* "Food intolerance: a major factor in the pathogenesis of irritable bowel syndrome," *Lancet,* ii (1982), 1115–17

12. Rowe, A. H., Rowe, A. and Young, E. J. "Bronchial asthma due to food allergy alone in ninety-five patients," *JAMA,* 169:1 (1953), 1158–62

13. See also "Food Allergy" references.

Tea and Coffee

1. Bolton, S. and Null, G. "Caffeine: psychological effects, use and abuse," *J. Orthomol. Psychiat.,* 10:3 (1981), 202–11

*2. Greden, J. F. "Coffee, tea and you," *Sciences,* (January 1979)

3. Greden, J. F. "The tea controversy in colonial America," *JAMA,* 236:1 (1976), 63–6

4. Ruenwongsa, P. and Pattanavibag, S. "Decrease in the activities of thiamin pyrophosphate-dependent enzymes in rat brain after prolonged tea consumption," *Nutrition Reports International,* 27:4 (1983), 713

5. Victor, B. S., Greden, J. F. and Lubetsky M. "Somatic manifestations of caffeinism," *J. Clin. Psychiat.,* 42:5 (1981), 185–8

6. Greden, J. F., Fontaine, R., Lubetsky, M. and Chamberlin, K. "Anxiety and depression associated with caffeinism among psychiatric in-patients," *Am. J. Psychiatry,* 135:8 (1978), 963–6

7. Greden, J. F., Victor, B. S. Fontaine, P. and Lubetsky, M. "Caffeine-withdrawal headache: a clinical profile," *Psychosomatics,* 21:5 (1980), 411–18

8. Greden, J. F. "Anxiety or caffeinism: a diagnostic dilemma," *Am. J. Psychiatry,* 131:10 (1974), 1089–92

9. Borgman, R. F. and Peller, H. J. "Relationship of nutrition, caffeine consumption and cigarette smoking in problem drinkers: a prospective study in South Carolina," *J. S. Carolina Med. Assoc.,* (August, 1982) 426–30

10. Sagnella, G. A., MacGregor, G. A. "Characteristics of a Na-K-ATPase inhibitor in extracts of tea," *Am. J. Clin. Nutr.*, 40 (1984), 36–41

11. Morck, T. A., Lynch, S. R. and Cook, J. D. "Inhibition of food iron absorption by coffee," *Am. J. Clin. Nutr.*, 37 (1983), 416–20

12. Disler, P. B., Lynch, S. R., Charlton, R. W., *et al.* "The effect of tea on iron absorption," *Gut*, 16 (1975), 193–200

13. Solomons, N. W. and Cousins, R. J. "Inhibitors of zinc absorption (coffee)" in N. W. Solomons and I. H. Rosenberg (eds.) *Absorption and Malabsorption of Mineral Nutrients*, 161p. Alan R. Liss, New York, 1984

Alcohol, Smoking and Tranquilizers

1. Royal College of Physicians, *Smoking or Health*. Pitmans Medical, London, 1977

2. Royal College of Physicians, *Health or Smoking*. Pitmans Medical, London, 1983

3. Symposium Report, *Alcohol and Child Development*. Institute of Alcohol Studies, 12 Caxton Street, London SW1, 1983

4. Thomson, A. D. "Alcohol and nutrition," *Clinics and Endocrinology and Metabolism*, 7 (1978), 405–28

5. Glen, A. I. M., Glen, E. M. T., MacDonnell, L. E. F. and Skinner, F. K. "Essential fatty acids and alcoholism" in S. Davies and A. Stewart (eds.) *Essential Fatty Acids in Clinical Medicine*, proceedings of the fifth conference of the British Society for Nutritional Medicine. John Wiley & Sons, Chichester, 1987

*6. Stoppard, M. *Quit Smoking*. Ariel Books, BBC, London, 1982

*7. Trickett, S. *Coming off Tranquillizers*. Thorsons, 1986

Drug-Nutrient Interactions

1. Roe, D. A. *Drug-Induced Nutritional Deficiencies*. AVI Publishing Co. Inc., Westport, Connecticut, 1976

2. Krauser, M. B. and Mahan, L. V. "The interaction between drugs, nutrients and nutritional status," *Food, Nutrition and Diet Therapy*, pp. 452–65. W. B. Saunders, Philadelphia, 1979

3. Garrison, R. H. "Drug-nutrient interaction," in J. Bland (ed.) *Yearbook of Nutritional Medicine 1984–85*, pp. 93–112. Keats, New Canaan, Connecticut, 1985

Free Radicals and Lipid Peroxidation

1. Levine, S. A. and Kidd, P. M. *Anti-oxidant adaptation—its role in free radical pathology,* Biocurrents Division, Allergy Research Group, 400 Preda Street, San Leandros, California 94577. 1985

2. Bland, J. "Anti-oxidants in nutritional medicine" in J. Bland (ed.) *Yearbook of Nutritional Medicine 1984–85,* pp. 213–38. Keats, Connecticut, 1985

*3. Kenton, L. *Ageless Ageing*. Century, London, 1986

4. Levine, S. A. and Kidd P. M. "Anti-oxidant adaptation: a unified disease theory," *J. Orthomol. Psychiat.*, 14:1 (1985), 19–38

5. Florence, T. M. "Cancer and ageing: the free radical connection," *Int. Clin. Nut. Rev.,* 4:1 (1984), 6–19

6. Cranton, E. M. and Frackelton, J. P. "Free radical pathology in age-associated diseases: treatment with EDTA chelation, nutrition and anti-oxidants," *J. Holistic Medicine,* 1:6 (spring/summer 1984)

7. Dormandy, T. L. "An approach to free radicals," *Lancet,* ii (1983), 1010–14

Environmental Poisons

*1. Schroeder, H. A. *The Poisons Around Us*. Indiana University Press, London, 1974

2. Vander, A. J. *Nutrition, Stress and Toxic Chemicals*. University of Michigan Press, Ann Arbor, 1981

*3. Ottoboni, M. A. *The Dose Makes the Poison—A Plain-Language Guide to Toxicology.* Vincente Books, Berkeley, California, 1984

*4. Makower, J. *Office Hazards*. Tilden Press, Washington DC, 1981

*5. Zamm, A. V. and Gannon, R. *Why Your House May Endanger Your Health*. Simon & Schuster, New York, 1980

6. Calabrese, E. J. *Nutrition and Environmental Health: The Influence of Nutritional Status on Pollutant Toxicity and Carcinogenicity,* Vol.1, *The Vitamins*. John Wiley & Sons, Chichester, 1980.

7. Calabrese, E. J. *Nutrition and Environmental Toxicity: The Influence of Nutritional Status on Pollutant Toxicity and Carcinogenicity,* Vol. 2, *Minerals and Macronutrients*. John Wiley & Sons, Chichester, 1981

8. DHSS. *Pesticide Poisoning—Notes for the Guidance of Medical Practitioners*. HMSO, London, 1983

9. *Report of the Working Party on Pesticide Residues 1977–1981*. The ninth report of the steering group on food surveillance. HMSO, 1982

10. Waldbott, G. L. *Health Effects of Environmental Pollutants*. 2nd edn. C. V. Mosby Co., St. Louis, 1978

Food Allergy

GENERAL REVIEWS

1. Joint report of the Royal College of Physicians and the British Nutrition Foundation (1984). "Food intolerance and food aversion." *J. Roy. Coll. Phys. Lond.*, 18:2 (April 1984), 2

2. *Adverse Reactions to Food*. American Academy of Allergy and Immunology Committee on Adverse Reactions to Foods, US National Institute of Allergy and Infectious Diseases. NIH publication no. 84-2442, July 1984

*3. Randolph, T. G. and Moss, R. W. *Allergies—Your Hidden Enemy.* Lippincott & Crowell, New York, 1980 (in UK, Turnstone Press, Wellingborough, 1981)

*4. MacKarness, R. *Not All in the Mind*. Pan Books, London, 1976

*5. Rapp, Doris J. *Allergies and the Hyperactive Child*. Cornerstone Library, (Simon & Schuster), New York, 1979

*6. Rapp, Doris J. *Allergies and Your Family.* Sterling Publishing, New York, 1980

*7. Buist, Robert. *Food Intolerance; What It Is and How to Cope With It*. Harper & Row, Sydney, Australia, 1984

8. Breneman, J. C. *Basics of Food Allergy.* Charles C. Thomas, Springfield, Illinois, 1978

9. Lessof, M. H. (ed.) *Clinical Reactions to Foods*. John Wiley & Sons, Chichester, 1983, 220pp

10. Dickey, L. D. (ed.) *Clinical Ecology.* Charles C. Thomas, Springfield, Illinois, 1976

PAPERS

11. Scott, B. B. and Losowsky, M. S. "Coeliac disease: a cause of various associated diseases?" *Lancet,* ii (1975), 956–7

12. Sarri, K. M. and Keyrilainen, O. "Immunological disorders of the eye complicating coeliac disease," *Lancet,* i (1984), 968–9

13. Editorial. "Infertility in coeliac disease" *Lancet,* i (1983), 453–4

14. Stewart, J. "Asymptomatic coeliac disease in adults," *J. Irish Med. Assoc.*, 67:15 (1974), 415–16

15. Manku, M. S., Horrobin, D. F. and Morse, N. "Reduced levels of prostaglandin precursors in the blood of atopic patients: defective delta-6-desaturase function as a biochemical basis for atopy," *Prostaglandins Leucotriens Med.*, 9 (1982), 615–28

16. Horrobin, D. F. and Manku, M. S. "Essential fatty acids in clinical medicine," *Nutrition and Health,* 2 (1983), 127–34

17. Morley, J., Bray, M. A., Beets, J. L. and Paul, W. "Regulation of allergic responses by prostaglandins: a review," *J. Roy. Soc. Med.*, 73 (1980), 443–7

18. Naeije, N., Bracamonte, M., Michael, O., Sergysels, R. and Duchateau, J. "Cross-desensitization between aspirin and benzoate in asthma," *Lancet,* ii (1983), 1035–6

19. Freedman, B. J. "Asthma induced by sulphur dioxide, benzoate and tartrazine contained in orange drinks," *Clin. Allergy,* 7 (1977), 407

20. Walker, W. A. and Isselbácher, K. J. "Uptake and transport of macromolecules by the intestine: possible role in clinical disorders," *Gastroenterology,* 67 (1974), 531

21. Zioudrou, C., Streaty, R. A. and Klee, W. A. "Opioid peptides derived from food proteins: the exorphins," *J. Biol. Chem.*, 254 (1979), 2446–7

22. Zioudrou, C. and Klee, W. A. "Possible roles of peptides derived from food proteins in brain function" in R. J. Wurtman and J. J. Wurtman (eds.) *Nutrition and the Brain,* Vol. 4, pp. 125–52. Raven Press, New York, 1979

23. Morley, J. E. "Food peptides—a new class of hormones?" *JAMA,* 17 (1982), 2379–80

24. Morley, J. E., Levine, A. S., Yamada, T., Gebhard, R. L., Prigge, W. F., Shafrer, R. B., Goetz, F. C. and Silvis, S. E. "Effect of exorphins on gastrointestinal function, hormone release and appetite," *Gastroenterology,* 84 (1983), 1517-23

25. Paganelli, R., Atherton, D. J. and Levinsky, R. J. "Differences between normal and milk-allergic subjects in their immune responses after milk ingestion," *Arch. Dis. Child.*, 58 (1983), 201–6

26. Cunningham-Rundles, C., Brandeis, W. E. Pudifin, D. J., Day, M. K. and Good, R. A. "Autoimmunity in selective IgA deficiency: Relationship to anti-bovine protein antibodies, circulating immune complexes in clinical disease," *Clin. Exp. Immunol.*, 45 (1981), 299–304

27. Massa, M. C., Quinby, S., Palumbo, P. and Schroeter, A. L. "Immune complexes and diabetes mellitus," *New Engl. J. Med.,* (8 Oct. 1981), 894

28. Darlington, L. G., Ramsay, N. W. and Mansfield, J. R. "Placebo-controlled blind study of dietary manipulation therapy in rheumatoid arthritis," *Lancet,* i (1986), 236–8

29. Coombs, R. R. A. and Oldham, G. "Early rheumatoid-like joint lesions in rabbits drinking cows' milk," *Int. Arch. Allergy Appl. Immunol.,* 64 (1981), 287

30. Walport, M. J., Parke, A. L. and Hughes, G. R. V. "Food and connective tissue diseases," *Clinics in Immunol. and Allergy,* 21:1 (1982), 113–20

31. Parke, A. L. and Hughes, G. R. V. "Rheumatoid arthritis and food: a case study," *BMJ,* 282 (1981), 2027–9

32. See also "Migraine etc.," "Children's problems," "Arthritis etc.," "Nutritional psychiatry," "Eczema etc.," and "Gastrointestinal conditions" references

33. Campbell, M. B. "Neurological manifestations of allergic disease," *Ann. of Allergy,* 31 (1973), 485

34. Hall, K. "Allergy of the nervous system: a review," *Ann. Allergy,* 36 (1976), 49

35. Dees, S. C. "Allergic epilepsy," *Ann. Allergy,* 9 (1951), 446

36. Miller, J. L. "Evidence that idiopathic epilepsy is a sensitization disease," *Am. J. Med. Sci.,* 168 (1924), 635

37. Adamson, W. B. and Sellers, E. D. "Observations on the incidence of the hypersensitive state in 100 cases of epilepsy," *J. Allergy,* 5 (1933), 315–23

38. Fein, B. T. and Kamin, P. B. "Allergy, convulsive disorders and epilepsy," *Ann. Allergy,* 26 (1968), 241

39. Feingold, B. F. "Dietary management of nystagmus," *J. Neurol. Transmission,* 45 (1979), 107–15

40. Editorial. "The housedust mite and atopic dermatitis," *Lancet,* ii (1982), 806–7

41. Chandra, R. K. and Baker, M. "Numerical and functional deficiency of suppressor T-cells precedes development of atopic eczema," *Lancet,* ii (1983), 1393–4

42. Harper, J., Staughton, R. and Byrom, N. A. "Atopic eczema after viral infection," *BMJ,* 284 (1982), 117

43. Atherton, D. J., Soothill, J. F., Sewell, M. and Wells, R. S. "A double-blind controlled cross-over trial of an antigen-avoidance diet in atopic eczema," *Lancet,* i (1978), 401–3

44. Evans, R. W., Fergusson, D. M., Allardyce, R. A. and Taylor, B. "Maternal diet and infantile colic in breast-fed infants," *Lancet,* i (1981), 1340–2

45. Jenkins, H. R., Pincott, J. R., Soothill, J. F., Milla, P. J. and Harries, J. T. "Food allergy: the major cause of infantile colitis," *Arch. Dis. Child.*, 59 (1984), 326–9

46. Rebhun, J. "Duodenal ulceration in allergic children," *Ann. Allergy,* 34 (1975), 145

47. Rea, W. J. "Environmentally triggered cardiac disease," *Ann. Allergy,* 40 (1978), 243–51

48. Bernstein, C. and Klotz, S. D., "Allergy and the heart in clinical practice," *Ann. Allergy,* 8 (1950), 336

49. Ginsberg, R., Bristow, M. R., Kantrowitz, N., Baim, D. S. and Harrison, D. C. "Histamine provocation of clinical coronary artery spasm: implications concerning pathogenesis of variant angina pectoris," *Am. Heart J.*, 102 (1981), 819

50. Rea, W. J. "Recurrent environmentally triggered thrombophlebitis. A five-year follow-up," *Ann. Allergy,* 47 (1981), 338

51. Rea, W. J. "Environmentally triggered small vessel vasculitis," *Ann. Allergy,* 38 (1977), 245

52. Davies, D. F. *et al.* "Food antibodies and myocardial infarction," *Lancet,* i (1974), 1012

53. Rowe, A. H. and Rowe, J. A. "Chronic ulcerative colitis: atopic allergy in its aetiology," *Am. J. Gastroenterol.*, 34 (1960), 49

54. Breneman, J. C. "Food allergy as a cause of gall bladder disease" in *Basics of Food Allergy,* pp. 67–9. C. C. Thomas, Springfield, Illinois, 1978

55. Williams, B. "Palindromic rheumatism, the request," *Med. J. Aust.*, 2 (1972), 390–1

56. Caffrey, E. A., Sladen, G. E., Isaacs, P. E. and Clark, K. G. A. "Thrombocytopenia caused by cows' milk," *Lancet,* ii (1981), 316

57. Powell, N. B., Powell, E. B., Thomas, O. C., Queng, J. T. and McGovern, J. P. "Allergy of the lower urinary tract," *J. Urol.*, 107 (1972), 631

58. Vesey, S. "Orange juice and enuresis," *Lancet,* ii (1962), 1387

59. Law-Chin-Yung, L. and Freed, D. L. J. "Nephrotic syndrome due to milk allergy," *Lancet,* i (1977), 1056

60. Wray, D. "Aphthous stomatitis is linked to mechanical injuries, iron and vitamin deficiencies and certain HLA types," *JAMA,* 247:6 (1982), 774–5

61. Randolph, T. G. "Masked food allergy is a factor in the development of, and persistence of, obesity," *J. Lab. Clin. Med.*, 32 (1947), 1547

62. Green, R. G. "Diet and otitis media," *Can. Fam. Physician*, 29 (1983), 15–16

63. Marx, M. B. "Bruxism in allergic children," *Am. J. Orthodontics*, 77 (1980), 48–9

64. Dean, A. M., Dean, F. W. and McCutchan, G. R. "Interstitial keratitis caused by specific sensitivity to ingested foods," *Arch. Opthalmol.*, 23 (1940), 48–9

65. Buchbinder, E. M., Block, K. J., Moss, J. and Guiney, T. E. "Food-dependent, exercise-induced anaphylaxis—a case report," *JAMA*, 250:21 (1983), 2973–4

66. Randolph, T. G. "Fatigue and weakness of allergic origin (allergic toxemia) to be differentiated from 'nervous fatigue' or neurasthenia," *Ann. Allergy*, 3 (1945), 418

Gastrointestinal Conditions

GENERAL REVIEWS

1. Bouchier, I. A. D. *Gastroenterology*. 3rd ed. Baillière Tindall, London, 1982

2. Bouchier, I. A. D., Allan, R. N., Hodgson, H. J. F. and Keighley, M. R. B. *Textbook of Gastroenterology*. Baillière Tindall, London, 1984

3. Winick, M. (ed.) *Nutrition and Gastroenterology*. John Wiley & Sons, Chichester, 1980

4. Hemmings, W. A. (ed.) *Antigen Absorption by the Gut*. MTP, Lancaster, 1978

5. Hunter, J. O. and Alun Jones, V. *Food and the Gut*. Baillière Tindall, London, 1985

*6. Workman, E., Alun Jones, V., Hunter, J. O. *The Allergy Diet*. Martin Dunitz, London, 1985

PAPERS

6. Wray, D., Vlagopoulos, T. P. and Siraganian, R. P. "Food allergens and basophil histamine release in recurrent aphthous stomatitis," *Oral Surgery, Oral Medicine, Oral Pathology*, 54:4 (1982), 388–95

7. Editorial. "Aphthous stomatitis is linked to mechanical injuries, iron and vitamin deficiencies, and certain HLA types," *JAMA*, 247:6 (1982), 774–5

8. Tyldesley, W. R. "Recurrent oral ulceration and coeliac disease—a review," *Brit. Dent. J.*, 151 (1981), 81–3

9. Wray, D., Ferguson, M. M., Mason, D. K., Hutcheon, A. W. and Dagg, J. H. "Recurrent aphthae; treatment with vitamin B12, folic acid and iron," *BMJ,* 31 May 1975, 490–3

*10. Yudkin, J. "Sugar and disease," *Nature,* 239 (1972), 197–9 (X-ray negative dyspepsia and sugar)

11. Hunter, J. O. "The dietary management of Crohn's disease," in J. O. Hunter and V. Alun Jones (eds.) *Food and the Gut,* pp. 221–37. Baillière Tindall, London, 1985

12. Sturniolo, G. C., Molokhia, M. M., Shields, R. and Turnberg, L. A. "Zinc absorption in Crohn's disease," *Gut,* 21 (1980), 387–91

13. Skogh, Sundquist, T. and Tagesson, C. "Vitamin A in Crohn's disease," *Lancet,* i (1980), 766

14. Alun Jones, "Irritable bowel syndrome" in J. O. Hunter and V. Alun Jones (eds.), *Food and the Gut,* pp. 208–20. Baillière Tindall, London, 1985

15. Dronfield, M. W., Malone, J. D. G. and Langman, M. J. S. "Zinc in ulcerative colitis: a therapeutic trial and report on plasma levels," *Gut,* 18 (1977), 33–6

16. Andresen, A. F. R. "Ulcerative colitis: an allergic phenomenon," *Am. J. Dig. Dis.,* 9 (1942), 91

17. Lucey, M. R., "Recurrent pellagra in Crohn's disease," *Lancet,* ii (1982), 559

18. Rowe, A. H. and Rowe, A. "Chronic ulcerative colitis and regional enteritis: their allergic aspects," *Ann. Allergy* 12 (1954), 387

19. Manning, A. P., Heaton, K. W., Harvey, R. F. and Uglow, P. "Wheat fibre and irritable bowel syndrome: a controlled trial," *Lancet,* ii (1977), 417–18

20. Alun Jones, V., McLaughlan, P., Shorthouse, M., Workman, E. and Hunter, J. O. "Food intolerance: a major factor in the pathogenesis of irritable bowel syndrome," *Lancet,* ii (1982), 1115–17

21. Stephen, A. M. "Effect of food on the intestinal microflora" in J. L. Hunter and V. Alun Jones (eds.) in *Food and the Gut,* pp. 57–77. Baillière Tindall, London, 1985

22. Holti, G. "Candida allergy and irritable colon syndrome" in H. I. Winner and R. Hurley (eds.), *Symposium on Candida Infections,* pp. 73–81. E. & S. Livingstone Ltd., London, 1966

23. Neeman, A., Avidor, I. and Kadish, U. "Candidal infection of benign gastric ulcers in aged patients," *Am. J. Gastroenterol.,* 75 (1981), 211–13

24. Kodsi, B. E., Wickremesinghe, P. C. *et al.* "Candida esophagitis—a prospective study of twenty-seven cases," *Gastroenterology,* 71 (1976), 715–19

25. Sclafer, J. "Brulures gastriques par allergie mycosique," First International Congress for Allergy, S. Karger AP, Basel and New York, 1951. p. 961–4

26. Sclafer, J. "A l'allergie à candida albicans (clinique, diagnostic, traitement)" *Semaine Hopital Paris,* 33:6 (1957), 1329–39

27. See also "Food Allergy" references.

28. Chamberlin, D. T. and Perkin, H. J. "The level of ascorbic acid in the blood and urine of patients with peptic ulcer," *Am. J. Dig. Dis.,* 5 (1938–9), 493

29. Kokkonen, J., Fimila, S. and Herva, R. "Impaired gastric function in children with cows' milk intolerance," *European Journal of Paediatrics,* 132 (1979), 1–6. *Children Ann. Allergy,* 34 (1975), 145

30. Breneman, J. C. "Allergic elimination diet is the most effective gall bladder diet," *Ann. Allergy,* 26 (1968), 83

31. Cummings, J. H. "Fermentation in the human large intestine: evidence and indications for health," *Lancet,* i (1983), 1206–9. McEvoy, A., *BMJ,* 287 (1983), 789–93

Cardiovascular Disease

1. Shaper, A. G. *et al.* "Risk factors for ischaemic heart disease: the prospective phase of the British Regional Heart Study," *J. Epidemiology and Community Health,* 39 (1985), 197–209

2. Yudkin, J. "Diet and coronary thrombosis. Hypothesis and fact," *Lancet,* ii (1957), 155–62

3. Voors, A. W., Johnson, W. D. and Schuman, M. S. "Additive statistical effects of cadmium and lead on heart-related disease in a North Carolina autopsy series," *Arch. Environmental Health,* 37 (1982), 98–102

4. Leary, W. P. and Reyes, A. J. "Magnesium and sudden death," *SA Med. Jour.,* 64 (1983), 697–8

5. Ornish, D. *et al.* "The effects of stress management training and dietary changes in treating ischaemic heart disease," *JAMA,* 249 (1983), 54–9

6. Preuss, H. G. and Fournier, R. D. "The effects of sucrose ingestion on blood pressure," *Life Sciences,* 30 (1982), 879–86

7. Rouse, I. L., Beilin, L. J., Armstrong, B. K. and Vandongen, R. "Blood-pressure lowering effect of a vegetarian diet:

controlled trial in normotensive subjects," *Lancet,* i (1983), 5–10

8. Hofman, A., Hazebroek, A. and Valkenburg, H. A. "A randomized trial of sodium intake and blood pressure in newborn infants," *JAMA,* 250 (1983), 370–3

9. Brown, J. J. *et al.* "Salt and hypertension," *Lancet,* i (1984), 456

10. MacGregor, G. A., Smith, S. J., Markandu, N. D., Banks, R. A. and Sagnella, G. A. "Moderate potassium supplementation in essential hypertension," *Lancet,* ii (1982), 568–70

11. Wilcox, R. G., Bennett, T., Brown, A. M. and MacDonald, I. A. "Is exercise good for high blood pressure?" *BMJ,* 285 (1982), 767–9

12. Seltzer, C. C. "The effect of smoking on blood pressure," *Am. Heart J.,* 87 (1974), 558–64

13. McCarron, D. A., Morris, C. D., Henry, H. J. and Stanton, J. L. "Blood pressure and nutrient intake in the United States," *Science,* 224 (1984), 1392–8

14. Belizan, J. M. *et al.* "Reduction of blood pressure with calcium supplementation in young adults," *JAMA,* 249 (1983), 1161–5

15. Whitescarver, S. A., Ott, C. E., Jackson, B. A., Guthrie, G. T. and Kotchen, T. A. "Salt-sensitive hypertension: the contribution of chloride," *Science,* 223 (1984), 1430–2

16. Melbey, C. L., Melbey, P. C. and Hinder, G. C. "The rationale for incorporating non-pharmacological therapy in the treatment of borderline-mild hypertension," *J. Appl. Nutr.,* 36 (1984), 63–79

17. Lewis, B. "Disorders of lipid transport" in D. J. Weatherall, J. G. G. Ledingham, and D. A. Warrell (eds.) *Oxford Textbook of Medicine,* pp. 9, 58–9, 70. *OUP,* 1983

18. Buckley, B. M. and Bold, A. M. "Managing hyperlipidaemias," *BMJ,* 285 (1982), 193–4

19. Duffield, R. G. M. *et al.* "Treatment of hyperlipidaemia retards the progression of symptomatic femoral atherosclerosis," *Lancet,* ii (1983), 639–42

20. Miettimen, E. A. *et al.* "Fatty-acid composition of serum lipids predicts myocardial infarction," *BMJ,* 285 (1982), 993–6

21. Jain, R. C. "Onion and garlic in experimental atherosclerosis," *Lancet,* i (1975), 1240

22. Riales, R. and Albrink, M. J. "The effect of chromium chloride supplementation on glucose tolerance and serum lipids, including high density lipoproteins of adult men," *Am. J. Clin. Nutr.* 34 (1981), 2672–8

23. Williams, P. T. *et al.* "Coffee intake in elevated cholesterol and apolipoprotein B levels in men," *JAMA*, 253 (1985), 1407–11

24. Ginter, D. "Cholesterol: vitamin C controls its transformation to bile acids," *Science*, 179 (1973), 702–4

25. Sanders, T. A. B. and Ellis, F. R. "Serum cholesterol and triglyceride concentrations in vegans," *Proceedings of the Nutrition Society*, 36 (1977), 43a

26. Ames, R. P., and Hill, P. "Improvement of glucose tolerance and lowering of glyco-haemoglobin and serum lipid concentration after discontinuation of anti-hypertensive drug therapy," *Circulation*, 65 (1982), 899–904

27. Williams, P. T., Wood, T. D., Haskell, W. L. and Vranizan, K. "The effects of running mileage and duration on plasma lipoprotein levels," *JAMA*, 247 (1982), 2674–9

28. Durrington, P. N., Manning, A. P., Bolton, C. H. and Hartog, M. "The effect of pectin on serum lipids and lipoproteins, whole-gut transit time and stool weight," *Lancet*, ii (1976), 394–6

29. Hutchison, K. *et al.* "The effects of dietary manipulation on vascular status of patients with peripheral vascular disease," *JAMA*, 249 (1983), 3326–30

30. Yudkin, J., Szanto, S. and Kakkar, V. V. "Sugar intake, serum insulin and platelet adhesiveness in men with and without peripheral vascular disease," *Postgrad, Med. J.*, 45 (1969), 608–11

31. Haeger, K. "Long-time treatment of intermittent claudication with vitamin E," *Am. J. Clin. Nutr.*, 27 (1974), 1179–81

32. Barboriak, J. J., el Ghatit, A. Z., Shetty, K. R. and Kalkfleish, J. H. "Vitamin E supplements and plasma high density lipoprotein cholesterol," *Am. J. Clin. Path.*, 77 (1982), 371–2

Cancer

1. Ames, B. "Dietary carcinogens and anti-carcinogens," *Science*, 221 (1983), 1256–64

2. Tannenbaum, S. R. M. "Nitroso compounds: a perspective on human exposure," *Lancet*, 1 (1983), 629–32

3. Salonen, J. T. *et al.* "Risk of cancer in relation to serum concentrations of selenium and vitamins A and E: matched case-control analysis of prospective data," *BMJ*, 1 (1985), 417–20

4. Committee on Diet, Nutrition and Cancer. *Report on Diets and Nutrition in Cancer.* National Academy Press, Washington DC, 1982

*5. Salaman, M. *The Cancer Answer*. Stratford Publishing, Menlo Park, California, 1984.

Arthritis, Osteoporosis and Other Problems with Bones and Joints

1. Whedon, D. G. "Osteoporosis," *N. Eng. J. Med.*, 305 (1981), 397

2. Gallagher, J. C. and Riggs, B. L. "Current concepts in nutrition: nutrition and bone disease," *N. Eng. J. Med.*, 298 (1978), 193

3. Albanese, A. A., Lorenze, E. J., Wein, E. H. and Carroll, L. "Effects of calcium and micronutrients on bone loss of pre- and post-menopausal women." Scientific exhibit presented to the American Medical Association in Atlanta, Georgia, 24–26 January 1981

4. Nordin, B. E. C., Horsman, A., Crilly, R. G., Marshall, D. H. and Simpson, M. "Treatment of spinal osteoporosis in post-menopausal women," *BMJ*, 16 February 1980, 451

5. Gonzales, E. R. "Premature bone loss found in some nonmenstruating sportswomen," *JAMA*, 248 (1982), 513

6. Editorial. "Lactase deficiency in osteoporosis," *Lancet*, i (1979), 86

7. Frithiof, L. *et al*. "The relationship between marginal bone loss and serum zinc levels," *Acta, Med Scand.*, 207 (1980), 67

8. Parke, A. L. and Hughes, G. R. V. "Rheumatoid arthritis and food: a case study," *BMJ*, 282 (1981), 2027

9. Little, C. H., Stewart, A. G. and Fennessy, M. R. "Platelet serotonin release in rheumatoid arthritis: a study in food-intolerance patients," *Lancet*, ii (1983), 297

10. Hicklin, J. A., McEwen, L. M. and Morgan, J. E. "The effect of diet in rheumatoid arthritis," *Clin. Allergy*, 10 (1980), 463

11. Simkin, P. A. "Oral zinc sulphate in rheumatoid arthritis," *Lancet*, ii (1976), 539

12. Walker, W. R. and Keats, D. M. "An investigation of the therapeutic value of the 'copper bracelet': dermal assimilation of copper in arthritic/rheumatoid conditions," *Agents Action*, 6 (1976), 454

13. Machtey, I. and Ouaknine, L. "Tocopherol in osteoarthritis: a controlled pilot study," *J. Am. Geriat. Soc.*, 26 (1978), 328

14. General Practitioner's Research Group. "Calcium pantothenate in arthritis conditions," *Practitioner,* 224 (1980), 208–210

15. Stein, H. B., Hasan, A. and Fox, I. H. "Ascorbic-acid-induced uricosuria: a consequence of megavitamin therapy," *Ann. Intern. Med.*, 84 (1976), 385

16. Editorial. "Green-lipped mussel extract in arthritis," *Lancet,* 1 (1981), 85

19. Broadhurst, A. D. "Tryptophan and rheumatic diseases," *BMJ,* 13 August 1977, 456

20. Ellis, J. M. *et al.* "Response of vitamin B6 deficiency and the carpal tunnel syndrome to pyridoxine," *Proc. Natl. Aca. Sci.*, 79 (1982), 7494

Disorders of the Respiratory System

1. Pang, L. Q. "The importance of allergy in otolaryngology," *Clin. Ecol.*, 1:1 (1982), 53

2. Congven, P. J. *et al.* "Vitamin status in patients with cystic fibrosis," *Archives of Disease in Childhood,* 56 (1981), 708–14

3. Dodge, J. A. and Vassa, J. G. "Zinc deficiency syndrome in a British youth with cystic fibrosis," *BMJ,* 1 (1978), 411

4. Morrow Brown, H. *The Allergy and Asthma Reference Book*. Harper & Row, London, 1985

*5. Rapp, D. *Allergy in the Family.* Sterling Publishing Company, New York, 1980

Disorders of the Urinary System

1. Shah, P. J. R., Green, N. A. and Williams, G. "Unprocessed bran and its effect on urinary calcium excretion in idiopathic hypercalciuria," *BMJ,* 2 (1980), 426

2. Rao, P. N., Prendivile, V., Buxton, A., Moss, D. G. and Blacklock, N. J. "Dietary management of urinary risk factors in renal stone formers," *British Journal of Urology,* 54 (1982), 578–83

3. Prien, E. L. and Gershoff, S. F. "Magnesium oxide—pyridoxine therapy for recurrent calcium oxalic calculi," *Journal of Urology,* 112 (1974), 509–12

4. Kasidas, G. P. and Rose, A. "Oxalate content of some common foods: determination by enzymatic method," *Journal of Human Nutrition,* 34 (1980), 255–66

5. Yudkin, J., Kang, S. S. and Bruckdorfer, K. R. "The effects of high dietary sugar," *BMJ,* 2 (1980), 1396

6. Sandberg, D. H., MacIntosh, R. N., Bernstein, C. W., Carr, R. and Strauss, J. "Severe steroid-responsive nephrosis associated with hyper-sensitivity," *Lancet,* 1 (1977), 388–91

7. Howanietz, H. and Lubec, G. "Idiopathic nephrotic syndrome, treated with steroids of five years. Found to be allergic reaction to pork," *Lancet,* 2 (1985), 450

8. Pirotzky, E., *et al.* "Basophil sensitization in idiopathic nephrotic syndrome," *Lancet,* 1 (1983), 358–61

9. Powell, N. B., Powell, E. B., *et al.* "Allergy of the lower urinary tract," *Journal of Urology,* 107 (1972), 631

Eczema, Dermatitis and Other Problems of Skin, Hair and Nails

1. Campbell, A. J., McEwen, G. C. "Treatment of brittle nails and dry eyes," *British Journal of Dermatology,* 105 (1981), 113

2. Ferrandiz, C., Henkes, J., Peyri, J. and Sarmiento, J. "Acquired zinc deficiency syndrome during total parenteral alimentation—clinical and histopathological findings," *Dermatologica,* 163 (1981), 255–66

3. Miller, J. A., Darley, C. A., Karkavitsas, K., Kirby, J. D. and Munro, D. D. "Low sex-hormone-binding globulin levels in young women with profuse hair loss," *British Journal of Dermatology,* 106 (1982), 331–6

4. Feiwel, M. and Fielding, J. "Hair-fall in blood-donors," *Lancet,* i (1967), 84–5

5. Shuster, S. "The aetiology of dandruff and the mode of action of therapeutic agents," *British Journal of Dermatology,* 111 (1984), 235–42

6. David, T. J., Wells, F. E., Sharpe, T. C. and Gibbs, A. C. C. "Low serum zinc in children with atopic eczema," *British Journal of Dermatology,* 111 (1984), 597–601

7. Atherton, D. J., Sewell, M., Soothill, J. F., Wells, R. S. and Chilvers, C. E. D. "A double-blind, controlled cross-over trial of an antigen-avoidance diet in atopic eczema," *Lancet,* i (1978), 401–3

8. Manku, M. S., Horrobin, D. F., Morse, N. L., Wright, S. and Burton, J. L. "Essential fatty acids in the plasma phospholipids of patients with atopic eczema," *British Journal of Dermatology,* 110 (1984), 643–648

9. Wright, S. and Burton, J. L. "Oral evening primrose oil improves atopic eczema," *Lancet,* 2 (1982), 1120–2

10. Michaelsson, G. and Edqvist, L. E. "Erythrocyte glutathione peroxidase activity in acne vulgaris, the effects of selenium and vitamin E treatment," *Acta. Derm. Venereol.,* 64 (1984), 9–14

11. Cunliffe, W. J., Burke, B., Dodman, B. and Gould, D. J. "A double-blind trial of a zinc sulphate/citrate complex and tetracycline in the treatment of acne vulgaris," *British Journal of Dermatology,* 101 (1979), 321

12. Michaelsson, F. "Zinc in relation to some skin diseases" in K. M. Hambidge and P. J. Aggett (eds.) *Zinc in Human Medicine—Symposium*. TIL Publications Ltd. Isleworth, 1984

13. Crutcher, N. *et al*. "Oral nystatin in the treatment of psoriasis," *Arch Dermatol.,* 120 (1984), 435–6

Diseases of the Eyes

1. Campbell, A. and MacEwen, C. G. "Systemic treatment of Sjogren's syndrome and the Sicca syndrome with efamol (evening primrose oil), vitamin C and pyridoxine" in D. F. Horrobin (ed.) *Clinical Uses of Essential Fatty Acids*. Eden Press Inc., London, 1982

2. See index for zinc, Vitamin A, cataracts, etc.

Diabetes Mellitus

*1. Philpott, D. H. and Kalita, D. K. *Victory over Diabetes*. Keats, New Canaan, Connecticut, 1983

*2. Anderson, J. *Diabetes—A Practical New Guide to Healthy Living*. Martin Dunitz, London, 1983

PAPERS

3. British Diabetic Association. "Dietary recommendations for diabetics for the 1980s—a policy statement," *Human Nutrition: Applied Nutrition,* 36a (1982), 378–94

4. Helderman, J. H. *et al*. "Prevention of the glucose intolerance of thiazide diuretics by maintenance of body potassium," *Diabetes,* 32 (1983), 106–11

5. Coeling, H., Bennink, H. J. T. and Schreurs, W. H. P. "Improvement of oral glucose in gestational diabetes by pyridoxine," *BMJ,* 3 (1975), 13–15

6. Moles, K. V. and McMullen, J. K. "Insulin resistance in hypomagnesaemia: Case report," *BMJ,* 2 (1982), 262

7. Offenbacher, E. G. and Xavier Pi-Sunyer, F. "Beneficial effect of chromium-rich yeast on glucose tolerance on blood lipids in elderly subjects," *Diabetes,* 29 (1980), 919–25

8. Vacca, J. B., Henke, W. J. and Knight, W. A. "The exocrine pancreas in diabetes mellitus," *Annals. Int. Med.*, 61 (1964), 242–7

9. McNair, P. *et al*. "Hypomagnesaemia, a risk factor in diabetic retinopathy," *Diabetes*, 27 (1978), 1075–7

10. Bhatt, H. R., Linnell, J. C. and Matthews, D. M. "Can faulty vitamin B12 (cobalamin) metabolism produce diabetic neuropathy?" *Lancet*, ii (1983), 572

Hypoglycemia

*1. Saunders, J. and Ross, H. M. *Hypoglycemia*. Clinical Books, Los Angeles, 1980

*2. Dufty, W. *Sugar Blues*. Abacus Press, Tunbridge Wells, 1980

*3. Budd, M. *Low Blood Sugar*. Thorsons, Wellingborough, 1983

4. O'Keffe, S. J. D. and Marks, V. "Lunchtime gin and tonic: a cause of reactive hypoglycaemia," *Lancet*, i (1977), 1286–8

5. Long, P. A., Abell, D. A. and Beischer, N. A. "Importance of abnormal glucose tolerance (hypoglycaemia and hyperglycaemia) in the aetiology of pre-eclampsia," *Lancet*, ii (1977), 923–5

6. Virkkunen, M. "Reactive Hypoglycaemic Tendency Among Arsonists," *Acta. Psychiatr. Scan.*, 69 (1984), 445–52

7. Gorman, J. M. *et al*. "Hypoglycaemia and panic attacks," *Am. J. Psychiatry*, 141 (1984), 101–2

8. Stebbing, J. B., Turner, M. O. and Franz, K. B. "Reactive hypoglycaemia and magnesium," *Magnesium Bulletin*, 2 (1982), 131–4

9. Anthony, D. *et al*. "Personality disorder and reactive hypoglycaemia: a quantitative study," *Diabetes*, 22:9 (1973), 664–75

10. Lishman, W. A. *Organic Psychiatry: The Psychological Consequences of Cerebral Disorder*, pp. 631–41. Blackwell, Oxford, 1978

11. Harris, S. "Hyperinsulinism and dysinsulinism," *JAMA*, 83 (1924), 729

Menstrual Problems

PREMENSTRUAL SYNDROME

1. Dalton, K. *Premenstrual Syndrome and Progesterone Therapy.* Heinemann, London, 1984

2. Abraham, G. E. "Nutrition and the premenstrual tension syndromes," *Jour. Appl. Nutrition,* 36 (1984), 103–24

3. Abraham, G. E. and Lubran, M. N. "Serum and red cell magnesium levels in patients with premenstrual tension," *Am. J. Clin. Nutr.,* 34 (1981), 2364–7

4. Abraham, G. E. and Hargrove, J. T. "The effect of vitamin B6 on premenstrual symptomatology in women with premenstrual tension syndrome: a double-blind cross-over study," *Infertility,* 3 (1980), 155–67

5. Piesse, J. W. "Nutrition factors in premenstrual syndrome," *Int. Clin. Nut. Rev.,* 4 (1984), 54–81

6. Chakmakjian, Z. H., Higgins, C. E. and Abraham, G. E. "The effect of nutritional supplement, 'Optivite for Women,' on premenstrual tension syndromes: (II). The effect of symptomatology using a double-blind, cross-over design," *Jour. Appl. Nutrition,* 37 (1985), 12–17

MENORRHAGIA (HEAVY PERIODS)

7. Lithgow, D. M. and Politzer, W. M. "Vitamin A in the treatment of menorrhagia," *SA Med. J.,* 51 (1977), 191

8. Cohen, J. D. and Ruben, H. W. "Functional menorrhagia: treatment with bioflavonoids and vitamin C," *Curr. Ther. Res.,* 2 (1960), 539

9. Taymor, M. L., Sturgis, S. H. and Yahia, C. "The etiological role of chronic iron deficiency in production of menorrhagia," *JAMA,* 187 (1964), 323

10. Samuels, A. J. "Studies in patients with functional menorrhagia: the antihaemorrhagic effect of the adequate repletion of iron stores," *Israel J. Med. Sci.,* 1 (1965), 851

DYSMENORRHEA (PAINFUL PERIODS)

11. Butler, E. B. and McKnight, E. "Vitamin E in the treatment of dysmenorrhea," *Lancet,* i (1955), 844

12. Shafer, N. "Iron in the treatment of dysmenorrhea: A preliminary report," *Curr. Ther. Res.,* 7 (1965), 365

13. Abraham, G. E. "Primary Dysmenorrhea," *Clin. Obstet. Gynaecol.* 21:1 (1978), 139

Side-Effects of the Pill

1. Tomkin, S. Y. "Vitamins and oral contraceptives" in M. H. Briggs (ed.) *Vitamins in Human Biology in Medicine* pp. 29–64, CRC Press, Boca Raton, Florida, 1981

*2. Seaman, B. and Seaman, G. *Women and the Crisis in the Sex Hormones*. Bantam Books, New York, 1977

*3. Grant, E. C. G. *The Bitter Pill—How Safe is the Perfect Contraceptive?* Elmtree Books/Hamish Hamilton Ltd., London, 1985

4. Luhby, A. L., Davis, P., Murphy, M. *et al.* "Pyridoxine and oral contraceptives," *Lancet*, ii (1970), 1083

5. Prasad, A. S. *et al.* "Effect of oral contraceptives on nutrients III vitamins B6, B12 and folic acid," *Am. J. Obstet. Gynaecol.* 125 (1976), 1063

6. Briggs, M. H. "Megadose vitamin C and the metabolic effects of vitamin C," *BMJ*, 283 (1981), 1547

7. Butterworth, C. E. *et al.* "Improvement in cervical dysplasia associated with folic acid therapy in users of oral contraceptives," *Am. J. Clin. Nutr.*, 35 (1982), 73–82

8. Smith, J. C. and Brown, E. D. "Effects of oral contraceptive agents on trace element metabolism—a review" in A. S. Prasad (ed.) *Trace Elements in Human Health and Disease* Vol. 11, pp. 315–45. Academic Press, New York.

*9. Flynn, A. and Brooks, M. *A Manual of Natural Family Planning*. George Allen and Unwin, London, 1984

Infertility

*1. Stanway, A. *Why us?—A Commonsense Guide for the Childless*. Thorsons, Wellingborough, 1984

2. Calloway, D. H. "Nutrition and reproductive function of man," *Nutrition Abstracts and Reviews, Reviews in Clinical Nutrition,* 53:5 (1983), 361–82

3. Piesse, J. "Zinc and human male infertility," *International Clinical Nutrition Reviews,* 3:2 (1983), 4–6

4. Jungling, M. L. and Bunge, R. G. "The treatment of spermatogenic arrest with arginine," *Fert. Ster.* 27 (1976), 282

5. Editorial "Infertility in coeliac disease," *Lancet*, i (1983), 453–4

6. Wynn, A. and Wynn, M. "The prevention of handicap of early pregnancy origin," p. 14. Foundation for Education and Research in Childbearing, 27 Walpole St. London, SW3. 1981 p. 14

Preconceptional Care

1. Laurence, K. M. "Dietary approaches to the prevention of neural tube defects," *Nutrition and Health,* 2 (1983), 181–9

2. Editorial. "Vitamin A and teratogenesis," *Lancet,* i (1985), 319–20

3. Editorial "Valproate and malformations," *Lancet,* ii (1982), 1313–14

4. Schoental, R. "Mycotoxins and foetal abnormalities," *Intern. J. Environ. Studies,* 17 (1981), 25–9

5. Wynn, M. and Wynn, A. *Lead and Human Reproduction*. Clear Charitable Trust, 2 North Down Street, London NW1, *Bri. J. Obst. Gynaecol.* 89 (1982), 892–5

6. Flynn, A. *et al.* "Zinc status of pregnant alcoholic women: a determinant of foetal outcome," *Lancet,* i (1981), 572

7. Smithells, R. W. *et al.* "Further experience of vitamin supplementation for prevention of neural tube defects recurrences," *Lancet,* i (1983), 1027–31

8. Fraser, F. C., Hansom, C. and Czeizel, A. "Increased frequency of neural tube defects in siblings of children with other malformations," *Lancet,* ii (1982), 144–5

9. Golding, J., Sladden, T. "Congenital Malformations and Agricultural Workers," *Lancet,* ii (1983), 1393

10. Buamah, P. K. *et al.* "Serum copper concentrations significantly less in abnormal pregnancies," *Clin. Chem.,* 30 (1984), 1676–7

11. "Alcohol consumption, pregnancy and low birth weight," *Lancet,* i (1983), 663–5

12. Evans, H. J. *et al.* "Sperm abnormalities and cigarette smoking," *Lancet,* i (1981), 627–9

13. Zimmerman, N., Gifford, W. H. and Grey, B. "Potato Scab and Teratogeny," *Lancet,* ii (1975), 990–1

14. Wibberley, D. G. *et al.* "Lead levels in human placenta from normal and malformed births" *J. Med. Genetics,* 14:5 (1977), 339–45

15. Hurley, L. S. "Trace metals in mammalian development," *John Hopkins Med. J.,* 148 (1981), 1–10

16. Editorial "Diabetes and malformation," *Lancet,* ii (1982), 587–8

17. Frishncho, A. R., Matos, J. and Flegel, P. "Maternal nutritional status and adolescent pregnancy outcome," *Am. J. Clin. Nutr.,* 38 (1983), 739–46

18. Wynn, M. and Wynn, A. "The importance of nutrition around the time of conception in the prevention of handicap" in E. C. Bateman (ed.) *Proceedings of the British Dietetic Association Study Conference*. John Libby, London, 1981

19. Kalter, H. Warkany. "Congenital malformations: etiologic factors and their role in prevention," *N. Engl. J. Med.*, 308 (1983), 424–31 and *N. Engl. J. Med.*, 308 (1983), 491–7

20. Wynn, M. and Wynn, A., "The influence of nutrition on the fertility of women," *Nutrition and Health*, 1 (1982), 7–13

21. Pfeiffer, C. C. "The role of zinc, manganese, chromium and vitamin deficiencies in birth defects" in J. Rose (ed.) *Nutrition and Killer Diseases—The Effects of Dietary Factors on Fatal Chronic Diseases*, pp. 148–169. Noyes, New Jersey, 1982

22. Wynn, M. and Wynn, A. *Prevention of Handicap and Health of Women*, p. 247. Routledge and Kegan Paul, London, 1979

*23. *Guidelines for Future Parents*. Foresight, the Association for the Promotion of Preconceptional Care, The Old Vicarage, Church Lane, Witley, Godalming, Surrey, GU8 5DN

Pregnancy and Breast-Feeding

PREGNANCY

1. Nichols, B. L. and Nichols, V. N. "Nutrition in pregnancy and lactation," *Nutrition Abstracts and Reviews—Reviews in Clinical Nutrition*, 53:4 (1983), 259–73

2. Beaufils, M. *et al.* "Prevention of pre-eclampsia by early antiplatelet therapy," *Lancet*, i (1985), 840–2

3. "Toxemia of pregnancy: the dietary calcium hypothesis," *Nutrition Reviews*, 39:1 (1981), 124

4. Clieger, J. A. *et al.* "Abnormal pyridoxine metabolism in toxemia of pregnancy," *Annals of New York Academy of Sciences*, 166 (1969), 288

5. Long, P. A., Abell, D. A. and Beischer, N. A. "Importance of abnormal glucose tolerance (hypoglycaemia and hyperglyceamia) in the etiology of pre-eclampsia," *Lancet*, i (1977), 923–35

6. Erskin, K. J., Iversen, S. A. and Davies, R. "An altered ratio of 18:11 (9,11) to 18:11 (9,12) linoleic acid in plasma phospholipids as a possible predictor of pre-eclampsia," *Lancet*, i (1985), 554–6

*7. Brewer, T. H. *Metabolic Toxemia of Late Pregnancy—A Disease of Malnutrition*. Keats, Connecticut, 1982

8. Hammar, M., Larsson, L. and Tegler, L. "Calcium treatment of leg cramps in pregnancy," *Acta. Obstet. Gynaecol. Scand.*, 60 (1981), 345–7

9. Page, E. W. and Page, E. T. "Leg cramps in pregnancy: etiology and treatment," *Obstet. Gynaecol.*, 1 (1953), 94–100

10. Weinstein, B. B., Wohlz, Mitchell G. J. and Sustendal, G. F. "Oral administration of pyridoxine hydrochloride in the treatment of nausea and vomiting of pregnancy," *Am. J. Obstet. Gynaecol.*, 47 (1944), 389

11. Merkel, R. L. "The use of menadione bisulfite and ascorbic acid in the treatment of nausea and vomiting of pregnancy: A preliminary report," *Am. J. Obstet. Gynaecol.*, 64 (1952), 416–18

12. Coeling, H., Bennink, H. J. T. and Schreurs, W. H. P. "Improvement of oral glucose tolerance in gestational diabetes by pyridoxine," *BMJ*, 3 (1975), 13–15

13. Hemminki, E. and Starfield, B. "Routine administration of iron and vitamins during pregnancy: review of controlled clinical trials," *Brit. J. Obstet. and Gynaecol.*, 85 (1978), 404–10

14. Campbell, D. M. and Gillmer, M. D. J. (eds.) *Nutrition in Pregnancy—Proceedings of the tenth Study Group of the Royal College of Obstetricians and Gynaecologists*. RCOG, London, 1983

15. See also "Preconceptional Care" references.

BREAST-FEEDING

*16. Stanway, P. and Stanway, A. *Breast is Best*. Pan Books, London, 1978

17. Whitehead, R. G. "Nutritional aspects of human lactation," *Lancet*, i (1983), 167–9

18. Nichols, B. L. and Nichols, V. N. "Nutrition in pregnancy and lactation," *Nutrition Abstracts and Reviews—Reviews in Clinical Nutrition*, 53:4 (1983), 259–73

19. Wilson, J. T. "Contamination of human milk by drugs and chemicals," *Nutrition and Health*, 2 (1983), 191–201

20. Kulangara, A. C. "The demonstration of ingested wheat antigens in human breast milk," *IRCS Medical Science: Elementary System, Biochemistry* etc. 8 (1980), 19

21. Matthew, D. J., Norman, A. P., Taylor, B., Turner, M. W. and Soothill, J. F. "Prevention of eczema," *Lancet*, i (12 Feb. 1977)

22. Sandstrom, B., Sederblad, A. and Lonnerdal, B. "Zinc absorption from human milk, cows' milk and infant formulas," *Am. J. Dis. Child.*, 137 (1983), 726–9

23. See also "Food Allergy" references.

Benign Breast Disease

1. Gonzalez, E. R. "Vitamin E relieves most cystic breast disease; may alter lipids, hormones," *JAMA*, 244 (1980), 1077–8

2. Check, W. "Benign breast lumps may regress through change in diet," *JAMA*, 241 (1979), 1221

3. Ernster, V. L. *et al.* "Vitamin E and benign breast 'disease': a double-blind, randomized clinical trial," *Surgery*, 97 (1985), 490–4

4. Preece, P. E. *et al.* "Evening primrose oil (Efamol) for mastalgia," in D. F. Horrobin (ed.) *Clinical Uses of Essential Fatty Acids*, pp. 147–54. Eden Press, London, 1982

5. Minton, J. P. *et al.* "Clinical and biochemical studies on methylxanthine-related fibrocystic breast disease," *Surgery*, 90 (1981), 299–302

Infections

1. Beisel, W. R., Edelman, R., Nouss, K. and Suskind, R. M. "Single-nutrient effects on immunological functions," *JAMA*, 245 (1981), 53–8

2. Chandra, R. K. "Nutrition, immunity and infection: present knowledge and future directions," *Lancet*, i (1983), 688–91

3. Beach, R. S., Gershwin, M. E. and Hurley, L. S. "Persistent immunological consequences of gestation zinc deprivation," *Am. J. Clin. Nutr.*, 38 (1983), 579–90

4. Hamblin, T. J., Hussain, J., Akbar, A. N., Tang, Y. C., Smith, J. L. and Jones, B. B. "Immunological reason for chronic ill health after infectious mononucleosis," *BMJ*, 2 (1983), 85–8

5. Gershwin, M. E., Beach, R. S. and Hurley, L. S. *Nutrition and Immunity*. Academic Press, Orlando, 1985

6. Good, R. A. "Nutrition and immunity," *Journal of Clinical Immunology*, 1:1 (1981), 3–11

7. Duchateau, J., Delepesse, G. *et al.* "Beneficial effects of oral zinc supplementation on the immune response of old people," *Am. J. Med.*, 70 (1981), 1001–4

8. Djorksten, D. *et al*. "Zinc and immune function in Downs syndrome," *Acta. Paediatrica Scand.*, 69 (1980), 183–7

Candidiasis

1. Schafer, J. "Brulures gastriques par allergic mycosoque" in *Proceedings of the First International Congress for Allergy,* pp. 961–4. S. Karger AG, Basel and New York, 1952

2. Ruiz-Moreno, G. "Eczematoid monolid of the eyelids (Candida)," *Annals of Allergy,* March–April 1947, 132–6 (in French)

3. Kourilsky, R., Burtin, P., Monnier, F. and Ternynck, T. "L'állergie à candida albicans," *Société Médicale des Hopitaux de Paris,* 10 April 1959, pp. 391–4 (in French)

4. Holti, G. "Candida allergy" in H. I. Winner and R. Hurley (eds.) *Symposium on Candida Infections,* pp. 73–81. E. & S. Livingstone Ltd., London, 1966

5. Holti, G. "Management of pruritis and urticaria," *BMJ,* 1 (1967), 155–8

6. Holti, G. "Some skin hazards and allergy problems in dentistry," Lecture given to the North of England Odontological Society, 13 January 1969. *Newcastle Medical Journal,* xxx (7 March 1969), 9pp

7. Truss, C. O. "Tissue injury induced by candida albicans: mental and neurological manifestations," *J. Orthomol. Psychiat.*, 7:1 (1978), 17–37

8. Truss, C. O. "Restoration of immunologic competence to candida albicans," *J. Orthomol. Psychiat.*, 9:4 (1980), 287–301

9. Truss, C. O. "The role of candida albicans in human illness," *J. Orthomol. Psychiat.*, 10:4 (1981), 228–38

10. Truss, C. O. *The Missing Diagnosis*. PO Box 26508, Birmingham, Alabama 35226, USA, 1983

*11. Crook, W. G. *The Yeast Connection* 2nd edn. Professional Books, PO Box 3494, Jackson, Tennessee, 38301, USA. 1984

12. Krause, W., Matheis, H. and Woolfe, K. "Fungaemia and funguria after oral administration of candida albicans," *Lancet,* i (1969), 598–9

13. Crook, W. G. "Depression associated with candida albicans infections," (letter), *JAMA,* 251:22 (1984), 2928

14. Candida Albicans Conference, Dallas, 10 July 1982. Tape proceedings of the twelve-hour conference available on cassette from Creative Audio, 8751 Osborne, Highland, Indiana 47322, USA

15. The Yeast-Human Interaction Conference, San Francisco, March 1985. Twenty-one hours of recorded conference proceedings available on cassette from Creative Audio (see above)

16. Rosenberg, E. W., Belew, P. W., Skinner, R. B. and Crutcher, N. "Crohn's disease and psoriasis," (letter) *N. Engl. J. Med.*, 308:2 (1983), 101

17. Higgs, J. M. and Wells, R. S. "Chronic mucocutaneous candidiasis: associated abnormalities for iron metabolism," *Brit. Med. J. Dermatol.*, 86:8 (1972), 83–102

18. Meeman, A., Avidor, I. and Kadish, U. "Candidal infection of nine gastric ulcers in aged patients," *Am. J. Gastroenterol.*, 75 (1981), 211–13

19. Truss, C. O. "Metabolic abnormalities in patients with chronic candidiasis—the acetaldehyde hypothesis," *J. Orthomol. Psychiat.*, 13:2 (1984), 66–93

20. Galland, L. "Nutrition and candidiasis" *J. Orthomol. Psychiat.*, 14:1 (1985), 50–60

21. Shuster, S. "The aetiology of dandruff and the mode of action of therapeutic" *Brit. J. Dermatol.*, 111 (1984), 235–242

Disorders of the Central Nervous System

1. Harrell, R. F., Kapp, R. H. *et al.* "Can nutritional supplements help mentally retarded children? An exploratory study," *Proceedings of the National Academy of Science* (USA) 78:1 (1981), 574–8

2. Coleman, M. and Abbassi, V. "Downs syndrome and hypothyroidism: coincidence or consequence?" (letter) *Lancet,* i (1984), 569

3. Koch, R., Share, J. and Graliker, B. "The effects of cytomel on young children with Downs syndrome: A double-blind longitudinal study," *J. Paediatr.*, 66 (1965), 776–8

4. Wynn, A. (editorial). "Nutrition and Downs syndrome," *Nutrition and Health,* 3 (1984), 5–7

5. Allan, R. B. "Nutritional aspects of epilepsy—a review of the potential of nutritional intervention in epilepsy," *Int. Clin. Nutr. Rev.* 3:3 (1983), 3–9

6. Joost, T. L. *et al.* "Epileptic-type convulsions in magnesium deficiency," *Aviation, Space and Environmental Medicine,* (1979), 734–5

Migraine and Related Headaches

1. Hanington, E., Jones, R. J., Aness, J. A. L. and Wachowicz, B. "Migraine: A platelet disorder," *Lancet,* ii (1981), 720–3

2. Egger, J., Carter, C. M., Wilson, J., Turner, M. W. and Soothill, J. F. "Is migraine food allergy? A double-blind controlled trial of oligoantigenic diet treatment," *Lancet,* ii (1983), 865–9

3. Monro, J., Carini, C. and Brostoff, J. "Migraine is a food-allergic disease," *Lancet,* ii (1984), 719–21

4. Grant, E. C. G. "Food allergies in migraine," *Lancet,* i (1979), 966–9

Children's Problems

1. Egger, J., Carter, C. M., Graham, P. J., Gumley, D. and Soothill, J. F. "Controlled trial of oligoantigenic treatment in the hyperkinetic syndrome," *Lancet,* i (1985), 540–5

2. David, O. J., Hoffman, S. P., Sverd, J., Clark, J. and Voeller, K. "Lead and hyperactivity. Behavioural response to chelation: a pilot study," *Am. J. Psychiatry,* 133:10 (1976), 1155–8

3. Needleman, H. L. *et al.* "Deficits in psychologic and classroom performance of children with elevated dentine lead levels," *New Engl. J. Med.,* 300 (1979), 689–95

4. Howard, J. M. H. "Clinical import in small increases in serum aluminium," *Clin. Chem.,* 30:10 (1984), 1722–3

5. Rimland, B. and Larson, G. E. "Hair mineral analysis and behaviour: an analysis of fifty-one studies," *J. Learning Disabilities,* 16:5 (May 1983)

6. Silbergeld, E. K. and Anderson, S. M. "Artificial food colours and childhood behaviour disorders," *Bulletin of the New York Academy of Medicine,* 2nd series, 58:3 (1982), 275–95

7. Dickerson, J. W. T. "Diet and Hyperactivity," *J. of Human Nutrition,* 34 (1980), 167–74

8. Weiss, B. *et al.* "Behavioural responses to artificial food colours," *Science,* 207 (1980), 1487–9

9. Swanson, J. M. and Kinsbourne, M. "Food dyes impair performance of hyperactive children on a laboratory learning test," *Science,* 207 (1980), 1485–7

10. Rimland, B. "The Feingold diet: An assessment of the reviews by Mattes, by Kavale and Forness and others," *J. of Learning Disabilities,* 16:6 (1983), 331–3

11. Brenner, A. "The effects of megadoses of selected B complex vitamins on children with hyperkinesis: Controlled studies with long-term follow up," *J. Learning Disabilities,* 15:5 (1982), 258–64

*12. Colquhoun, V. and Bunday, S. "A lack of essential fatty acids as a possible cause of hyperactivity in children," *Med. Hypothesis,* 7 (1981), 673–9

13. Pihl, R. O. and Parkes, M. "Hair element in learning disabled children," *Science,* 198 (1977), 204–6

*14. Rapp, D. J. *Allergies in the Hyperactive Child.* Cornerstone, Simon and Schuster, New York, 1979

15. Cott, A. *The Orthomolecular Approach to Learning Disabilities.* Academic Therapy, San Rafael, California, 1977

*16. Crook, W. G. *Can Your Child Read? Is He Hyperactive?* Professional Books, Jackson, Tennessee, 1973

17. Barnes, B. and Colquhoun, V. *The Hyperactive Child.* Thorsons, Wellingborough, 1984

18. Zaleski, A., Shokeir, M. K. and Gerrard, J. W. "Enuresis: Familial incidents and relationship to allergic disorders," *Can. Med. Ass. J.,* 106 (1972), 30

19. Tseng, R. Y. L., Mellon, J. and Bammer, K. *The Relationship Between Nutrition and Student Achievement, Behaviour, and Health—A Review of the Literature.* California State Department of Education, Sacramento, California, 1980

*20. Feingold, B. F. *Why Your Child is Hyperactive.* Random House, New York, 1974

21. Tucker, D. M., Sanstead, H. H. *et al.* "Iron status in brain function: serum ferritin levels associated with asymmetries of carticol electro-physiology and cognitive performances," *Am. J. Clin. Nutr.,* 39 (1984), 105–13

22. Lozoff, B. *et al.* "Behavioural abnormalities in infants with iron deficiency anaemia" in E. Pollitt and R. L. Leibel (eds.) *Iron Deficiency, Brain Biochemistry and Behaviour,* pp. 183–94, 195–208. Raven Press, New York, 1982

*23. Schauss, A. *Diet, Crime and Delinquency.* Parker House, Berkeley, California, 1980

24. Thatcher, R. W. *et al.* "The effects of low levels of cadmium and lead on cognitive functioning in children," *Arch. Environ. Health,* 37:3 (1982), 159–66

25. Hansen, J. C., Christensen, L. B. and Tarp, U. "Hair lead concentrations in children with minimal cerebral dysfunction," *Danish Medical Bulletin,* 27 (1980), 259–62

26. Botez, M. I. "Hypotonia and Folate Deficiency in Children," *J. Paediat.,* 96 (1980), 774

27. Templeton, L. *The Right Food for your Kids—A Parent's Guide to Healthy Eating for Children.* Century, London, 1984

*28. Ash, J. and Roberts, D. *Happiness is Junk-Free Food.* (Recipes) Thorsons, Wellingborough, 1986

*29. Lebrecht, E. *Sugar-Free Cakes and Biscuits—Recipes for Diabetics and Dieters.* Faber & Faber, London, 1985

30. Schoenthaler, S. J. "Alabama diet—behaviour programme: an empirical evaluation at Coosa Valley Regional Detention Center," *Int. J. Biosocial Res.,* 5:2 (1983), 78–87

31. Schoenthaler, S. J. "The Los Angeles Probation Department diet—behaviour programme: an empirical analysis of six institutional settings," *Int. J. Biosocial Res.,* 5:2 (1983), 88–9

32. Schoenthaler, S. J. "The effects of citrus on the treatment and control of anti-social behaviour: a double-blind study of an incarcerated juvenile population," *Int. J. Biosocial., Res.* 5:2 (1983), 107–17

33. Schauss, A. "Nutrition and anti-social behaviour," *Int. Clin. Nutr. Rev.,* 4:4 (1984), 172–7

34. See also "Food Allergy" references.

Nutrition in Old Age

1. Exton-Smith, A. N. "Nutrition of the elderly," *Brit. Jour. Hosp. Med.,* (1971) 639–46

2. Editorial. "Old people's nutrition," *BMJ,* 2 (1974), 212–13

3. Morgan, A. G. *et al.* "A nutritional survey of the elderly: blood and urine vitamin levels," *Internat. J. Vit. Nutr. Res.,* 45 (1975), 448–62

4. Morgan, A. G. *et al.* "A nutritional survey of the elderly: haematological aspects," *Internat. J. Vit. Nutr. Res.,* 43 (1973), 461–71

5. Addis, G. M. and Runcie, J. "Water-soluble vitamin deficiency in the elderly," *Medical Laboratory Sciences,* 42 (1985), 90–1

6. Goodwin, J. S., Goodwin, J. M. and Garry, P. J. "The association between nutritional status and cognitive function in a healthy elderly population," *JAMA,* 249 (1983), 2917–21

7. Roe, D. A. *Geriatric Nutrition*. Prentice-Hall, New Jersey, 1983

*8. Kenton, L. *Ageless Ageing*. Century, London, 1986

9. Watkin, D. M. *Handbook of Nutrition, Health and Ageing*, Noyes, New Jersey, 1983

10. DHSS. *Nutrition and Health in Old Age*. Report on Health and Social Subjects No. 16, HMSO, London, 1979

Nutritional Psychiatry

*1. Cheraskin, E. and Ringsdorf, W. M. *Psycho-dietetics*. Bantam Books, 1974

*2. Fredericks, C. *Psycho-nutrition*. Grosset & Dunlap, New York, 1976

*3. Newbold, H. L. *Meganutrients for your Nerves*. Berkeley Publishing Corporation, New York, 1975

*4. Schauss, A. *Diet, Crime and Delinquency*. Parker House, Berkeley, 1980

5. Wurtman, R. J. and Wurtman, J. J. (eds.) *Nutrition and the Brain*, Vols. 1–6. Raven Press, New York, 1977–83

6. Wurtman, R. J. "Behavioural effects of nutrients," *Lancet*, i (1983), 1145–7

7. Crowdon, J. M. "Neuro-transmitter precursors in the diet: their use in the treatment of brain diseases" in R. J. Wurtman and J. J. Wurtman (eds.) *Nutrition and the Brain*, vol. 3, pp. 117–81. Raven Press, New York, 1979

8. Colby–Morley, E. "Neuro-transmitters and nutrition," *J. Orthomol. Psychiat.*, 12:1 (1983), 38–43

9. Lonsdale, D. and Shamberger, R. J. "Red cell transketolase as an indicator of nutritional deficiency," *Am. J. Clin. Nutr.* 33 (1980), 205–11

10. Kawai, C., Wakabayashi, A., Matsumura, T. and Yui, Y. "Reappearance of beri beri heart disease in Japan—a study of twenty-three cases," *Am. J. Med.* 69 (1983), 383–6

11. Carney, M. W. P., Williams, D. G. and Sheffield, B. F. "Thiamine and pyridoxine levels in newly-admitted psychiatric patients," *Brit. J. Psychiat.*, 135 (1979), 249–54

12. Carney, M. W. P., Ravindran, A., Rinsler, M. G. and Williams, D. G. "Thiamine, riboflavin and pyridoxine deficiency in psychiatric in-patients," *Brit. J. Psychiat.*, 141 (1982), 271–2

13. Rudin, D. O. "The three pellagras," *J. Orthomol. Psychiat.*, 12:2 (1983), 91–110

14. Hoffer, A. "Mechanism of action of nicotinic acid and nicotinamide in the treatment of schizophrenia" in D. Hawkind

and L. Pauling (eds.) *Orthomol. Psychiat., Treatment of Schizophrenia,* pp. 202–62. W. H. Freeman & Co., San Francisco, 1973

15. Gilka, L. "The biochemistry of schizophrenias," *J. Orthomol. Psychiat.*, 7:1 (1978), 6–16

16. Rudin, D. O. "Choroid plexus and systems disease in mental illness I, a new brain attack mechanism," *Biol. Psychiat.*, 15 (1980), 517–39

17. Rudin, D. O. "The choroid plexus and systems disease in mental illness II, systemic lupus erythematosus—a combined transport dysfunction model for schizophrenia," *Biol. Psychiat.*, 16 (1981), 373–98

18. Rudin, D. O. "The choroid plexus and systems disease in mental illness III, the exogenous peptide hypothesis of mental illness," *Biol. Psychiat.*, 16 (1981), 489–512

19. Rudin, D. O. "The major psychoses and neuroses as omega-3 essential fatty acid deficiency syndrome: substrate pellagra," *Biol. Psychiat.*, 16:9 (1981), 837–50

20. Rudin, D. O. "The dominant diseases of modernized societies as omega-3 essential fatty acid deficiency syndrome: substrate beri beri," *Med. Hypotheses,* 8 (1982), 17–47

21. Adams, P. W., Rose, D. P., Folkard, J., Wynn, V., Seed, M. and Strong, R. "Effect of pyridoxine hydrochloride (vitamin B6) upon depression associated with oral contraception," *Lancet,* i (1973), 897–904

22. Khaleeleddin, K. and Philpott, W. H. I "The clinical report of ecologic and nutritional disorders in chronic mental and physical degenerative diseases," II "The significance of B6 and methionine metabolic disorders in mental disease." xxxx *J. Applied Nutr.*, 32:2 (1980), 37–52

23. Wilcken, D. E. L., Wilcken, B., Dudman, N. P. B. and Tyrell, R. T. A. "Homocystinuria—the effects of betaine in the treatment of patients not responsive to pyridoxine," *N. Engl. J. Med.* 309:8 (1983), 448–53

24. Pfeiffer, C. C., Sohler, A., Jenney, C. H. and Iliev, V. "Treatment of pyroluric schizophrenia (malvaria) with large doses of pyridoxine in a dietary supplement of zinc," *J. Orthomol. Psychiat.*, 3:4 (1974), 292–300

25. Hoffer, A. and Osmond, H. "Malvaria: a new psychiatric disease," *Acta. Psychiat. Scand.*, 39 (1963), 335–7

26. Easlove, M., Silverio, T. and Minenna, R. "Severe riboflavin deficiency: a previously undescribed side-effect of phenothiazines," *J. Orthomol. Psychiat.*, 12:2 (1983), 113–15

27. Pinto, J., Huang, Y. and Rivlin, R. "Inhibition of riboflavin metabolism in rat tissues by chlorpromazine, imipramine and amtriptyline," *J. Clin. Invest.*, 67:5 (1981), 1500–6

28. Evans, D. L., Edelsohn, C. A. and Golden, R. N. "Organic psychosis without anaemia or spinal cord symptoms in patients with vitamin B12 deficiency," *A. J. Psychiat.*, 140 (1983), 218–21

29. Van Tiggelin, C. J. M., Peperkamp, J. P. C. and Tertoolen, J. F. W. "Vitamin B12 levels of cerebro-spinal fluid in patients with organic mental disorder," *J. Orthomol. Psychiat.*, 12 (1983), 305–11

30. Reading, C. M. "X-linked dominant manic-depressive illness: linkage with Xg blood group, red-green colour blindness and vitamin B12 deficiency," *J. Orthomol. Psychiat.*, 8:2 (1979), 68–77

31. Carney, M. W. P. "Investigation into serum folate and B12 concentrations in psychiatric in-patients with particular reference to schizophrenia" in G. Hemmings and W. A. Hemmings (eds.) *Biological Basis of Schizophrenia* pp. 117–26. MTP Press, Lancaster, 1978

32. Editorial. "Folate responsive schizophrenia," *Lancet,* i (1975), 1283–4

33. Reynolds, E. H., Carney, M. W. P. and Toone, B. K. "Methylation and mood," *Lancet,* ii (1984), 196–8

34. De Liz, A. J. "Large amounts of nicotinic acid in vitamin B12 and the treatment of apparently irreversible psychotic conditions found in patients with low levels of folic acid," *J. Orthomol. Psychiat.* 8:2 (1979), 63–5

35. Naylor, G. J., Smith, A. H. W. "Vanadium: a possible aetiological factor in manic-depressive illness" *Psycholog. Med.*, 11 (1981), 249–56

36. Editorial. "Vanadium in manic-depressive illness," *Lancet,* ii (1981), 511–12

37. Naylor, G. J., Smith, A. H. W., Bryce-Smith, D. and Ward, N. I. "Elevated vanadium-content of hair and mania," *Biol. Psychiat.* 19:5 (1984), 759–63

38. Cohen, B. M., Lipinski, J. F. and Altesman, R. I. "Lecithin in the treatment of mania: double-blind placebo-controlled trials," *Am. J. Psychiat.*, 139:9 (1982), 1162–4

39. Horrobin, D. F. and Manku, M. S. "Possible role of prostaglandin in E1 in the affective disorders and alcoholism," *Brit. Med. J.*, 1 (1980), 1363–6

40. Horrobin, D. F. "Prostaglandins, essential fatty acids and psychiatric disorders: a background view," in D. F. Horrobin

(ed.) *Clinical Uses of Essential Fatty Acids,* pp. 167–74. Eden Press, Montreal, 1982

41. Lieb, J. "Linoleic acid in the treatment of lithium toxicity and familial tremor," *Prostaglandins Med.*, 4 (1980), 275–9

42. Holman, T. "Nutritional approaches to manic-depressive illness," *Int. Clin. Nutr. Rev.*, 3:4 (1983), 4–6

43. Burnett, F. M. "A possible role of zinc in the pathology of dementia," *Lancet,* i (1981), 186–8

44. Lishman, W. A. *Organic Psychiatry: The Psychological Consequences of Cerebral Disorder.* Blackwell Scientific Publications, Oxford, 1978

45. Juan, D. "A Review—clinical significance of hypomagnasemia," *Surgery,* 91:5 (1982), 510–17

46. Politt, E. and Leibel, S. (eds.) *Iron Deficiency: Brain Biochemistry and Behaviour.* Raven Press, New York, 1982

47. Pfeiffer, C. C. *Zinc and Other Micronutrients* pp. 204–5, 77, 17, 178–9, 208–9. Keats, Connecticut, 1978

48. Shapiro, I. M., Sumner, A. J., Spitz, L. K., Cornblath, D. R., Uzzell, B., Ship, I. I. and Bloch, P. "Neuro-physiological and neuro-psychological functions in mercury-exposed dentists," *Lancet,* i (1982), 1147–50

49. Naylor, G. J. and Smith, A. H. W. "Vanadium: a possible aetiological factor in manic-depressive illness," *Psychology Med.*, 11 (1981), 249–56

50. *See* also "Hypoglycemia" references.

51. Walinder, J., Skott, A., Carlsson, A. and Roos, D. E., "Potentiation of the antidepressant action of clomipramine by tryptophan," *Arch. Gen. Psychiat.*, 33 (1976), 1384–9

52. Lehmann, J., Persson, S., Walinder, J. and Wallin, L. "Tryptophan malabsorption in dementia, improvement in certain cases after tryptophan therapy as indicated by mental behaviour and blood analysis," *Acta. Psychiat. Scand.*, 64 (1981), 123–31

53. Crowdon, J. H. "Neurotransmitter precursors in the diet: their use in the treatment of brain diseases" in R. J. Wurtman and J. J. Wurtman (eds.) *Nutrition and the Brain* Vol. 3, pp. 117–81. Raven Press, New York, 1979

54. Gelenberg, A. J., Wojcik, J. D., Crowdon, J. H., Sved, A. S. and Wurtman, R. J. "Tyrosine for the treatment of depression," *Am. J. Psychiat.*, 137:5 (1980), 622–3

55. Buist, R. A. (editorial). "The therapeutic predictability of tryptophan and tyrosine in the treatment of depression," *Int. Clin. Nutr. Rev.*, 3:2 (1983), 1–3

56. *See* also "Problem Child" references.

Index

About the Authors

Dr. Stephen Davies was born in Cardiff, Wales in 1948. He was educated at Rugby School, Jesus College, Oxford and Westminster Medical School, London. He obtained his degree in physiology and biochemistry from Oxford in 1970 and qualified as a doctor in 1973. Since that time he has worked within the National Health Service and spent eighteen months in Canada, working in deprived areas where he acquired his interest in nutrition. He is a consultant physician with a major interest in nutrition. He is director of a research unit that looks into the role that diet and nutrition play in the prevention and management of illness.

He has published papers on the role of trace elements and toxic elements in health and disease, and is founding chairman of the British Society for Nutritional Medicine, an association formed to provide an educational forum for medical doctors on the subject of nutrition. He is on the editorial board of a number of international journals, and is medical adviser to a number of health-orientated organizations. (Hyperactive Children's Support Group, Foresight, the Association for Preconceptional Care, etc.). He is a fellow of the American College of Nutrition.

Dr. Alan Stewart qualified from Guy's Hospital, London, in 1976, and spent five years specializing in hospital medicine. He became a member of the Royal College of Physicians (MRCP UK). For the last seven years he has had a major interest in nutrition, and is a founding member of, and Information Officer for, the British Society for Nutritional Medicine. He is married with two children and lives in Sussex.

He is also medical advisor to the Premenstrual Tension Advisory Service.